Working Ethically in Child Protection

T0265066

In their day-to-day practice, social work and human services practitioners frequently find themselves in confusing ethical quandaries, trying to balance the numerous competing interests of protecting children from harm and promoting family and community capacity. This book explores the ethical issues surrounding child protection interventions and offers a process-oriented approach to ethical practice and decision making in child protection and family welfare practice. Its aim is to prepare students and early career professionals for roles in the complex and challenging work of child protection and family support.

Beginning with a critical analysis and appreciation of the diverse organisational and cultural contexts of contemporary child protection and ethical decision-making frameworks, the authors outline a practical 'real-world' model for reshaping frontline ethical practice. Moving away from a focus on the child apart from the family, the authors recognise that child safeguarding affects the lives, not just of children, but also of parents, grandparents and communities. *Working Ethically in Child Protection* eschews dominant rational-technical models for relational ones that are value-centred and focus on family well-being as a whole.

Rather than a single focus on assessing risk and diagnosing deficit, this book recognises that our child protection systems bear down disproportionately on those from disadvantaged and marginalised communities and argues that what is needed is real support and practical assistance for poor and vulnerable parents and children. It uses real-world case examples to illustrate the relevant ethical and practice principles, and ways in which students and practitioners can practise ethically when dealing with complex, multifaceted issues.

Bob Lonne has extensive experience as a social worker in various child protection roles in Australia. With Nigel Parton, Jane Thomson and Maria Harries, he co-authored *Reforming Child Protection*. In 2008, he was appointed as the foundation Chair at the Queensland University of Technology, Brisbane, Australia. He was the National President of the Australian Association of Social Workers from 2005 to 2011.

Maria Harries has had a 45-year career in practice, teaching and research where she has held numerous senior positions. Her focus has been on mental health and the well-being of children and families. She has taught and consulted extensively on ethics in governance and clinical practice.

Brid Featherstone is Professor of Social Work at the Open University, UK. With Sue White and Kate Morris, she has written *Re-imagining Child Protection: Towards humane social work with families*. She has a particular interest in engaging fathers and gender issues in child protection.

Mel Gray has extensive experience in the field of ethics having completed her PhD in this area and authored several book chapters and journal articles on social work ethics. She also edited, with Stephen Webb, the highly successful *Ethics and Value Perspectives in Social Work* (2010).

Working Ethically in Child Protection

Bob Lonne, Maria Harries,
Brid Featherstone and Mel Gray

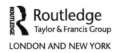
Routledge
Taylor & Francis Group

LONDON AND NEW YORK

First published 2016
by Routledge
2 Park Square, Milton Park, Abingdon, Oxon OX14 4RN

and by Routledge
711 Third Avenue, New York, NY 10017

Routledge is an imprint of the Taylor & Francis Group, an informa business

© 2016 B. Lonne, M. Harries, B. Featherstone and M. Gray

British Library Cataloguing-in-Publication Data
A catalogue record for this book is available from the British Library

Library of Congress Cataloging in Publication Data
Lonne, Bob, author.
Working ethically in child protection / Bob Lonne, Maria Harries, Brid Featherstone, and Mel Gray.
p. ; cm.
Includes bibliographical references and index.
I. Harries, Maria, author. II. Featherstone, Brid, author. III. Gray, Mel, 1951- , author. IV. Title.
[DNLM: 1. Child Welfare--ethics. 2. Ethics, Professional. WA 310.1]
HV713
362.7--dc23
2015007303

ISBN: 978-0-415-72933-8 (hbk)
ISBN: 978-0-415-72934-5 (pbk)
ISBN: 978-1-315-85102-0 (ebk)

Typeset in Sabon
by GreenGate Publishing Services, Tonbridge, Kent

Contents

Illustrations

Figures

Tables

Foreword   The Ethics of Work for "the Cruelty"

In the late nineteenth century, the newly formed New York Society for Prevention of Cruelty to Children (arguably the world's first agency for child protection; see www.nyspcc.org) sought "to rescue little children from the cruelty and demoralization which neglect, abandonment and improper treatment engender." In NYSPCC's own account of its history, this mission to *rescue* or *save* children arose during a time of massive immigration and urbanization and of the worst excesses of the industrial revolution: "Public and private service systems were overwhelmed, riots were frequent, crime was rampant, and the child cruelty and exploitation they engendered was as common as the sixteen-hour work day."

The agents of NYSPCC and the comparable societies that soon emerged in other states had statutory authority to take custody of children who were victims of violence, found in a state of destitution, or accused of participation in a crime. Such action generally resulted in institutionalization of children, who were seldom returned to their parents (Levine & Levine, 1992). Police were directed to assist the NYSPCC agents, and the agents themselves were authorized to participate in prosecution of adults charged with mistreating children. NYSPCC's charter called for the agency "to aid...in the enforcement of the laws intended for [children's] protection and benefit" and "to secure...the prompt conviction and punishment of all persons violating such laws..., especially [those who]...cruelly ill treat and shamefully neglect...little children of whom they claim the care, custody or control."

Thus, the NYSPPC agents experienced no ambivalence in their work. NYSPPC was a law enforcement agency intended to rescue children, not to help families. The agents often pursued their mission zealously:

> The agents roamed the streets looking for children who appeared neglected or abused or who were out of school. They then imperiously summoned people to their offices, threatened to arrest families or to remove their children, and interviewed neighbors and relatives to collect incriminating evidence. And when they entered homes, they sometimes seized whiskey bottles or even told people they found objectionable to leave the premises.
>
> (Levine & Levine, 1992, pp. 210–211)

This vigorous enforcement of middle-class American norms of childrearing was neither circumspect nor even-handed:

> Although there were clearly cases of horrific abuse…, more typically, the child savers judged the immigrant homes using white, upper-class norms. The child savers, for example, were horrified by the immigrants' use of garlic in cooking and their habit of drinking wine with dinner, and they decided that these were adequate bases for removing children. Appalled by what they perceived as the deviant lifestyles of immigrant families, the child savers sought to "improve" these families by insisting that children be quiet and clean, dress well, and eat "good" food, not traditional immigrant cuisine.
>
> (Huntington, 2014, p. 75)

Applying such standards through aggressive scrutiny of life in the tenements of New York City, NYSPCC removed thousands of children each year and placed them in long-term institutional care (Huntington, 2014; Levine & Levine, 1992). It is hardly surprising then that NYSPCC's expansive and powerful—but selectively applied and largely unregulated—efforts to protect children were the subject of fear and dread among impoverished, immigrant parents in New York City in the late nineteenth century. (Similar strategies and reactions were observed in other U.S. cities at the time.) It should come as no surprise then that the awkwardly named New York Society for Prevention of Cruelty to Children (a name derived from earlier organizations for humane care of animals) became popularly known simply as "the Cruelty" (Levine & Levine, 1992).

In that context, the principal ethical problem for the NYSPCC agents was whether to continue in the work. There was no pretense that they were improving family welfare. They were instead striving to punish parents and other caregivers whom they regarded as mistreating children. Even when they were not seeking primarily to apply the retributive force of the criminal law, they were "saving" children in ways that were perceived by parents as cruel and punitive and that often subjected children to institutional conditions that they too regarded as products of "the Cruelty."

Indeed, the absence of a truly protective impulse in the child protection system created a situation in which often there were only losers, whether the perspective was that of parents, children, or the broader community. That situation prevailed in both concept and reality until the creation of the contemporary child protection system in the United States in the mid-1960s as the product of the extraordinary efforts of Henry Kempe and his colleagues at the University of Colorado. The resulting rapid adoption, dissemination, and application of mandated reporting laws probably contributed, at least indirectly, to new cultural norms signaling the unacceptability of either hitting or sexually exploiting children. However, the mandated reporting laws were based on erroneous assumptions about the frequency and complexity of the problem, and the system as a whole created or exacerbated ethical dilemmas by mixing coercion, voluntariness, and both beneficent and retributive goals (Melton, 2005).

Indeed, there is ample evidence to suggest that, in the aggregate, the formal child protection system may make a bad situation worse. Whatever the motives of the workers themselves and the body politic whom they serve, no one can seriously doubt that the knock on the door by a representative of Child Protective Services (CPS) is often perceived by parents and their neighbors as an unwelcome visit by the Cruelty, even if that label has passed from common usage.

Parents' fears are confirmed in many respects by data on the operation of the system. In the United States, for example, in Federal Fiscal Year 2013, state and county child welfare agencies received 3.5 million referrals about 6.4 million children who were believed to be victims of child maltreatment (U.S. Department of Health and Human Services, 2015). Almost 40 percent of the officially recorded referrals were screened out, so that no action (not even an investigation) was taken. That percentage is surely a gross underestimate of the actual screen-outs, because it does not include referrals that were not logged as such. Only about one in six recorded referrals resulted in a finding that abuse or neglect had occurred. Even among those "founded" referrals, one in three families received no "services" other than an investigation to determine whether maltreatment had occurred. It is likely that many—probably most—of those families who were recorded as having received help in fact were offered a group parent education class or some other "treatment" that had little, if any, relation to the needs that brought them to the attention of the CPS.

Consider in that regard that almost 80 percent of referrals to the CPS were for suspected neglect—usually multi-problem circumstances for both the affected families themselves and their communities. In such instances, parents rarely intentionally withhold resources for children. Instead, because of broader material deprivation and a multitude of personal and social challenges for parents and their neighbors, adverse circumstances multiply in a way that the care for children may be inadequate. In such a situation, common sense easily challenges the notion that children's safety will be enhanced by a law-enforcement-style investigation to determine whether legally cognizable neglect has occurred. Moreover, if the allegation of neglect is substantiated and a "service" is provided, it is apt to be a single-factor, inexpensive, office-based intervention that is unlikely to improve children's well-being and safety. If there is no good reason to believe that an intervention will work, it won't! Meanwhile, whatever vestiges remain of parents' belief that they can make a difference for their family are apt to be erased.

In such a context (consistent in general terms with the situation in most wealthy countries; see Lonne et al., 2008), child welfare professionals may struggle with the "old" ethical dilemma of whether to participate in a system that may often do more harm than good—or, conversely, to remain a bystander when threats to children's safety and well-being remain. If professionals do choose to be participants in—even employees of—the CPS, then they inevitably—and frequently—will face complex "new" moral decisions as they grapple with conflicting goals and uncertain predictions. Thus Bob Lonne and his colleagues are striving to make child welfare professionals' work easier—and child protection clients' lives less stressful and more dignified—through the publication of this book. These are noble goals.

Ultimately, however, the answer to the "ethics problems" in the CPS is a new system that is ethically coherent and responsive to current realities. Ethical problems would be greatly reduced if there were universal structures and processes to provide neighborly voluntary assistance to parents in preserving their children's security and assuring adequacy of care (cf. Kimbrough-Melton & Melton, 2015; Melton, 1996). The pursuit of such a new framework for child protection policy and practice has long been a project for Lonne and his colleagues (e.g., Lonne et al., 2008). Achievement of this goal is, however, a formidable challenge that will require sustained effort, maybe for decades, by visionary people of goodwill (cf. Metrikin-Gold, 2015).

In the meantime, if the harms embedded in contemporary child protection systems are to be kept in check, then the them-and-us thinking that has long characterized such policies and practices must be greatly reduced. Hence, in a manner reminiscent of Katz's (2002) sensitive and influential writing on relationship-based ethics in health practice, Lonne and his colleagues call on child welfare professionals to be hospitable toward the children and parents who are least likely to be shown due respect (cf. Melton, 2014). Lonne et al. (2008) show that even the children and parents who are on or outside the margins of the community both deserve and benefit from thoughtful, authentic expressions of humility, caring, and respect.

Such an approach is courageous, demanding, and redemptive. It requires a Solomonic exercise of power in decisions touching on the most sensitive dimensions of the lives of the most vulnerable people. Widespread adoption of such an attitude may go far toward the policy transformation that is needed in the long term. In the meantime, it will be an important step toward humanizing a system that far too often has felt like Cruelty—that has been more concerned with "dutifully record[ing]...incidents in...files" than with diligent action to fulfill children's rights to personal security and to protection of their family environments in strong communities (cf. *DeShaney v. Winnebago County Department of Social Services*, 1989 [J. Blackmun, dissenting]).

Gary B. Melton
University of Colorado School of Medicine
and Colorado School of Public Health

References

DeShaney v. Winnebago County Department of Social Services (1989). 489 U.S. 189.

Huntington, C. (2014). *Failure to flourish: How law undermines family relationships*. New York: Oxford University Press.

Katz, J. (2002). *The silent world of doctor and patient*. Baltimore, MD: Johns Hopkins University Press (original work published 1984).

Kimbrough-Melton, R. J., & Melton, G. B. (2015). "Someone will notice, and someone will care": How to build strong communities for children. *Child Abuse & Neglect*, 41, 67–78.

Levine, M., & Levine, A. (1992). *Helping children: A social history*. New York: Oxford University Press.

Lonne, B., Parton, N., Thomson, J., & Harries, M. (2008). *Reforming child protection*. London: Taylor & Francis.

Melton, G. B. (1996). The child's right to a family environment: Why children's rights and family values are compatible. *American Psychologist*, 51, 1234–1238.

Melton, G. B. (2005). Mandated reporting: A policy without reason. *Child Abuse & Neglect*, 29, 9–18.

Melton, G. B. (2014). Hospitality: Transformative service to children, families, and communities. *American Psychologist*, 69, 761–769.

Metrikin-Gold, B. D. (2015). Personal reflections about the work of the U.S. Advisory Board on Child Abuse and Neglect. *Child Abuse & Neglect*, 41, 3–18.

U.S. Department of Health and Human Services, Administration for Children and Families, Administration on Children, Youth, and Families, Children's Bureau (2015). *Child Maltreatment 2013*. Retrieved from http://www.acf.hhs.gov/programs/cb/research-data-technology/statistics-research/child-maltreatment

Preface

The 2009 publication *Reforming Child Protection* identified a range of areas where child protection systems in Anglophone countries were failing and highlighted the need for embedding ethics into child protection policy and practice. In this book, we seek to address the thorny question of how we practise ethically in an environment where much of the work to be done is controlled by statutes and the organisations in which we work have strict rules and protocols surrounding practice requirements. This is as it should be; such is the important responsibility of protecting the safety of children and families in society. Concomitantly in this 'safeguarding environment', as professionals we are duty bound to be ethical; that is, to treat clients with respect, to ensure equity, fairness and justice, and to practise relationally. We favour a dialogical approach to ethical decision making since we believe strongly that the best solutions lie in our relational engagements with our clients, peers, managers and co-workers. Nowhere are good communication skills more needed than in ethical decision making given that this is an area bereft of hard-and-fast answers and solutions. Ethical conundrums are best thought through in dialogue with others, within the bounds of strong relationships, where all involved are equally committed to ethical outcomes. Thus, what we hope to achieve with this book is to open up spaces for dialogue on what it means to work ethically in child protection. We believe strongly that achieving this rests on a relational respective, where clients are seen as part of a 'web of care', wherein their strongest supports lie. People are relational and social beings; they are embedded in social relationships and thinking relationally is recognition of this. Thus, our plea with this book is that due recognition be given to the role and resources of families and communities in serving the best interests of children everywhere.

Acknowledgements

We are extremely grateful to, and wish to acknowledge the generosity of, Emeritus Professor Ian Thompson for enabling us to use the DECIDE ethical framework, which he and his team developed and which we have adapted herein. His *Nursing Ethics*, co-authored with Kath Melia and Kenneth Boyd, has been widely used across the healthcare disciplines in the training of care, protection and justice workers across the world. The model, which has been central to the ethics syllabus in many universities, has also been used by the authors of this book. We thank Ian for encouraging us to focus on the very practical nature of ethics in child protection to better understand the more 'heady' arena of moral thought; hence, we have nuanced the framework to add a central place for relational practice.

Abbreviations

AFA	Alliance for Forgotten Australians
CA	capabilities approach
CLAN	Care Leavers Australia Network
COAG	Council of Australian Governments
CPP	child protection plan
CREATE	The CREATE Foundation Australia
DMT	decision-making technologies
FIN	Family Inclusion Network Australia
FGC	family group conference
FRG	Family Rights Group England
GCSE	General Certificate of Secondary Education
LAC	looked after children
MDGs	Millennium Development Goals
MR	mandatory reporting
NCCPR	National Coalition of Child Protection Reform
NPM	new public management
NSPCC	National Society for the Prevention of Cruelty to Children
PTSD	post-traumatic stress disorder
UNCRC	United Nations Convention on the Rights of the Child
UNHCR	United Nations High Commissioner for Refugees
UK	United Kingdom
USA	United States of America

Part 1

Ethical theory and historical frameworks for practice

Chapter 1 **The ethical landscape in child protection**

People involved in caring for the welfare and safety of children make choices and decisions that have profound consequences, and nobody would argue against the need to be ethical in this work. Indeed, to do so would be unorthodox and unprofessional as well as immoral. All people working in the caring professions 'sign off' on a commitment to act ethically and most organisations have codes of ethics and codes of conduct with which employees are expected to comply along with their particular profession's ethical code. In various countries, there are significant sanctions applied to employees or self-employed professionals who are found to have acted unethically. In this book, we explore the ethical issues involved in this very difficult though rewarding area of work. We offer insights from the work over the centuries by human beings concerned with the most profoundly important questions that confront us as human beings: what does it take 'to be good'? 'What makes a good person'? How do we know that we are 'doing good'? How do we weigh up what 'is good'? On what basis do 'good people' act towards others? What are 'good people's responsibilities' towards others, especially those suffering hurt and harm? We also draw from the considerable literature that has specifically concerned itself with the issues for children, young people and families and we have a particular interest in exploring the implications of the research evidence of adverse intervention for the ethics of contemporary practice.

Challenges and rewards of child protection work

As attested throughout this book, child protection work is not for the fainthearted; it is intellectually and emotionally demanding, and sometimes exceedingly stressful. It entails relating to others with integrity and thinking through fraught human interactions, while simultaneously wending one's way through a complex web of legal, organisational and ethical requirements. It can involve dealing with confronting events and egregious behaviours, particularly where children and other vulnerable people have suffered greatly. Such cases can expose practitioners to secondary trauma as the result of involvement with confronting matters that offend one's moral sensibilities. Personal costs can result.

All the while, in this work, there is an imperative of assuring others' safety through considering all the relevant factors when making assessments and decisions regarding the protection of children. At times, working effectively with service users involves making inquiries into matters they find painful and wish to avoid, asking awkward questions that can appear intrusive, and broaching subjects that trigger grief and trauma reactions. Practitioners can feel as though there is not enough time or resources to do the job properly; they are often under pressure to get things done quickly with insufficient space provided for proper engagement with service users. The work also involves being on the receiving end of others' displeasure or anger, acting with grace and humility while 'under fire' and giving 'bad' or 'unwelcome' news about events, assessments and the use of statutory authority. Understandably, practitioners may often feel overwhelmed and exhausted by these demands.

Many child protection and family welfare professionals report high levels of work stress (Lonne *et al.*, 2012). In many countries, the media has added to this stress, blaming practitioners for making the 'wrong' decisions as to whether or not to remove children. Retaining the capacity for equanimity, so central to ethical practice when one is feeling 'under siege' and fearful of failure and the very public consequences that entails, is no easy matter. There is clearly a huge vulnerability associated with the work given the public perception of the 'moral failure' of those mandated to protect children, especially when a child dies or is seriously injured (Hollis and Howe, 1986).

However, this work is also immensely rewarding. While it exposes practitioners to others' pain and trauma, and perhaps their own, it nonetheless entails being centrally involved in healing and recovery for service users. It can entail deep connection with others in relationships that are growth producing for all, and enable practitioners to discover and develop themselves – making them richer and wiser for the experience (see Chapters 11 and 12). Perhaps most importantly, this relational work can enable practitioners to feel elation, satisfaction and immense self-worth from travelling with others on their life-changing journeys. The rewards gained from joining with service users who undergo profound change and betterment should not be underestimated as they go to the fundamental motivations for practitioners in the helping professions: caring for others; being there when needed; helping others who are in a fix; experiencing emotional and spiritual connections; and furthering social justice – 'making the world a better place'. Helping others brings 'its own rewards'.

This work, which some see as a vocation, involves the head and the heart, thinking and feeling on one's feet as new information comes to hand, questions come to mind and emotional reactions occur. It can be a roller-coaster experience for all concerned. These sorts of inter- and intra-personal environments and relational demands require much from practitioners. This forms a critical part of the landscape in which ethics are required in day-to-day practice. So, while ethical decision making is a logical process, it also entails managing the emotional aspects through reflective and reflexive thinking. Further, neither the intellect nor the emotions should dominate to the point where they hinder sound relational and ethical practice. Throughout this book we seek to address the presenting issues in a balanced way that recognises the need for logical reasoning and emotional engagement.

Ethical practice in child protection

Fundamental to understanding the ethical challenges facing those working in child protection and family welfare is an appreciation of client vulnerability, unequal power relationships and the centrality of relationship in effective ethical practice. Children are generally less powerful than adults, but, as we identify throughout this book, the adults involved have often suffered or are suffering greatly themselves. Herein lies a central ethical tension requiring the most careful engagement with issues of power and powerlessness, and responsibility and choice. Most organising principles in child protection practice involve power relationships between the powerful and not so powerful. The potency of statutory powers to enter the 'sacred' domain of families, investigate them and remove children is weighty. These legal powers are generally located in large, seemingly impervious, bureaucracies, the collective strength of which sits in marked contrast to the vulnerability of those who experience their power. Professional status locates power and authority in certain individuals rather than others.

The evidence is clear that most of the families and communities targeted by statutory child protection and family welfare systems are among the least powerful in society, with little access to powerful allies. Poverty, unemployment, ethnic minority status, mental illness, ill health, alcohol and drug addictions, disability and cultural dislocation define some of the major demographics for those who come under the 'gaze' of child protection services (Gilbert *et al.*, 2009a, 2009b). Increasing debate concerning inequality in child protection and family welfare, along with the health inequalities literature, talks to the profound injustices in a public policy world that leaves the social determinants of disadvantage and involvement in child welfare largely unacknowledged (Bywaters, 2015). In this book, we suggest too little attention has been paid to the explicit power differentials between 'at risk' cohorts and the bureaucracies legislated to intervene in their lives when a child's safety is in question. Recognising these power differentials is an essential first step in finding a balance to enable children's well-being and safety to be ensured while not further threatening or indeed compounding the vulnerability of their families and communities.

Practitioners are acutely aware of the relevant legislation that underpins their work and the demands of legal compliance. But what do we mean by ethics? How do we understand the requirements of ethical practice? Codes of ethics are well established, of course, as well as organisational codes of practice. However, these often provide little guidance in a practice world of immense complexity and which is often highly risk averse. To highlight some the features of this practice world, let us consider the following example of contemporary practice.

Case example: distance and danger

This is a story from England. While carrying its own specifics, it epitomises some themes around the increasing distances between statutory practitioners and families and communities. It also emphasises the omnipresent focus on risk and danger that characterises practitioner and family interactions lending them a choreographed quality that can impede the possibilities for truthful and healing encounters.

Jo has been qualified as a social worker for two years. She works from a new office in the centre of town, based above the 'one stop shop' access point for local authority services. Most days she visits families in their homes, driving to a large social housing estate where many of those on her caseload live. Jo visits the estate in her car. She has never walked around it, shopped there or stopped for a coffee, sandwich or a drink. Indeed, there are few places to buy food and drink on the estate. She has noticed that the corner shop has just closed and some of her families have complained to her that the supermarket is two bus rides away. There is a children's centre and she has visited it for meetings but she has no time to be involved in any of the activities run there (activities that are ceasing at an alarming rate because of cuts in government spending).

When she visits family homes, she is very aware of the importance of seeing and talking to the children and occasionally tries to take them out for a trip to town on their own. The importance of engaging directly with children has been drummed into her at training events where successive child deaths have been held up as salutary warnings about the dangers of not doing so. She has been told repeatedly that children can become invisible especially if workers are too caught up with the needs of parents or immobilised by their angry and resist-ant behaviour. So she works very hard to adopt a firm and consistent approach with parents. She is always aware of the dangers of being too trusting of their accounts or becoming too involved with them. After all, her job is to be there for the child. She is careful to keep conversations with parents very clearly focused on the children's welfare and not let matters stray onto problems par-ents might say they have with each other unless of course it is domestic abuse. She knows that such abuse can have very damaging impacts upon children and should be dealt with decisively, often through getting the perpetrator to leave. She is also aware of the need to see the contents of cupboards and fridges and also to check bedrooms.

Source: Featherstone *et al.* (2013)

Featherstone and colleagues (2013, 2014a, 2014b) have questioned the effects of this system design and the underpinning ethos on children, families and practitioners themselves. While boxes are ticked and the 'right' people are seen and talked to, we suggest there is too high a price being paid by children, families and practitioners. Although the system is ostensibly all about them, children and young people seldom self-refer in England and tell researchers that when they are troubled, they prefer to seek help from those they know and trust (or helplines where they can remain anony-mous). They tell of their fear of talking to child protection workers as they may lose control over what is done and how. Research with their parents and wider family networks suggests encounters that are experienced as frightening and deficit-focused. Moreover, their distrust of services can be furthered when they see practitioners oper-ating within an instrumental approach that treats them as means rather than ends. Thus, they are considered only insofar as their actions/inactions impact upon chil-dren, not as people in their own right. They know and resent it when no attempt is made to understand them as relational, emoting beings and there is apparently little appreciation of their everyday struggles in a context of little money and neighbour-hoods with rapidly disappearing facilities.

Parents who can afford little for themselves and, indeed, forego things to ensure children have birthday presents can find it quite painful when child protection workers take their children out for treats. It is therefore not that surprising that they become angry and resentful when they pick up that the intent of such activities, on the part of workers, is to assess for abuse. Indeed, we also know from children themselves that they can experience this kind of practice very ambivalently. We understand that the phrase 'I'm only here for the child' heard from many child protection workers supports the performance of a moral identity in a confusing and frightening landscape where there are multiple vulnerabilities and risks. However, for all its rhetorical and moral potency, it reflects, in our view, a profound and damaging misrecognition of children's relational identities and needs across the life course (Featherstone *et al.*, 2014b).

This case study highlights the complexities of work that is subject to strong legal and organisational mandates where there are multiple stakeholders. What values inform and underpin this ethical practice in general, and in our work with vulnerable children and families in particular? What does it mean to act ethically? And how does one act ethically on behalf of all the people one serves if the needs of some conflict with those of others? How do we protect children and concurrently care for their families and communities? Is this possible? How do we conceptualise and understand the notion of ethics, and how do we incorporate such an understanding in our work with children, young people and families? What ethical or decision-making guides do practitioners use when making decisions that involve quandaries relating to conflicting needs and competing interests? And, how might an understanding of the history of ethical thinking assist in conceptualising ethics in child protection practice nowadays? These are the questions this book seeks to address.

There have been profound demographic and social changes within and between cultures and countries over recent times, with inevitable impacts upon the well-being and safety of children and families. On the international stage, there are ongoing conflicts and associated traumas leading to family disintegration, the abandonment and displacement of children and families, massive increases in people seeking refuge, increased detention of children and young people in camps and other centres, and the sexual and financial exploitation of children and young people (UNHCR, 2013). Within our countries, we have witnessed these events along with other massive social changes, including increased reporting of domestic violence, alcohol and other drug misuse, intergenerational poverty, and growing economic disparities with their associated health and welfare consequences for children and families.

At the sociological and philosophical levels, we are witnessing the not so new, but expanding understanding of the relevance of vital social factors, such as race, culture and gender in the ways public and social policy worlds are organised (McRoy, 2004; Swift, 1995). Research literature – particularly informed by, and on behalf of, the populations who have been severely disadvantaged and sidelined by the lack of such understanding – can no longer be ignored (Buckley *et al.*, 2011a). Indeed, many scholars present a compelling argument that existing child welfare laws must be understood 'within an oppression framework' (Curtis and Denby, 2011, p. 112), and that justifications for many past and ongoing child welfare practices are morally and ethically indefensible (Bessant, 2013). It has long been known that children who populate out-of-home care statistics continue to come from the most disadvantaged social groups in society (Bywaters *et al.*, 2014; Pelton, 1989). They are Indigenous, from single-parent (generally female) households, have little, if any, contact with their fathers, are poor and otherwise alienated and powerless, and generally show very poor outcomes from care (Lonne *et al.*, 2009; McRoy, 2008). Research demonstrates consistently how risk factors, such as poverty and social inequality, rather than racial and gender bias alone, continue to drive disparities in child protection reporting and removal rates among different racial and ethnic groups (Drake *et al.*, 2011).

At the family and community levels, we witness an ever-escalating number of children reported to be living in adversity, to be at risk of abuse, or to have been neglected within, or harmed by, members of their own families (Gilbert *et al.,* 2009b, 2012). In the majority of instances, these families are themselves in turmoil. Previous government policies and practices have been blamed for some of this turmoil, in part because programmes have been 'siloed', and failed to acknowledge the centrality of children in the services provided to families in distress (Arney and Scott, 2013). These 'failed' policies include the forced removal of Indigenous children in many countries – often in the name of child protection; the institutionalisation of children and young people seen to be at risk; the lack of public policy support for struggling families; the labelling of 'bad mothers'; and alcohol, drug, disability and mental health systems' failure to recognise the needs of children in the families coming to their attention. The latter problem is increasingly associated with the machinery of government failing to integrate its human services and view the needs of children and families holistically (D. Scott, 2006). This book examines several ethical frameworks to assist workers as they engage in contemporary practice in this tumultuous arena.

Some challenges confronting ethical practice

At an organisational level, the demands on workers are reported as extreme, some referring to this situation as a 'crisis' (Mansell *et al.*, 2011; McCosker *et al.*, 2014; E. Scott, 2006; Shireman, 2003). Remaining calm, thoughtful, nonjudgmental and ethically poised in these 'toxic' environments is extremely challenging (Smith, 2014). Ever-increasing numbers of people with diverse training from different disciplinary backgrounds are involved in the arena of practice called child protection, though in some jurisdictions (such as England) it is the domain of social workers. Increasingly, the mantra 'child protection is everyone's business' is being adopted by policy makers (COAG, 2009). Clearly, then, an integrated system of service provision to children and families depends on reaching a shared understanding, despite our varying disciplinary perspectives, and informing policy makers and the public accordingly as to what ethical practice in child protection entails.

However, not all areas of agreement reached by policy makers are necessarily 'good for children or families'. For example, a very powerful narrative in many Anglophone countries, as we discuss in Chapter 5, is that of child rescue (Featherstone *et al.*, 2014a; Scott and O'Neil, 2003). This narrative speaks to a narrow duty of care to children but excludes families and begs the question of whether the duty to care for a child – perceived to be 'at risk'– always overrides other considerations – or even for that matter, what the child wants. Removing children from their families has not always proved the best option. Indeed, many texts and public policy documents contain reports from adults taken into state care as children that this was anything but 'in their best interests'; the outcomes for many of them were disastrous as enquiries on abuse in care attest (Hill, 2007; Parliament of Australia Senate Community Affairs Committee, 2004; Penglase, 2005). There is powerful and robust research, and evidential reports, demonstrating the failures of a duty of care 'best interests of the child' *rescuing* approach, which left children in a state of anomie, detached from familial and cultural connection. In this book, we challenge the 'child rescue' model and situate ethical decision making in a complex narrative of relational practice, where relationships and community networks – nodes of connection – are central to good outcomes for children and families (Melton *et al.*, 2002).

Ethical practice is not simply about how workers relate to children and families or each other and their employers, or how they respond to the needs of their constituencies, it is also about how policies are made and implemented, and whether or not this promotes respect and justice, and contributes to the creation of a society that cares (Thompson *et al.*, 2006). Ethical practice is contingent on a network of services and policies working in tandem with one another; it is not just about individual organisations and practitioners. It cannot be achieved in an environment that disregards the prime values of respect for people and social justice; it is contingent on context.

People have differing views on what respect looks like and where justice fits when children are living in adverse environments. Decisions have to be made as to whether or not to remove them from their families, especially when intervention focuses on the child leaving, with families left unsupported in coping with their failure and loss. Injustice has been perpetrated in the name of the primal ethical commitment to the child with irrefutable statistical evidence of unjust Indigenous child removals under the policy of assimilation. Indigenous peoples all over the world have not yet recovered from this and continue to be overrepresented in child protection statistics (Roberts, 2002).

We seek to provide some clarity on ethical issues in child protection in this book, exploring the tensions and examining the skills and competencies required for child protection workers to survive and thrive in this value-charged space, or what Donald Schön (1990) referred to as the 'swampy lowland' (p. 3), where messy and confusing problems defy easy solutions. We review recent scholarship and research on how practitioners and policy makers involved in the broad arena of child safety and protection understand and manage the challenges in these chaotic environments. We attempt to provide ethical frameworks and 'professional toolboxes' to prepare practitioners for these complexities and sensitivities. We examine how ethical practice in child protection is framed by employers, practitioners and service users, what recipients of child protection services say about the assistance they have received and how these might be incorporated in ethical and legal decision making.

We offer an ethical decision-making framework that enables practitioners to acknowledge and deal with the contextual complexities, some of which we have alluded to thus far, cognisant that professional codes of ethics, despite their explicit principles, can only take us so far; they cannot tell practitioners what to do in specific situations or how to manage 'harsh practice environments' (Gray, 2010a, p. 1). Paradoxically, despite the volumes of literature on the increased complexities in, and demands of, child protection and family welfare practice, there is little concrete guidance on what this means for ethical practice.

In our broad ethical decision-making framework, we avoid the 'tyranny of principles' (Jonsen and Toulmin, 1988) and acknowledge the central place of power and power relations. We highlight considerations relating to gender, culture, race and other social factors impacting on service provision. We reflect on the best principles to guide practitioners with a *duty to protect* children, where poor decisions have serious consequences, and we highlight the essential place of care, respect and relationship in this important area of work (Gray and Stofberg, 2000; Marcellus, 2005). Most importantly, we incorporate the understanding that ethics is not just about how workers make decisions about what to do about children and families; ethical practice is not just about the exercise of 'pure rationality' or what Platt and Turney (2014) call 'technical-rational models of decision making'. Also it is more than self-reflection and interpersonal and professional dialogue. It is about creating a just and caring world, and having compassion for the suffering of others.

We have endeavoured to situate the ethical guidance provision through our central decision-making framework in practice by providing case examples from our own practice, the experiences of service users and practitioners, and research data to demonstrate and amplify the very practical nature of ethical decision making. We link this, where possible, to moral and philosophical thought that helps us grapple with the realities of everyday decision making in the complex organisational, legal and political world of child protection practice. Ethics is a practical discipline, not just an intellectual endeavour, as Aristotle observed over 2000 years ago (Thompson *et al.*, 2006). Its goals are practical: to make sound decisions that do not harm the very people we are trying to help.

The DECIDE model is not a rigid framework but suggests a process for ethical decision making and relevant questions for different circumstances and contexts. It comprises six stages, discussed fully in Chapters 4 and 12:

- Define the problem;
- Ethical review;
- Consider options;
- Investigate outcomes;
- Decide on action; and
- Evaluate results.

As outlined above, the process takes place within relationship-centred and relational practice and provides guidance for reflective and reflexive practice (see Chapters 4, 8, 11 and 12). We have placed case examples and reflective questions at key points in the book to help readers work through practice-related issues, thereby developing ethical decision-making skills.

Developing this book

All four authors are qualified social workers educated in various international locations, who have longstanding collective experience working in child protection and family welfare across many countries. We describe ourselves as practitioners, researchers and educators. We have all published and taught child welfare practice and ethical reasoning to diverse discipline groups. Our professional experience spans direct practice, policy and management in government, non-government and community services for a range of services for vulnerable children, families and communities. This book is informed by our deep knowledge of the research and literature but, most importantly, by our experiences and those, articulated and otherwise, of vulnerable children and families who are the receivers of services. We seek to highlight the issues involved in practising ethically in this fraught area, identify the low level of priority this is afforded within dominant discourses, and provide momentum to the embedding of ethics within child protection and family welfare policy and practice frameworks. We are passionate and committed to improving practice and outcomes for service users.

We have a broad and diverse audience in mind for people from various health and social care backgrounds, who work in organisations that perform a range of functions and roles to protect the well-being and safety of children. While our focus is child protection, we are mindful of the various protective approaches and systems found in different jurisdictions (see Chapters 5 and 6). Here the term *child protection* refers to legally mandated, largely involuntary service delivery approaches and systems, with *child welfare* being an approach more oriented toward voluntary services. We use the term *child protection and family welfare* to describe these integrated approaches, recognising that most systems incorporate both aspects within their service mix.

As in our earlier text *Reforming Child Protection* (Lonne *et al.*, 2009), we locate our work as stemming primarily from our Australian and English perspectives, noting we have used a diverse array of research and scholarship from around the world to highlight the often ubiquitous themes and issues addressed and the vexed and systemic nature of the 'wicked problems' child protection presents (ARACY, 2009a, 2009b). However, we do not assert that the matters and problems we discuss are found or present themselves to the same extent in every jurisdiction. We note the differences across cultures and countries in language used for receivers of services, and the encumbered meanings that can ensue; *service users* is the term primarily used here, although *client* is sometimes employed, and *stakeholders* is used to describe those with a material interest in child protection decision-making outcomes. In general, we have used the terms *children, families* and *communities* acknowledging that, although the term *young person* is used in many parts of the world, the terms *child* and *children* are seen as generic for these key constituents. *Single parents* has been used rather than sole parents. We have also used *carers* rather than caregivers, and *kinship carers* rather than kin carers. We provide greater detail of our choices later (for example in Chapters 5, 7 and 13), foreshadowing here how we have dealt with language descriptors. We have used *Indigenous* and *Aboriginal* to describe First Nations peoples, but acknowledge these terms are not used in every country or culture. We have also used the terms *black*, *white* and *Asian* to describe various ethnicities and races, while acknowledging that these terms are used in the United Kingdom and can be inappropriate in other cultures. Finally, we have used *practitioners* when discussing the broad cohort involved in child protection and family welfare practice, *child protection workers* or *workers* when we talk about those who are specifically engaged in the work of child protection, and *professionals* when referring to those who are educated within a particular discipline and who are expected to comply with a specific ethical framework.

The book's structure

This book is presented in four parts, each of which contains a number of chapters:

Part 1   Ethical theory and historical frameworks for practice;
Part 2   The context of child protection practice;
Part 3   Professional ethics and ethical child protection and family welfare practice;
Part 4   Practising ethically.

Each part and chapter provides the foundation for those following, culminating in the final chapter which highlights the public nature of ethical decision making and looks forward to anticipated developments. Each chapter grounds the ideas presented in the world of contemporary practice and the implications for practitioners, children, families and organisations. We conclude each chapter with reflective questions for the reader. The final two parts provide robust case examples to situate, and make palpable and clear, the relevance of the issues and options we discuss for the everyday realities of practice decisions in complex workplaces.

Part 1 explores frameworks for ethical practice and provides an overview of the DECIDE model. Chapter 2 focuses on the foundations of moral and ethical theory that inform ethical decision making, highlighting core historical ethical perspectives and their potential for reductionism when applied to child protection and family welfare practice. Chapter 3 describes some new and emerging theories, often built on the theories named in the previous chapter, which highlight care, relationship and context in helpful ways for practice. In Chapter 4, we present an ethical decision-making framework to guide practitioners within what we have already described as a complex organisational, legal, relational and political environment. This framework is not revolutionary but is based on a model that has been developed, applied, described and adapted for diverse disciplines by Professor Ian Thompson and colleagues (2006).

Part 2 critically examines the ideologies and discourses underpinning complex child protection systems and that drive their policies and practices. Evidence is presented of the contemporary crisis within child protection and family welfare systems worldwide. Chapter 5 reviews social constructions and understandings of children, families and the state; examines developments, such as early intervention to protect children and support families; and describes the impact of neoliberal ideologies on child protection and broader welfare systems. Chapter 6 discusses the social and public policies that have influenced professional practice and interventions with children and families. The contested nature of the politics and policy environments is examined along with key theories guiding practice. Thereafter, in Chapters 7 and 8, the growing evidence from a variety of stakeholders that protective interventions are not meeting the needs of children, parents, families and communities well enough is introduced. System outcomes are critiqued and the disturbing conclusion reached that the state is too often a poor parent and grandparent to children, with profound intergenerational impacts affecting many who have experienced intrusive interventions into family and community life.

Part 3 focuses on how we use this complex contextual information to refine ethical judgment and decision making. Chapter 9 examines the legal and organisational imperatives involved in ethical practice, and Chapter 10 discusses key ethical principles, such as the best interests of the child, and equity and fairness. We use case examples to examine the complexity of ethical decision making in the realities of child protection and family welfare practice.

The final part focuses on practising ethically as a relationship-centred and relational approach in which health and social care practitioners use a holistic perspective – captured in our integrated framework, the DECIDE model (Chapters 4 and 12). The use of power and authority, and application of duty of care forms the subject of Chapters 13 and 14 with their focus on cross-cultural practice in response to circumstances of difference and diversity, and handling information ethically. Chapter 15 revisits the overall thesis of the book and summarises the core themes and principles examined, such as the centrality of power, vulnerability and relational practice. It concludes by examining important issues and emerging trends, and highlighting the role practitioner-led advocacy can play in the ongoing reform of child protection worldwide.

We undertook the tasks we set ourselves in this book with excitement and trepidation, mindful of the politics of care work, and need for systemic change. Through building ethics into child protection policy and practice frameworks, we believe a system that respects human dignity and worth, is serious about social justice, and values relationships will eventuate. We realise our views may be contested by others and look forward to dialogue about practising ethically in child protection.

Reflective questions

1   Contemplate what you believe works well in child protection policy and practice, and what does not work well.
2   How well do you think approaches to protecting children and supporting families help them to change their life circumstances for the better?
3   What is your personal approach to incorporating ethics into your practice?
4   What do you see as the major ethical issues in child protection?

Chapter 2   **Established ethical frameworks**

Child protection work entails professionally challenging and personally confronting roles and tasks as it:

> raises complex moral and political issues which have no one right technical solution. Practitioners are asked to solve problems every day that philosophers have argued about for the last two thousand years ... Moral evaluations can and must be made if children's lives and well-being are to be secured. What matters is that we should not disguise this and pretend it is all a matter of finding better checklists or new models of psychopathology – technical fixes when the proper decision is a decision about what constitutes a good society.
>
> (Dingwall *et al.*, 1983, p. 244)

Working ethically in child protection places ethical concerns at its heart and means acting with integrity, where assessments and decisions, and decisions and actions, align with our values and ethical frameworks. As Dingwall *et al.* (1983) observed, though this entails an intellectual process of rational decision making to discern the relevant facts, assess the risks, and develop suitable options, it is also a process of emotional engagement and connection with people who may be fearful and anxious about the power of the worker or who have indeed harmed their children and are anxious to avoid scrutiny. While planning possible supports and interventions is critical, opportunities for relational connection occur in situations where intense emotions and tensions are at play, and events often move quickly. Such is the fraught environment where ethical child protection practice lies. Effective practice, though, requires prior knowledge of the key ethical principles and the major approaches to ethical decision making so that practitioners are well-prepared and able to engage 'in the moment' (Varela, 1999) with children, parents, family members, carers and others, but are also able to 'think on their feet' and make ethically sound and just decisions.

Ethics

Ethics is a tool used to enhance understanding, develop awareness and deepen knowledge on moral matters. It does not aim to provide definitive answers regarding what is right or wrong, but helps people to develop the ability to think through moral problems, reach informed decisions about them and take appropriate action. These skills include the ability to define a question precisely, state an answer clearly, explain a position accurately, find the relevant arguments, examine every argument critically, make a decision anticipating possible consequences, and act on it. It is important to emphasise, however, that:

> *ethical propositions are statements of value related to action* ... Value-statements may draw on abstract or ideal notions but at the same time they necessarily carry with them implications for the way in which individuals act and the relationship between people as members of social groups.
>
> (Hugman and Smith, 1995, p. 2; emphasis added)

Working ethically in child protection means engaging in a rational process of deliberation on ethical matters, which necessarily involve less deliberative emotional and intuitive, as well as deliberative, engagement. Moral philosophy is especially concerned with critical reflection on morality and moral issues; this is a cognitive-rational process that involves clarifying the meaning of moral language to understand its intent and advancing theories about morality and their application to moral and ethical problems, such as those child protection practitioners deal with on daily basis. Ultimately, the study of ethics as it relates to child protection has the potential to aid in the making of intelligent moral choices and sound ethical decisions. Philosophical thinking about ethical problems includes making choices between alternative positions based on their anticipated consequences and being able to provide a sound rationale for the choices and decisions we make. It attests the need for a deep understanding of morality so that individuals might choose or commit themselves to behave morally and take responsibility for others.

The ethical theories discussed in this and the next chapter show how moral philosophers have debated morality and ethics to discern a deeper understanding of what makes people moral, and how to entreat them to behave ethically in respecting the interests of others. Moral philosophers disagree as to whether individuals are naturally caring, or self-interested – and therefore have to be made to care about others. The central question is whether people are by nature moral beings – as Aristotle (1954) believed in his naturalistic ethics – or whether they have to be made to be moral through the enforcement of moral rules and principles (non-naturalistic ethics of which utilitarianism is an example). Are individuals first moral, then social? Does ethics follows morality or vice versa? Those who believe individuals have to be made to be moral believe ethics is largely a normative domain associated with the modernist project of searching for 'golden rules' of conduct (Bauman, 1993; Kelemen and Peltonen, 2001). This is the approach taken by most systems of professional ethics, which are dominated by deontological and utilitarian approaches (Gray and Lovat, 2006). In child protection these approaches are visible in the emphasis placed on risk assessments and decisions to maximise the child's best interests, safeguard the child's safety and achieve the best outcomes for the child based on the argument that this is in everyone's best interests. There are other approaches, however, that counsel the importance of embracing the complexity and messiness attached to intervening in the lives of others, and the dangers of seeking or proclaiming certainty about what is the 'right' thing to do and what might be the 'right' outcome and, crucially, the importance of engaging in ongoing dialogue about means and ends (Featherstone *et al.*, 2014b; Thompson *et al.*, 2006).

All professional encounters that concern and affect the welfare of others have a moral component, and this is very evident in child protection where practitioners operate in very fraught contexts, with uncertain or ambivalent societal mandates, and where the stakes for all concerned can be extremely high. Practitioners can draw on various ethical perspectives to think through ethical dilemmas in child protection and family welfare work, such as when or whether to remove children, deciding on what is in the child's best interests, being clear on whose interests are being served, and so on. These various ethical approaches, though often apparently in tension with one another, can work alongside each other to help child protection practitioners maximise the good and minimise harm (a utilitarian approach) while doing their duty and following their values, principles and codes (a deontological approach). Houston (2010) has argued that although different schools of ethics have been hard to reconcile they need to be considered in a world where practitioners have to engage with legal requirements, procedural rules, the future consequences of decision making, issues that have a bearing on professional integrity, and situations of care. Thus deontology (rules) and consequentialism (consequences of one's actions) need to be integrated into understandings of care (ethics of care) and professional integrity and careful contingent judgments (virtue ethics). Houston argues for a form of discourse ethics to underpin this project as, for him, communication and inter-subjective engagement are the only media through which actors can reach morally binding decisions. This is echoed by Amartya Sen (2005), who argues 'the status that … ethical claims have must be ultimately dependent on their survivability in unobstructed discussion' (p. 160). The critical point is that moral philosophy and ethical theory 'enlarges our thinking on and understanding of moral issues; creates a dialogical space for debate and discussion with others; and enhances [our] ability to justify the ethical decisions [we] make' (McAuliffe, 2010, p. 44).

Ethical perspectives for child protection

In this section we briefly examine the ethical perspectives most relevant to child protection matters. Though often in tension with one another, collectively these perspectives expand our thinking on ethical issues and allow us to consider them from multiple viewpoints. Chapters 2 and 3 highlight the philosophical and practice tensions within and between the following disparate theories, and show how discussions about ethics are enriched by diverse influences.

1   The *deontological* perspective is concerned with our duties and obligations towards others, sometimes referred to as a duty-based morality. Since it also concerns rules and principles, it has also often been referred to as a rule-based morality. It is concerned with the means by which we achieve moral ends, such as respecting others, self-determination, and privacy and confidentiality. It looks to ethical codes and decision-making frameworks to assist in determining what to do to achieve the best possible ends (Banks, 2006, 2008; Congress, 2010; Dolgoff *et al.*, 2009; Lonne *et al.*, 2004; McAuliffe, 1999, 2010). The first deontological thinker was Immanuel Kant, whose *universalist-rationalist* approach has been widely embraced by social work; that is to say Kant believed the same moral rules applied to all people everywhere and we could solve moral problems through logical reasoning.

2   Ethical theories that are concerned with ultimate purposes or end states are known as *teleology*. These theories hold that the ends justify the means. Though each has a slightly different view of ends, all are concerned with consequences – *consequentialism* and *utilitarianism* – or ultimate ends – *virtue ethics*.

   a   A *consequential* perspective pays special attention to the consequences of particular decisions or actions rather than duties, obligations or rules, so decisions would be justified on the basis of anticipated outcomes. Hence removing a child would be justified if the child were at risk of significant abuse on the basis that the child would be safe away from the abusive parent, that is, if the worker were to anticipate the consequences of 'not removing the child' would result in further abuse and neglect. However, consideration of the consequences could result in non-removal in certain circumstances and, indeed, throughout this book we argue for the importance of thinking about the longer-term consequences of removal and the often very damaging implications.

   b   *Utilitarianism* is a particular consequential perspective that seeks to do, or decide, what will benefit the majority of people in a particular situation. It seeks to find a way to benefit the greatest number of people, that is to say, to minimise harm and maximise good. Therefore, it would sacrifice the interests of a single individual if it meant that a lot of people would benefit from the decision or action.

   c   *Virtue ethics* is concerned with moral disposition or motivation. It holds that *doing the right thing* – doing what is morally right – comes from following the virtues (Clark, 2006a; Gray and Lovat, 2007; Houston, 2003; McBeath and Webb, 2002). In virtue ethics doing the right thing in some circumstances might be not telling the truth, whereas, strictly speaking, in the rule-based deontological perspective the rule is to always tell the truth regardless of consequences. In virtue ethics, we are more inclined to think that the right thing to do depends on the circumstances or consequences rather than blindly following rules.

3   Several approaches are known as *relational ethics*, by which we mean they are based in the relationships we have with others. Two key approaches relevant for child protection of this kind are the *ethics of care* and the *ethics of responsibility*. These approaches have been increasingly influenced by the *politics of care*, leading them to be influential in the policy arena that shapes child protection legislation and practice.

   a   The *ethics of care*, associated with feminist ethics, has also become a political theory about the nature of care in society and whose responsibility it is to care for others (Featherstone, 2001, 2010; Gray, 2010a; Hugman, 2005; Meagher and Parton, 2004; Orme, 2002, 2008; Parton, 2003). In analysing the notion of care, it distinguishes between what it means to give and receive care. In child protection what it means to ethically care will be affected by contemporary social norms and constructions of childhood, for example, our understandings of child development or gendered family roles and responsibilities. This is where feminist theory has contributed important insights regarding dominant assumptions about motherhood, such as women should take the major responsibility for caring for their families. The *ethics of care* reconceptualises the deontological notion of duty grounding it in relationships such that care emerges in the context of our relationships with others, our concerns about approaches that prioritise our duty of care to the child notwithstanding (see Chapters 4 and 10).

b   Lévinas's *ethics of responsibility* is concerned with our responsibilities and duties towards others. Lévinas referred to this as *the call of the other* (Tascón, 2010). It is, at root, a deontological theory that concerns our duty towards others with whom we have a relationship.

4   *Discursive* or *discourse ethics* draws on the work of Jürgen Habermas (1996), who built this theory on Kant's idea that, through reasoned communication, we could reach agreement on most things. Hence it has also been referred to as a *dialogical approach*. Dialogical in this context means talking through our problems, taking all information and everyone's interests into account in the particular circumstances, and applying logical and practical reasoning to reach a solution. For Habermas (1996), the only way to reach morally binding decisions is through communication, and what he called 'intersubjective engagement', that is, through conversing with others, sharing ideas and discussing implications. Habermas (1996) emphasised the intersubjective, interactional components of our encounters (Hayes and Houston, 2007; Houston, 2010; Lovat and Gray, 2008).

5   *Postmodern ethics* is also a *particularist* approach, but it differs from discourse ethics in that it debunks deontology's universal rules and principles. A postmodern approach suggests that each situation must be dealt with on a case-by-case basis (Rossiter, 2006; Rossiter *et al.*, 2000). It is commonly perceived that this leads to a highly *relativistic* form of ethics, where people make up the rules as they go, there being no rules to which we all agree or which we can apply to every situation. However, as we shall see in Chapter 3, this is a misconception (see Gray, 2010b).

In addition to the perspectives outlined above, practitioners need to consider the ethical implications of the social context in which decisions are being made. The lens through which each of us views the world has ethical implications. Here the social perspectives embraced by social care professions have an important influence on their practice.

Social perspectives include feminist, anti-oppressive and anti-racist, human rights and social justice approaches. Most codes of ethics are guided by humanitarian and democratic ideals, and promote values based on respect for the equality, worth and dignity of all people, through the promotion of human rights and social justice (IFSW, 2014). Social perspectives have important ethical implications based on, among other things, issues of gender, race, ethnicity, culture and religion, and attention to these factors is central to child protection (see Chapters 5, 6 and 13). We need to address the key issues in many jurisdictions, such as the fact that children from the poorest and most marginalised areas are most likely to be placed into care and separated from their families and communities. Underlying professional ethical principles within child protection and family welfare need to be considered in relation to the core values of respect, beneficence and justice (see Chapter 9). These values are sometimes treated as universal across the professions even though the emphases on central principles in various professional codes of ethics might vary considerably. For example, social work tends to highlight values associated with justice, and nursing has highlighted values associated with the duty of care.

In the remainder of this chapter, we examine the established ethical theories of deontology and teleology, exploring the respective place of utilitarianism, consequentialism and virtue ethics (see Figure 2.1).

Deontology

Kantian deontological ethics is a principle-based ethics wherein moral phenomena are seen as *rational*. Here reason is central and reasons motivate or predispose actions. Kant's ethical theory is grounded in the respect owed to individuals because they are *rational moral agents* and reasons are seen as more reliable than emotions when making moral judgments. This is not to say that Kant overlooks the importance of emotions; he merely believes they do not give the moral agent *reason* or cause for action. This is the work of moral principles: to guide people to act in a certain way such that acting in accordance with these principles will produce the most appropriate ethical responses. For example, when a practitioner respects the client she does this because it is the right thing to do in terms of the principles attached to her professional values and code of ethics. Likewise, with the principle of confidentiality, the practitioner's duty to the client provides the reason to act as this rule requires. The object of the action is to keep the client's confidence and the reason for the action, which accords with the rule that requires her to do so, is the principles of maintaining client confidentiality. Hence, this form of ethics is primarily concerned with finding objective moral rules and principles that apply to all people in all situations. In this example, we must always act in such a way as to safeguard client confidentiality. However, as we shall see, in child protection there are riders to this principle (as we discuss in this book) and many matters to take into account in balancing confidentiality with the duty to protect, including the harm that can result from breaching confidentiality.

Kant's principle of respect for persons, as an end in itself, is tied to his view of individuals as rational beings with autonomy and self-determination (the capacity to choose for themselves) (Gray and Stofberg, 2000). It is this condition of *human agency* that sets the object of moral requirement in place and limits the kinds of actions we can take. It is precisely this view of the individual which leads to attention being paid to responsibility as the flipside of duty or obligation, and to ethical decision making as a rational activity. Much attention is then focused on devising moral principles, codes of ethics and ethical decision-making frameworks to guide ethical practice (see Chapter 4). Importantly, however, what lies behind this is what Goldstein (1987) was at pains to emphasise and that is a commitment to, and seriousness about, morality. Once we understand the moral reasons behind what we do, we begin to appreciate the

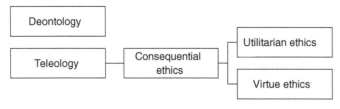

FIGURE **2.1** Established ethical theories

importance of following professional values, principles, rules and ethical codes, and do it not because we have to but because we want to.

Deontological approaches create a logic whereby professionals are duty-bound to follow their ethical code and where ethical practice without guiding principles is inconceivable. This allows for rational deliberation which comes into play in cases of conflict or uncertainty when our routine moral judgments fail us. While there is no denying the importance of principles when difficult ethical decisions have to be made, the possibility exists that other factors are equally important. Arguably, policy and practice in the contemporary Anglophone approach to child protection is dominated by a deontological, rules-driven approach to ethics. In this punitive, risk-aversive, managerial and politicised organisational environment of contemporary child protection, it has become increasingly difficult to maintain a broader ethical perspective; 'the practice of value' (Webb, 2006) is much more difficult than we realise (Lonne *et al.*, 2009). This, however, should not undermine the importance of professional principles and codes. Despite their imperfections, they can assist in focusing attention on, and guiding us in, the ethical aspects of practice decisions. Codes of ethics cannot solve problems or recognise contradictions, only practitioners can do this. At best, they are tools we can use, among others, to guide practice and they can be helpful tools if we use them well (Gray and Lovat, 2006).

However, some practitioners find a deontological principles- or rules-based approach too constraining, believing what's right or wrong depends crucially on the context in which the ethical issue arises. Areas where young people themselves express strong views on how they might best be protected can also challenge practitioners' beliefs about the 'right' way to proceed.

Teleology

While deontology is concerned with absolutist notions of duty and obligation, teleology's focus is on ultimate ends or purposes. Teleology began with Plato, but was extended by Aristotle (1954), who believed *everything exists for a reason*. He showed that being logical did not necessarily mean there was only a hard reality to be understood. He observed that everyone desired happiness but looked for it in many different ways, and some in the wrong places. Happiness was not to be found in wealth, pleasure and high social status. Rather, happiness, which he defined as the sense of harmony gained from living according to the virtues, came from behaving consistently with our human nature. Happy people were those who had worked this out or, as Aristotle put it, they engaged in well-reasoned behaviour. They thought before they acted, whether their behaviour conformed to the virtues of courage, prudence, respect, justice, and so on. Aristotle offered the basis for a naturalistic teleological theory, one grounded in human nature. For him, not only are humans born with an innate potential to 'be good' but given the right guidance, they will direct their abilities to the right ends because it is in their nature to do so.

In child protection, this might suggest that parents have the innate potential to care for their children because it is part of their fulfilment and happiness as human beings. With the right guidance (from a caring professional), a parent would provide their children with the best possible care. At times, however, everyone can find themselves unable to cope and, as a result, can be observed, according to this perspective, seeking happiness in the 'wrong places' (see discussion of Aristotelian virtue ethics below).

Consequential ethics

Unlike Aristotle's teleological theory that is concerned with ultimate ends and purposes, *consequentialism* – a term coined by G.E.M. Anscombe (1958) – concerns more immediate consequences. Here weight is given to the consequences of our moral decisions and actions, that is, the rightness or otherwise of an act is judged in terms of the ensuing consequences. Put another way, the right consequences ensue from the right decisions. In taking a consequential approach to ethics in child protection, the worker must choose to act in ways that maximise the child's safety. This approach would also suggest that clients should choose actions in their lives that lead to good outcomes. There is a potential ethical dilemma here because what is considered a 'good outcome' may vary considerably between worker and client, or even workers who take different ethical approaches and there is an important temporal consideration here in terms of consequences over the life course and intergenerationally. For example, though most ethical approaches take consequences into account, what they consider a 'good consequence' might vary. It is also hard to reliably anticipate the consequences of human actions and decisions. Disclosing something a client has told you in confidence may be justified if someone might be harmed by your silence. Importantly, consequentialism differs from deontology, where rightness or wrongness inheres in the means – the act or decision itself – rather than the ends – the consequences or outcomes of the actions associated with it.

Utilitarian ethics

Utilitarianism is a form of consequentialism concerned with the value of ends for the greater good. Hence, it is committed to maximising happiness by doing the greatest good for the greatest number. If one were to make a utilitarian judgment, one would seek the option that benefited the majority. Particularly influential on modern society has been Bentham's utilitarian theory, which, unlike Aristotle's optimistic view of human nature, contends that individuals are inherently oversupplied with self-interest and thus deficient in goodness or altruism. Hence they need to be coerced into looking after the interests of the majority.

In utilitarian ethics, moral intentions and acts could only result from social engineering, as they did not spring from an autonomous moral agent (as promoted in deontology). Thus it is important to devise foundational moral rules to ensure that people will look after the interests of the majority.

Though from different starting points, both deontology and utilitarianism share the modernist predilection for the search for universal moral rules and principles to prescribe or enforce standards of moral conduct. These theories hold that we can discern overriding universal moral principles that apply to everyone in all situations despite social, cultural, religious and other differences.

Utilitarianism sought to transform ethics into a social science establishing a social-scientific method for attaining ethical agreement as one of rational investigation, logical deliberation and democratic resolution. As a consequence, ethical decision making became a calculative business in which specialist ethics committees used checklists and computed scores. This made the power of such committees to rewrite the rights and wrongs of the past determinative in many instances. With the right software, the results of such a process could be fed into a computer and the final ethical decision produced electronically (see Reamer's 2001 Ethics Audit).

Virtue ethics

Virtue ethics continues in the Aristotelian tradition and was subsequently developed in the philosophy of St Thomas Aquinas and recent Thomistic thinkers, such as Alasdair MacIntyre and Martha Nussbaum. Aquinas (1225–1274) warned that if we cannot ground morality in human nature, or in divine law, then it can only be a matter of consensus that arises from shared moral attitudes resulting from 'continuing implicit negotiation, bargaining and compromise' (Harman, in Rasmussen and Den Uyl, 1991, p. 8). Habermas's (1996) discourse ethics pick up on the nature of such 'negotiation, bargaining and compromise'. His theory of communicative rationality rests on the Kantian idea that people can reach consensus through logical, rational discussion (see Chapter 3). However, feminists have argued there is more to the story:

> Virtue theory insists that it is misguided to expect reason to be able to establish some infallible moral doctrine which is compulsory and often counter to human nature and emotions. Perhaps morality is not about conforming to rules, but more about being trained to see problematic situations in a moral way. Morality may not be the rational control of the emotions but, more appropriately, the cultivation of desirable emotions.
>
> (Phoca and Wright, 1999, p. 123)

Virtue ethics, captured aptly here by Phoca and Wright (1999), is a branch of moral philosophy that critiques ethical theories which emphasise reason, logic and rationality as the cornerstone of ethical behaviour. Virtue ethicists see these rational approaches as reductive in their presumptions about the overriding importance of duties, obligations, rules, principles, purposes and consequences in moral behaviour. Do we keep a client's confidence merely because it is our duty to do so? Virtue ethicists think not. We keep confidentiality because it is the right thing to do, and because there is something intrinsic to our relationships with clients centred on mutuality and trust. There is a give and take within relationships that has little to do with consciously and rationally applying rules and principles. Bauman (1993) and Lévinas (1998) refer to it as the 'call of the other', a responsibility we feel not out of duty or obligation, but out of compassion and caring deeply. Thus 'something intrinsic' arises from a moral disposition, an innate tendency – something inherently human – that gets reinforced in the give and take of our relationships with others.

From a virtue ethics perspective, what makes a practitioner's behaviour ethical is the intention sitting behind it and the practitioner's desire to act virtuously – caring because it is good to care. It is our human capacity to reach out and respond to our clients that makes us want to behave ethically. Unlike Kant's reasons as motives, for virtue ethicists our innate tendencies propel us to act virtuously – to follow the virtues of honesty, kindness and care – and thus find the 'moral way' (Phoca and Wright, 1999). Murdoch (1970) emphasises the intrinsic nature of morality: it is good to be good merely because it is good to be good. We need no other reason than this – no universal principles or determining consequences.

Virtue ethicists criticise deontological rules-based approaches for failing to pay attention to the relational aspects of our moral behaviour. But Herman (1993) argues that Kantian moral theory can accommodate relationships, and it is precisely the deliberative intersubjective aspects of Kant's moral theory that Habermas (1996) develops in his discourse ethics (discussed in Chapter 3). If one were to see virtue ethics and the ethics of care (a related ethical theory discussed in Chapter 3) in Kantian terms, one would acknowledge that the fulfilment of human needs, including the need for care, is necessary to sustain oneself as a rational being and that the rule in operation is one of beneficence. In terms of Kant's theory, *everyone's needs count* because their fulfilment is an end that cannot be ignored. So the universal principle of beneficence prevents us from giving preferential treatment to those with whom we have close or good relationships while ignoring the needs of others.

What we see evolving here is the casting of ethical dispositions and actions in a very different way to the deontological focus on duties, obligations, principles and rules. According to virtue ethicists, intrinsic virtues, or traits of character, and particular moral attitudes and dispositions, can never ensue from simple rule-following or the mechanical application of principles. This is not to say deontologists were not mindful of the importance of practical reasoning, but it is rather to emphasise that people can learn to be moral through training, experience and practice; they can learn to be virtuous through processes demonstrating that following the virtues produces good outcomes. However, remember it is not good outcomes that make actors or their actions moral – as in consequential theories – but their motivations, intentions and dispositions. Hence, morality under virtue ethics has a motivational force that propels people to take action and it is the individual's moral character that is the 'stable reference point, not the action' (McBeath and Webb, 2002, p. 1026; see also Clark, 2006a). Virtue ethics makes the qualities of the individual's character, which are discernible from their actions, foundational. It is easy to see how this resonates for those who see 'use of self' and reflective practice as pivotal to good helping relationships (see Chapters 8 and 11).

The important difference in this approach to ethics is that contemporary Aristotelian virtue ethics provides a naturalistic account of morality as something which inheres in our human nature rather than in abstract principles. However, one of the sticking points for those who are sceptical about virtue ethics is how virtues are defined. Aristotle (1954) believed that virtues could be discerned by looking at the character traits of the virtuous person, or from observing what is needed for human flourishing. He believed there was a direct connection between following virtues and human happiness and well-being (Sen, above, thus called virtues 'capabilities' or capacities for human flourishing). By attributing morality to *human* nature, rather than to gender differences, virtue ethics enables feminists to focus on fundamental *human* interests and needs. This fits well with the strengths perspective, where professionals help people achieve their full potential by actualising their innate capacities (Gray, 2011) (see Chapter 6).

However, Aristotle's (1954) naturalistic philosophy went beyond the individual to discerning the kind of society needed for human flourishing, and fits well with value perspective on human rights and social justice. (It is the theory underlying Sen's capabilities approach.) These concerns are very different from those of *non-natural* ethics, like Kant's deontology, which 'depict ethics as something transcendentally pure and uncontaminated by the world of human desires' (Phoca and Wright, 1999, p. 124). However, when ethics are removed from this 'objective' level, they become closer to psychology or sociology, which can be problematic for feminists. For example, by grounding ethics in 'feminine' characteristics, as Noddings (2003) and others have done, feminists depict relationships, empathy, care and so on as 'women's special virtues'. As Phoca and Wright (1999) note, there is a danger in seeing women as 'innately supportive, non-competitive nurturers' (p. 125) as this can all too easily result in their being disregarded and feminist ethics once again being marginalised. Feminist virtue ethicists thus advocate a broader focus on character, disposition and the myriad factors needed for human flourishing (see Chapter 3).

Feminists highlight the importance of context. Hence ethics is not just about doing the right thing but also about being the sort of person who does the right thing (Tobin, 1994). Thus virtue ethics incorporates an appreciation and balancing of principles within the context of personal morality. Through an examination of a 'pure' Aristotelian view, this section provides the opportunity to reflect on the tensions for those caught in the headlights of child protection (those who are poor and marginalised and bear the brunt of stigma and discrimination) trying to pursue happiness in a world that places them at the bottom of Maslow's hierarchy.

With regard to parental responsibility, a virtue ethics approach would suggest that it is the child protection practitioner's responsibility to provide practical and moral guidance to service users. The crucial element in Aristotle's (1954) approach is the 'idea that living rationally intelligently is the natural end ... of a human being' (p. 35) and 'living rationally or intelligently creates well-being through the process of self-actualisation and maturation' (Rasmussen and Den Uyl, 1991, p. 36). Hence, *human flourishing* or *eudaimonia* is achieved through our own actions. For workers, then, the key concerns cohere around how to generate the conditions necessary to assist families to flourish (see Gupta *et al.*, 2014).

Unlike consequentialism, Aristotelian virtue ethics is not simply about consequences but, rather, about ultimate ends: being the best parent or worker you can be. Only we can do this: we must reach (actualise) our potential because that is what is in our nature: Only we can do what is necessary for our own flourishing:

> Actualizing our potentialities, finding fulfilment and wellbeing, is just what it is for us to be good. Our obligations arise in terms of our attaining this good. We must live in accordance with our nature – it is good for us to do so – this we all share. But, at the same time, each human being is different – unique – and so what is good for one sort of living thing may not be good for another.
>
> (Rasmussen and Den Uyl, 1991, p. 56)

This indicates the importance of considering the unique nature of each individual encountered in child protection practice in order to help them to discern what might be good for them. For Aristotle (1954) a person who knows what is right does what is right. Thus we don't need rigid principles. Moral principles can only serve as guides for action – provide us with the standards of successful living and tell us how certain courses of action will impact on our lives; as such they can provide guidelines for virtuous behaviour – guidelines but not definitive solutions. Nothing can substitute for the individual's responsible personal judgment: 'personal freedom, judgment, and responsibility are given pride of place in the Aristotelian project' (Rasmussen and Den Uyl, 1991, p. 30).

Rasmussen and Den Uyl (1991) continue: the value of the Aristotelian tradition is that it does 'not attempt to speak to every issue or circumstance. In practice, flexibility or indeterminacy translate into a recognition of the value of diversity, pluralism, and a basic commitment to individual judgment and responsibility' (p. 27); our *telos* [purpose] and rational nature generate an obligation to lead an examined life' (p. 29).

In Aristotelian ethics, primacy of place is given to the person 'to integrate the various elements of human behaviour into a coherent pattern of personal existence' (p. 39). This 'can be given more content if we consider human nature in conjunction with other factors that are part of human living (such as) … circumstances, personal attitudes, prudential judgment, habituation, cultural surroundings and values, risk and uncertainty' (p. 29).

In summary, all Aristotelians share certain basic beliefs: (i) *commitment to teleology* – the end point of being the best one can be; (ii) *eudaimonism* – the theory that people must strive to realise their nature, their capabilities, using their reason and intellect to work out how to reach their full potential – the point of human flourishing; (iii) *grounding of ethics in human nature* – in the actualisation of one's nature given values exist because of the needs and requirements of human beings; (iv) *primacy of reason over passion* – though rational desires are possible, reason can motivate someone to act; and (v) *rejection of reductive naturalism* – the theory that morality can be explained and maintained by a system of regulative rules, or in terms of purpose and consequence.

Conclusion

In conclusion, this chapter has examined the established ethical theories of deontology, teleology, consequentialism, utilitarianism and virtue ethics. It has shown how different ethical theories have different starting points and focus on alternative aspects of moral behaviour. The two key theorists are Kant and Aristotle, the former constructing a theory of deontology around extrinsic notions like duties and obligations, and the latter around intrinsic human characters and traits and how these lend themselves to following a path that leads to self-fulfilment and happiness. Chapter 3 discusses 'emergent' ethical theories that build on these ethical traditions, including the ethics and politics of care, dialogical or discourse ethics, and the postmodern ethics of responsibility. We explore how Habermas (1996) develops discourse ethics in the Kantian tradition, feminists develop the ethics of care in the tradition of virtue ethics, and Bauman takes a different tack from Kant in his postmodern ethics of responsibility that follows in the phenomenological tradition whereby ethics, or the desire to behave morally, flows from the 'call of the other'.

Reflective questions

1 Which of the deontological and teleological approaches to ethical decision making do you prefer and why?
2 What are the key ethical principles relevant to child protection?
3 How might a utilitarian approach be used within child protection practice?
4 What personal characteristics might a child protection worker who embraces a virtues ethic approach display?

Chapter 3   **Emergent ethical theories**

Relational ethics might be seen as an approach interested in what happens in the space between people in relationships; what Habermas (1996) might call an *intersubjective space*. Encompassing all aspects of relationships, it weaves a narrative thread that combines the notions of *ethics* as a set of moral principles with a narrative of *relation*. Relationships from this perspective are seen as co-constructed encounters with ethical and moral dimensions (Gabriel and Casemore, 2009). Hence, relational approaches to ethics are generally more process oriented and less formalised and rule bound. They are often situational and focus on the 'unpredictable, often subtle, yet ethically important moments [in practice]' (Ellis, 2007, p. 4). In this approach to ethics, Buber (1958) suggests, we are required to be true to our character and responsible for our actions *and their consequences for others*. This requires that we approach our decisions, actions and interactions mindfully (Gabriel, 2001, 2005; Gabriel and Casemore, 2009). Relational ethics insists on fairness in our interpersonal relationships and a balance between entitlement and obligation – give and take (Ford, 2008).

All relationships occur within a complex, multidimensional context that simultaneously influences, and is influenced by, our encounters with others (Gabriel and Casemore, 2009). The complexity of the child protection arena makes these approaches particularly relevant for practitioners who are making decisions *with* and *for* children and their families. When complex decisions are made regarding children and their future relationships with their families and communities, relational ethics are in play. The worker's task in this approach to ethics becomes to establish the conditions in their relationships with families for mutual respect, dignity and connectedness between people and the communities in which they live (Ellis, 2007). These underlying values require workers in child protection and family welfare to shift from a sole focus on what should be done – though this remains a central concern when children are in danger – to how might this best be done given the emotional bonds connecting parents, families, children and significant others, and their wider community support networks (see Chapters 5 and 11).

Relational ethics is mindful that you have stepped into a conversation, as it were, that has antecedents and consequences; it fits well with a narrative approach that seeks to understand how relationships are shaped over time so as to retell the story in a more empowering way for those involved (Ellis, 2007). Several emergent ethical theories draw on these relational ethics to move the focus to issues of care and responsibility, to questions of how we might best forge caring relationships that are fulfilling and satisfying, to meet our common human needs for love, recognition and mutual respect. Elements of the ethical theories discussed in Chapter 2 run through these newer approaches, which might best be seen as attempts to correct the prescriptive elements of earlier ethical perspectives and to take account of the issues they overlooked, such as gender and the politics of care. Here feminists have been prime contributors to an approach that has come to be known as the ethics of care.

Ethics of care

Relationships are central to feminist thinking about ethics. Hence, the feminist ethics of care casts the nature of ethics in a different way to the focus on duties and rules (deontology) or consequences and maximising the good or minimising harm (consequentialist-utilitarian). It is closer to, though different from, virtue ethics and its focus on moral character. While the feminist ethics of care attempts to provide a more complete view of morality and ethics, there are important philosophical problems that must be examined before we can determine whether it offers a better understanding of morality than existing approaches in ethics, particularly to those complex problems that child protection workers face in the harsh, risk-saturated environments in which they work, where value-based practice is becoming increasingly difficult.

There are two main strands to the feminist ethics of care. One stems from psychology starting with the developmental work of Carol Gilligan, and the other from that of political scientists Joan Tronto and Selma Sevenhuijsen.

Gilligan's (1982) groundbreaking work on *gender differences* in moral development significantly influenced the development of the feminist ethics of care. Gilligan discerned that, since most thinking on ethics had been done by men, including the psychological research on children's moral development, rational approaches predominated, while the relational, emotionally connected and nurturing aspects more usually attributed to women were completely absent. To redress this imbalance, her ethics of care perspective involved seeing ourselves as connected to others within a web of relationships (see Chapter 11). Rather than arising autonomously, she saw our sense of self as tied to our relationships and to our responsiveness to one another. The idea of *responsivity* separated ethics of care approaches from other normative approaches centred on responsibility; normative approaches focus on devising rules to ensure that people behave responsibly to one another. For ethics of care theorists it is not rules but relationships that determine human behaviour; feminist scholars 'hoped to find in women's "difference" a more humane model for public life' (Faludi, 1992, p. 359).

Noddings' (2003) ethics of care approach was rooted in the roles women assume in society. Rather than a form of virtue ethics, for Noddings, care concerns the *mutuality of the caring relationship*, which embodies a unique way of being responsive to the particular details of the caring situation through one's actions within it. For her, the *duty* of care (deontology) is not the same as the *ethic* of care. Care involves an emotional dimension; one is immersed in a caring relationship with the one being cared-for in a way that ensures he or she *feels* cared for. Without this one is merely acting out of duty or obligation. What this means within the child protection and family welfare context is that practitioners cannot avoid being immersed in the emotional entanglements of family relationships. Special skills are required to ensure respect and fairness for all involved. For Noddings, this means suspending evaluation in order to get the full story.

Davion (1993) draws attention to the *moral risks* involved in walking the tightrope between caring and protecting. In child protection this means ensuring parents who are assessed as abusive feel 'cared for' even when their child is being removed from their care. To maintain integrity in our relationships, we 'must be able to maintain deeply held convictions' (Davion, 1993, p. 163). Sometimes this means people need to end relationships for the sake of their own well-being. Examples might include the woman who chooses to leave a relationship with a partner who she still loves but who is behaving abusively towards her, or a worker who removes a child from his or her parents to ensure his or her safety, even though, in the process, a previously 'caring' relationship with a spouse or parent respectively might be jeopardised (see case example in Chapter 11).

Importantly, care is not just about concern for others but also includes care of the self. Davion (1993) believes the idea that individuals within caring relations are important in themselves is missing from Noddings's approach. The idea that the ideal self is 'developed in congruence with one's best remembrance of caring and being cared-for' (Noddings, 2003, p. 22) leaves little room for autonomy. Also, the practices of caring, trusting and empathising can frequently be harmful or manipulative since there is nothing self-regulating in these practices to prevent this. Thus, making care the core virtue raises problems, as do approaches that reinforce traditional women's roles, since they ignore other virtues and may hinder women's autonomy (Davion, 1993; Held, 1995; Keller, 1997; Koehn, 1998). But Meyers (in Keller, 1997) asserts:

> ... a person can be very much connected to others and still be autonomous ... friendships can enhance the autonomy competency, and thereby the self-respect, of someone who may be minimally autonomous to begin with. Finally, [she] ... issues one last challenge to the individualistic conception of autonomy by conceiving autonomy [as does Habermas] as an intersubjective activity.
>
> (p. 161)

Ultimately, however, care is not merely a private, relational, moral matter but also a political issue that relates more broadly to how national governments take care of their citizens, including the care and protection of children. How the burden of care is shared is the crucial question for feminists like Tronto (1993) and Sevenhuijsen (1998, 2000, 2003) for whom care is more than an ethical practice based on emotional connections in the private sphere of relationships.

Politics of care

Tronto (1993) and Sevenhuijsen (1998, 2000, 2003) believe that many feminist care ethicists overlook the role of care in broader social policy. They take the emotional bond of our relational connections to another level, drawing on feminist arguments about care as invisible, unpaid and undervalued women's work. They politicise care by highlighting its marginalisation and devaluation in Western society. For them, care is a complex moral and political issue: it is not merely a private interpersonal or familial matter but a public welfare concern. Furthermore, citizen–consumers have a democratic right to care and policy makers and care providers have a responsibility to listen to their concerns. For example, welfare recipients – usually described as passive and dependent in dominant discourses – are active care providers and 'normal citizens' (Bozalek et al., 2007) caring for themselves and others.

This is extremely important in child protection, which tends to focus on what parents do wrong rather than on what they do right. Child protection systems turn on the largesse of caring foster parents and kinship networks, as well as struggling parents trying against all odds to keep their families intact. Rather than see welfare benefits as a 'drain' on society, the politics of care reminds us that we owe people an obligation to care for them, and to care for those doing the caring. Hence Daly and Lewis (2003) see the politics of care in 'the activities and relations involved in meeting the physical and emotional requirements of dependent adults and children, and the normative, economic and social frameworks within which these are assigned and carried out' (p. 285).

An important issue is that the supply of care decreases as more women enter the labour force, the population ages, norms about family change, and so on, while demand for care increases. This has forced governments to think of alternative ways of providing care formally in the public sphere, since society can no longer rely solely on the family as a source of informal care, hence the expansion into new forms of (paid) care. The image of family solidarity prevalent in social policy has given way to a more realistic, gendered understanding of family, while the decreasing availability of private unpaid, family-based care has led to its expansion into the private market sector. Thus, when analysing new policies, it is essential to acknowledge the inevitable diversity of care provision in increasingly pluralistic societies.

The politics of care forces us to examine the relationship between justice and care. This is particularly relevant in child protection, where most clients have little choice. In short, justice and care are inseparable, rights to care are essential and care is a social obligation. Held (2006), however, sees care as more fundamental than justice, utility or virtue:

> ... caring relations should form the wider moral framework into which justice should be fitted. Care seems the most basic moral value ... Without care ... there would be no persons to respect and no families to improve ... Within a network of caring, we can and should demand justice, but justice should not push care to the margins, imagining justice's political embodiment as the model of morality, which is what has been done.
>
> (pp. 71–72)

The complex and contentious relationship between justice and care is further complicated in child protection by who we perceive as the client – the child, the parent or the family (see the case example in Chapter 11). Workers are constantly balancing individual and collective needs, interests and concerns.

Since the development of the autonomous adult human being requires nurture and care, there is a strong case for an ethics of care on the one hand and, given the constraints within which care is practised, for an impartial, fair and universal concept of justice on the other. This is important in light of the conditions in which externally determined standards, including child protection legislative requirements, are brought to bear on relationships of care, particularly when people have impaired decision-making capabilities. There must be an agreed standard of care for those in need to avoid paternalism, subjectivism and unfairness. Care must be connected to justice or it would become a random practice.

It is crucial, then, to acknowledge the inextricable links between the political 'rights and justice' agenda and the moral 'care' agenda, and to recognise the impact of each on the other. As Gray and Lovat (2007) note, even though we might have laws and procedures to ensure a just system wherein people have rights, without compassion there is no guarantee that these systems will function in a humane way. Neither justice nor care, by themselves, are sufficient. Justice says everyone is entitled to the same treatment but an ethics of care may lead to differential treatment as it may dictate that some people are needier of care than others based on situational and often subjective judgments. Thus an ethics of care is not necessarily just and a just system is not necessarily caring. Especially in child protection, the differential treatment of adults compared with children becomes possible in situations where a greater need for care for the abused child is identified. Hence, the need for laws and policies surrounding child protection to ensure fairness and equity. Without the moral underpinnings of a relational ethics approach, there is a danger the rule of law will win over compassion for parents and children struggling to do the best they can with the minimal resources they have at their disposal. As we see in the next approach, Habermas (1996) believes justice prevails through a discourse ethics.

Discourse ethics

At first glance, Habermas's (1996) discourse ethics might appear a misfit with relational approaches, since he follows in the Kantian tradition of deontology. However, he seeks to use communication as the method through which we negotiate a reasoned ethical approach to balance universals – like duties, rules and principles – with the practicalities of particular situations. Following Aristotle and Aquinas, Habermas's scentral thesis in his theory of communicative action and discourse ethics is that *by using our reasoning abilities, we can discover truth*. Habermas is a strong believer in the power of reason and rational discussion. Hence, Habermas situates morality in our *intersubjectivity*. He believes that Kant failed in his goal to find a universal foundation for ethics because of his focus on a subject-centred rationality. He believes that his notion of intersubjectivity can overcome the problems inherent in Kant. Our intersubjectivity derives from our social nature and the central role of communication. Habermas unfailingly believes that, by talking with one another, in time, we can overcome bias and prejudice through the application of *rational argumentation*.

Essentially, he believes that objectivity is possible; that through communicative rationality we can cooperate with one another, reach consensus and discover truth. Indeed, he believes that we are motivated to communicate because we are seeking the truth and, conversely, that truth can only be reached through communication. Thus the notion of discourse is central to Habermas's (1996) ethical theory. It is the means through which we understand the importance of the other. So Habermas tries to base a relational ethics in reasoned argumentation and communication rather than emotional connection as in the ethics of care.

Feminists have questioned the relevance of Habermas's (1996) theory of communicative action and discourse ethics to issues of power, privilege, status and access, the concerns of anti-oppressive practice. For them, a central limitation of Habermas's theory is its lack of understanding of the realities of power. Habermas's theory of communicative action is highly proceduralised and normative, and presumes an ideal state in which argument takes place. Importantly, Habermas sees the democratic process as directly linked to judicial institutionalisation, with political change arising from constitution writing and institutional reform, and not from the uprising of the oppressed. *What this means for child protection is that any change or improvement to policy and practice is likely to come through a deliberative policy-making process rather than service-user activism.* Nevertheless, he is a firm believer in the participatory processes of emancipatory practice and the power of discussion among people in particular real-life situations setting the parameters for the issues to be discussed and debated. To this extent, his ethical theory is somewhat akin to quests to find universal values and standards shared across widely divergent contexts, while at the same time paying attention to the exigencies of particular situations.

Habermas's (1996) dialogical or discourse ethics represent his quest to develop an ethical theory for pluralistic societies which no longer have a single, overarching moral authority (Gimmler, n.d.). His discourse ethics defines the subject as someone who is open and willing to listen and accept a position of dependence and intersubjective vulnerability, as the ground is set by our dialogical interactions. It is meant to follow from 'communicative interactions in which participants coordinate their plans of action consensually' (Warnke, 1995, p. 249). We can reach pragmatic solutions based on the interests and needs of those involved rather than rely on solely injunctions of the 'should' and 'ought' variety to define human interaction. By appealing to good reasons, we can generate 'local consensual knowledge that is only provisionally binding and that is grounded instead at the level of collective interaction' (Kester, 2004, p. 112). The principles of discourse can be applied in the form of argumentation rules for finding solutions for limited domains, for concrete questions and for different interests. While discourse ethics cannot provide norms for every moral conflict that might arise, it is, nevertheless, effective in providing tools for a communicative framework in which political and moral conflicts might be resolved.

Habermas's (1996) discourse ethics is a form of situational ethics, where rational and universal goals are still valued, since the requirements for communicative rationality would apply to all human beings everywhere: 'The idea is to win the assent of participants in a non-coercive and non-distorting, but regulated manner for the better judgements based on the best possible information and reasons, while integrating the perspectives of the participants' worldview and understanding' (Sewpaul, 2004, p. 225). Habermas believes that we can put aside our worldviews, and not be ruled by them, via self-reflective action, but we can never, nor should we try to, totally outgrow them. They are, after all, the substance that underlies the comprehensiveness of our shared response to reason.

The framework needed to embrace difference or to interact across boundaries comes from the interaction itself and our ability to *decentre* ourselves from our socio-historical perspective. Habermas (1996) expects individuals in particular contexts to take a disinterested perspective. His concept of decentring implies an ability to transcend personal needs and societal norms to consider moral problems abstractly (Endres, 1996). Thus Habermas presumes that people can, do, and will put aside their own needs and interests, as well as power issues, to engage in discursive exchanges and reasoned argument to reach consensus, once they have agreed on the norms and practices. Habermas believes that people's identities are formed and changed in such dialogical relationships. His method is pragmatic in the sense that it turns to the real needs of everyday conversation for its criteria.

However, Habermas (1996) overlooks nonverbal means of communication or the power of emotions, which are such an important part of people's conversations, especially in situations where long-held beliefs and attitudes are being challenged. This is particularly relevant to child protection work, where emotions escalate when abusive beliefs, attitudes and practices are highlighted and questioned by workers (see Chapters 4 and 8).

Habermas (1996) also presumes that people change their behaviour, or are responsive to, good reasons. There are many examples where people know intellectually that something is not good for them but still they continue this behaviour. Why, in any way, should people respond to reason? Often, tradition and culture carry more force than good reasons, and what makes an argument or reason good? Is it the consequences it achieves? Is it good if people agree with it? Or are there standards, values and interests that make some arguments and decisions better than others? What part does scientific evidence or expert knowledge play? Do facts based on scientific knowledge and professional expertise, or even procedural justice, take precedence over the 'fact' or reality of human experience? Do people necessarily change their interpretation of their experience when they are confronted with facts they didn't know before, or when they are challenged about their position? People agree to do things through subtle coercion even though they seemingly agree, such as remaining silent in exchanges where people are vociferously expressing an opposing view, or in child protection when a parent might seem to agree to undertakings required by a worker, even though they believe them to be coercive or unfair, and resist implementing any changes to their behaviour. Thus they profess one opinion publicly but engage in contrary behaviour privately. How do we know someone is not merely agreeing based on someone's persuasive ability or fear rather than true understanding? People can be enticed to do wrongful acts by persuasive individuals able to mount convincing or coercive arguments, as can sometimes occur in ritual abuse where there are multiple perpetrators, one of whom is dominant or charismatic.

Thus a severe limitation of Habermas's (1996) discourse ethics is that it 'contains no checks and balances – other than an ... appeal to reason' (Flyvbjerg, 2001, p. 95). Every society must have 'procedures for dealing with conflicts that cannot be resolved by argumentation' (Bernstein, in Flyvbjerg, 2001, p. 96). Furthermore, while our discursive interactions might help us in the search for self-knowledge and ultimate truth, 'a connected knowledge is grounded in our capacity to identify with other people'; our capacity for empathy enables us to 'both know and feel our connectedness with others' (Kester, 2004, p. 114). A dispassionate self, free from emotion and bias, able to argue on the basis of good reasons alone, is hardly the self of caring professions.

Habermas's (1996) discourse ethics typifies a modern view of values as foundational and universal, of the propensity to reach agreement on ethical issues, to make rational decisions and to adhere to a non-negotiable set of values. Habermas believes in rational argumentation, in the justification of some values over others and in the expectation that society and the professions ought to promote these agreed-upon values (and, on this score, social work agrees). This rather orderly picture of values and ethics and their rational moral foundation is what a postmodern ethics of responsibility overturns.

Postmodern ethics: an ethics of responsibility

An ethics of responsibility holds that moral responsibility is where morality begins. Given the autonomy of the self and morality as a personal issue (as proposed by deontology and teleology), in the ethics of responsibility, morality begins when 'the other' becomes the self's responsibility. It is rooted in relationships – in my encounter with the other. Being for the other is the point at which morality moves from a primarily personal pursuit to accepting responsibility for, and safeguarding the uniqueness of, the other person (Kelemen and Peltonen, 2001).

This thinking is closely akin to that of Bauman (1993), author of *Postmodern Ethics*, who sees modern ethics – as explicated in deontology and utilitarianism – as a normative domain, which tries to discern universal rules to ensure that people behave morally. The rules, duties and obligations of deontology seek to make individuals alike. For Bauman (1993) what distinguishes them and makes them into individuals is *responsibility*. If ethics is concerned with rules, 'the moral is what *resists* codification, formalization, socialization, [and] universalization ... The moral is what remains when the job of ethics ... has been done' (p. 54). In other words, once the code of ethics has been devised, the work of moral responsibility begins and morality, by its very nature, always involves a choice between what we believe to be right and wrong. This realisation is 'a cruel predicament' (p. 13) for when we accept our moral responsibility, we realise the gravity of the choices we have to make:

> [This] solitude marks the beginning of the moral act ... We are not moral thanks to society (we are only ethical or law-abiding thanks to it); we live in society, we *are* society, thanks to being moral. At the heart of sociality is the loneliness of the moral person. Before society, its law-makers and its philosophers come down to spelling out its ethical principles, there are beings who have been moral without the constraint (or luxury?) of codified goodness.
>
> (Bauman, 1993, p. 61; emphasis in the original)

Hence, Bauman (1993) believes it is in our nature to be moral. Rather than the constant focus on externally driven moral criteria, he brings us back to rethinking what it means to discern a deeper understanding of morality. He wants to lift the veil of illusion created by the sought for *certainties* of modern ethics and is at pains to point out that the business of ethics is transacted on murky grounds; life is messy and human behaviour is disorderly and unpredictable making it difficult to generate decision-making options and anticipate consequences rationally.

Hence, the starting point of postmodern ethics is the recognition of the ever-present uncertainty present in moral issues, and the ongoing tensions in matters of values, ethics and morals. We have to learn to deal with these tensions, to muddle through, to be morally responsible for others, to care for others unselfishly in situations we might not understand and for which there are no knowable solutions. Bauman's postmodern ethics is not about rational judgments, decisions and choices. It does not involve a weighing of all the factors involved or reasoned argumentation. It is a responsive form of ethics evoked by what is needed and called for by my responsibility for the other. For Bauman (1993), the emphasis placed on moral rules is deeply distrustful of the individual moral self's propensity to do or be good.

Central to Bauman's ethical theory – following the philosophy of Lévinas, whom Bauman regards as the first postmodern ethicist – is the notion of *moral responsibility*. For Bauman, 'responsibility' is the direct antithesis of the externally imposed deontological notion of 'duty' prominent in Kantian modern ethics. To understand what he means by moral responsibility, one has to understand that, for Bauman, morality precedes or transcends *being*. There can be no *being* without morality; there can be no *being for* or *being with* the other – the pillars of his notion of moral responsibility – without it: 'Morality is *before* ontology; *for* is before *with* ... Moral relationship comes *before* being' (Bauman, 1993, p. 71). By the same token, *being for* the other, or having moral regard for the other, precedes *being with* the other (i.e. showing the other love and care, bringing comfort to others and so on). Importantly for Bauman, morality comes from an internal wellspring. It cannot be socially engineered or externally imposed, as modern ethics would have us believe.

Moral responsibility involves being for the other whether or not the other is for me. It is unselfish. It includes respect for the other's autonomy, which means not interfering in any way with the other's freedom. There is no demand for repayment or mutuality or expectation of reciprocation, no owing me anything, no dues to be paid. Thus, in child protection, I as the worker must acknowledge the client's freedom to refuse my help or advice and if he or she accepts it, there should be no expectation of reciprocation or owing me anything because, for Bauman (1993), responsibility loses its moral content 'the moment I try to turn it around to bind the other' (p. 50). 'I' must be concerned for the other entirely for the other's sake. Morality thus creates an unequal relationship, and it is this which makes the encounter *with the other* a moral event. To remember the distinction it is best to think of *being for the other's sake*, not mine. Consequently in child protection, where unequal relationships are rife, if one enters into a relationship with a parent and maintains a focus on being there *for their sake* rather than one's own, the interaction will have a moral footing consistent with Bauman's ideas.

Conclusion

This chapter examined 'emergent' ethical theories, which help to extend our ethical thinking and discussion beyond the established approaches to ethics discussed in Chapter 2. Feminist insights into the ethics and politics of care were highlighted, including Habermas's (1996) discourse ethics from Kantian deontology and Aristotelian virtue ethics, and Bauman's postmodern ethics of responsibility. Each in its different way presents an ethical theory grounded in relationships, collectively referred to here as a relational ethics. This relational ethics forms the grounds of our approach to practising ethically in child protection developed in subsequent chapters, where our focus is on our ethical responsibility of caring for children, parents and families.

Reflective questions

1 What might be the benefits and limitations of using relational ethics in child protection?
2 Which of the relational ethics approaches to ethical decision making do you prefer and why?
3 How important are relationships when making ethical decisions in child protection?
4 How much opportunity do you think there is to adopt a dialogical approach in ethical practice in child protection?

Chapter 4   **Ethical decision making**

Ethics entails the reasons for, and principles by which, professionals make decisions on ethical matters, such as their duties and obligations towards others, and the best thing to do in particular situations. Although it may not always feel like it, ethical decision making is inherently a rational process involving conscious deliberations about matters at hand, notwithstanding that child protection and family welfare practice is inherently emotive. Additionally, ethical decision making requires a certain kind of reasoning to discern what ought to be done, which does not ensue merely by following standardised lists of values and principles, or codes of practice: 'The help that these offer is limited in the context of challenging dilemmas or conflicting interests; it is at this point that professional skills and judgment must be applied' (Smith, 2005, p. 8).

In the difficult arena of child protection, ethical decision-making processes and the decisions reached are often highly contested. In the analogous difficult arena of nursing, these have been referred to as 'the whirlwind of shifting clinical, situational and spiritual forces demanding quick decisions' (Corley *et al.*, 2005, p. 381). Hence, when factoring in these emotional and demanding forces, it seems simplistic to view ethical decision making as a purely rational process where practitioners simply follow their values, intuitions, beliefs, principles and understandings. As Hoggett (2005) notes: 'the idea of the human agent calmly making reasoned choices between ethical alternatives has been subject to considerable challenge' (p. 13). However, reason and calm are essential. Ethical decision making must take place in the context of orderly rational conversations with colleagues and others about how practitioners determine the good and right thing in complex circumstances entailing competing perspectives, values, interests, duties, obligations, consequences and interpretations of facts. Most importantly, it requires that practitioners appreciate the importance of doing the 'right thing' and valuing the virtue of good practice in which they are able to justify their decisions to themselves and others, particularly stakeholders (see Chapter 6).

This chapter outlines the complexity of this decision-making arena and provides a theoretical framework to guide practice-related thinking in situations that are highly emotive and challenging for children, families and communities. These situations generally result from accusations of harm or risk to children within their families, where the potential consequences are significant, such as the permanent removal of children from their families with life-long consequences for all concerned. The chapter outlines several helpful decision-making frameworks that have been developed and used in the field of human services. Building on the preceding chapters, it provides a new framework for conceptualising and balancing values and ethical principles across the variable and dynamic organisational and cultural contexts that frame child protection practice decisions. In particular, the chapter highlights the significance of:

- the moral character of decision makers;
- the rights and duties of practitioners and service users;
- the rights of all parties involved in child protection decisions;
- awareness of, and dealing with, the power dimensions of culturally complex and highly political service user-worker relationships; and
- mindfulness of the structural, political and cultural factors characterising the context in which practitioners fulfil their duty to protect children from harm.

Ethical principles and pressures of practice

Ethics is a practical discipline requiring the application of careful thought and reflexivity to questions of deep moral concern to children, families and communities. Because it deals with questions about values, rights, rules, principles, duties and obligations, discerning the 'right' thing to do in child protection and family welfare invariably involves a complex rational, emotional and relational process in which the practitioner's personal and professional values – and the values of all involved – often collide. Many diverse, sometimes contradictory, factors involving professional values and cultural perspectives have to be considered within ever-changing organisational environments marked by sometimes inflexible policies, procedures and legal prescriptions.

Practitioners making ethical decisions have their own values and beliefs grounded in their personal histories and professional experiences. They need to be able to contain their uncertainties and anxieties as they attempt to understand and negotiate often conflicting values. Simultaneously, they need to use their critical thinking skills to determine how their personal and professional values influence the decisions they make. Critically reflective practitioners constantly develop and review their values as they learn from past decisions and adapt to changing expectations.

Practitioners working with children and families, who are deemed to be 'at risk', generally do so with a deep sense of moral responsibility, where the moral consequences of their decisions weigh heavily personally, morally and legally, and decisions are not taken lightly (Hollis and Howe, 1987). This is especially true nowadays, where media attention and moral panics about professionals' failure to protect children proliferate, and decisions are viewed through an environment of 'scandal politics and ... prism of child deaths' (Ferguson, 2005, p. 90; see also Clapton et al., 2013; Harrison et al., 2014; Lonne and Parton, 2014). In many highly publicised cases of injury to, or the death of, a child, practitioners have been blamed for poor decisions, wrongful judgments and misguided actions. Many have expressed outrage at the public vilification of practitioners and the lack of appreciation of the vulnerability, risk and threat inherent in many child protection decisions.

Often overlooked, however, are the imbalances of power and authority in these pressurised organisational and practice environments (see Chapter 9); there is always an urgency to deciding on the best course of action to ensure the safety and protection of children (Mansell et al., 2011; Parton, 2006a; Shoesmith, 2013). Also overlooked is the practitioner's need for personal safety, and the ever-present threats of becoming victims of the culture of blame and moral panics surrounding child protection (Clapton *et al.*, 2013). Perhaps it is unsurprising that, worldwide, child protection practitioners are often hard to recruit, burn out rapidly and resign quickly (Littlechild, 2005; Lonne *et al.*, 2009; Stanley and Goddard, 2002; Stevens and Higgins, 2002). Many are ill-equipped ethically for the organisational priorities and regulatory mechanisms shaping child protection practice (Lonne *et al.*, 2004).

Some even question 'whether the present care system works to anyone's benefit' (Neuberger, 2005, p. 126), and call for a review of practices and a more respectful attitude towards child protection workers in a risk-averse society 'more concerned with stopping one child murder – however awful – than with supporting dozens if not hundreds of vulnerable youngsters via a system that places full trust in the judgment of professionals' (p. 126). Given the decreasing trust of professionals, it is all the more important that they are able to articulate the reasoning behind their decisions to ensure the safety of children (Kemshall, 2002; Neuberger, 2005; Parton *et al.*, 1997; Reder *et al.*, 1993).

Most practitioners are driven by a sense of moral duty to protect children and need as many tools as possible to do so effectively. These include the ethical principles to guide their judgments and decisions (deontological), their ethical reasoning as to their possible outcomes (consequential) and the virtue of prudence in not blindly following procedural rules (virtue ethics). Ethical decision making always involves care and forethought – prudence – about the lives of others, and it is essential that practitioners provide rational, coherent and well-considered accounts of their decisions. This is where ethical principles are crucial, not only in guiding decision making, but also in articulating and communicating the explicit reasons for the decisions made. Key principles guide those involved in the care and protection of children and young people: where do these principles come from?

1   the child's best interests;
2   maintaining a relational perspective;
3   safeguarding children;
4   best available evidence;
5   judicious information sharing;
6   protecting the client's interest; and
7   equity, fairness and consistency (see Chapter 10).

The primary ethical principles of duty of care, respect and justice are encapsulated in professional codes of ethics. In an increasingly pluralistic world, there is great variability between cultures about how to name, describe and operationalise principles, values and guidelines for ethical practice. Nevertheless, within a particular cultural milieu, such as child protection practice, codes of ethics usually attempt to ensure some universal consistency in the values and principles surrounding moral behaviour and ethical decision making. Yet, ethical principles and professional codes of ethics are limited in what they can achieve (Gray and Gibbons, 2007; McAuliffe, 1999). Practitioners need guidance in interpreting these principles and codes and are assisted in this by decision-making frameworks. The discussion that follows outlines several earlier models of decision making and provides a framework that seeks to integrate these within the contemporary pluralistic context of child protection practice.

Ethical decision-making process

As already observed, essentially ethical decision making is a rational problem-solving process that requires practitioners to provide sound moral reasons to justify the intervention choices they make, especially where ethical issues are involved. Furthermore, ethical decision-making processes require evaluations or judgments about the ethical aspects of complex practice situations that usually involve conflicting and competing interests. All ethical decision-making models suggest a process in which moral or ethical analysis is a central component of assessment and intervention. Most models of ethical decision making – usually incorporated in education for professional practice – minimally propose practitioners follow some form of template incorporating the following course of action:

1 *Determine the facts*: Obtain as much relevant and available information as possible on the situation in which the decision must be made.
2 *Understand the value issues involved and the moral aspects of the situation*: This requires an understanding of morality, a commitment to behave morally, an expectation that clients behave morally, and so on. The language used – of 'oughts' and 'shoulds' – portends the moral aspects being dealt with and reflects the normative ideas prompting ethical decisions. To summarise: rules, duties, obligations and principles are the concerns of deontology; virtues, character, moral education and the desire to make the right choice are within the lexicon of virtue ethics; and consequences (minimising harm and safeguarding children) provide a clue to consequential thinking.
3 *Consider professional ethical commitments*, such as duty of care, accountability to service users, the need for transparency and concern with social justice; each carry certain ethical principles about the way in which practitioners should respond to people, and the way in which they expect them to behave.
4 *Discern what constitutes 'good practice' and why*: Being open with clients, enabling them to be self-determining and protecting the confidentiality of the information they reveal helps practitioners develop trusting relationships with them, where they feel respected, listened to and empowered. However, relational values such as these – though pivotal – are difficult anchors for risk-saturated child protection practice (see Chapters 11 and 14).

Loewenberg and Dolgoff's (2000) ethical decision-making model is perhaps the best known and most oft-quoted model in human services practice. They examine the various ways in which moral or ethical decisions are generally made based *inter alia* on conscience or guilt arising from our innate moral sense; *moral pragmatism* or the practical judgments made about the most workable or realistic solution; *self-realisation* through personal or individual choice; *situational ethics* – taking a case-by-case approach; *religious ethics* or religious beliefs about morality; and *utilitarianism* and *communitarianism* reflecting a humanistic approach favouring the greater good. Their approach is grounded in a deontological perspective, that is, it is duty, rule and principle based. They introduce several devices to assist in decision making, including the *Hierarchy of Ethical Obligations*, where the duty of care, including the duty to save or protect children, takes precedence over all other duties; then comes the duty to respect client privacy, followed by the duty to maintain confidentiality, the duty to inform, the duty to report and the duty to warn.

Extrapolated to decision making in child protection, the duty of care toward children is, in their view, an overriding obligation and means that practitioners must prioritise protecting the child's best interests. However, this obligation often means there is a duty to inform, report or warn, and so less important would be the higher order duties on this hierarchy of safeguarding client privacy and confidentiality in their approach.

Most ethical frameworks are a variation of these principles and steps. Robinson and Reeser's (2000) 'least harms model' is based on the principle or rule of choosing the 'least harm' or 'lesser evil'– to the well-being of oneself and others – which is only fourth on Loewenberg and Dolgoff's hierarchy. This rule takes precedence over others and might, for example, involve hiding the truth or revealing confidential information in order to safeguard children. Congress's (1999) ETHIC decision-making model has similar steps in which the practitioner:

- Examines relevant personal, societal, agency, client and professional values;
- Thinks about the relevant ethical standards in the code of ethics which apply to the situation, as well as about pertinent legislation and decisions;
- Hypothesises about the possible consequences of the various courses of action;
- Identifies who will benefit and who will be harmed in light of professional commitment to the most vulnerable; and
- Consults with supervisors and colleagues about the most ethical choice.

A personalised process of ethical decision making based on Loewenberg and Dolgoff's (2000) model would entail the practitioner identifying: (i) their own personal values in relation to the ethical decision; (ii) societal values relevant to the ethical decision to be made; (iii) the relevant professional values, ethics and commitments; and (iv) possible ethical options available. These can be discerned by asking questions, informed by a duty of care and the various ethical theories available, such as the following:

- What principles or rules – or precepts of our professional code – apply to this situation (deontological)?
- Which of the possible ethical actions will protect the child's rights and those of others involved (rights-based)?
- Which course of action will protect society's rights and interests to the greatest extent possible (consequentialism and utilitarianism)?
- What can be done to minimise any conflicts between one's personal and professional values, the agency's policy and societal values?
- What can be done to minimise conflicts between the client's rights, the rights and welfare of others, and society's rights and interests?
- Which course of action will result in doing the 'least harm' possible (consequentialism)?
- Which course of action will result in maximising the good (utilitarianism)?
- Which course of action will result in doing the right thing (virtue ethics)?
- To what extent will the various courses of action be efficient, effective and ethical?
- To what extent have the short- and long-term ethical consequences of each possible decision or course of action been considered (consequentialism)?

Most models involve identifying the problem or dilemma and the potential issues involved; reviewing the code of ethics and relevant laws and regulations; consulting and obtaining advice when needed; considering possible and probable courses of action; enumerating the potential consequences of various decisions; and deciding on what appears to be the best course of action (see Chapter 12). They are meant to be applied within an ongoing reflective and reflexive process through which the worker's personal biases and actions, and the various factors influencing the decision, including client, professional, organisational and societal interests, are considered.

Ethical decision making in child protection

The number of ethical decision-making frameworks in the professional literature attests the ethical conundrums constantly faced in daily practice and the ongoing need to refine the frameworks we use in the context of changing values, beliefs and expectations about 'best practice'. There is ever-increasing evidence from various stakeholders on the poor outcomes of decision making about how to protect children. The past decade has seen growing interest in ethical challenges in child protection, along with much attention paid to the complexities of decision making (Congress and McAuliffe, 2006; Gray and Gibbons, 2007; Hugman, 2005; McConnell and Llewellyn, 2005; Meagher and Parton, 2004; Munro, 2011).

As already mentioned, child protection work is driven by an obligation to protect vulnerable children. International protocols, such as the United Nations Convention on the Rights of the Child (UNCRC), set out the broad parameters within which nation states seek to ensure rights-based child protection practice (see Chapter 5). However, broad policies, such as rights protocols and professional codes, cannot tell practitioners what to do when faced with the complex and intricate decisions they have to make daily. It is unsurprising that 'practitioners' personal moral frameworks are more frequently described as more influential [in their decision making] ... than professional norms and codes of ethics' (Asquith and Cheers, 2001, p. 16), a conclusion also reached by others (McAuliffe, 1999). An ethical decision-making framework seeks to bridge the gap between broad procedural policy regulations and professional codes, and the day-to-day exigencies of practice in maximising children's safety and well-being, and managing the tensions inherent therein.

Many child protection manuals focus on policies and procedures to identify predictors of risk, present risk assessment tools and propose a variety of checklists to determine 'the best interests of the child'. But they rarely mention ethics and value-based practice, and thereby they reflect the primary rational-bureaucratic policy framework in Anglophone countries focused on 'developing the law, procedures, audit, inspection and other forms of performance management' (Ferguson, 2004, p. 206). Yet, there is abundant evidence that this increase in proceduralisation is an escalating feature of contemporary practice (Munro, 2011). Rather than foregrounding ethical practice, this has contributed to problem-saturated, risk-dominated practices. Within such a context, practitioners seek guidance on managing the competing interests of children and families and the ever-demanding procedures and protocols governing their work.

However, risk-aversive, reactive and defensive practice environments do not necessarily mean the loss of moral legitimacy (Wallace, 2013). Risk assessments do not preclude a focus on children's and parents' needs and interests. On the contrary, they are designed to ensure 'the best interests of the child' are upheld. Within this context, an ethical framework is required that is built around the duty of care to children, alongside a relational, rights-based approach enabling practitioners to make accurate judgments about the best interests of children, while considering a range of matters. It is in this risk-averse environment of 'profound uncertainty' that a more comprehensive framework that is ethically valid, functionally accountable and re-awakens core commitments to the most vulnerable populations in society is needed (Webb, 2006).

Given the overriding focus on protecting the rights of children, it is inevitable that, when working with children and families, the principle of protecting children is more often than not driven by the deontological position – a 'duty to care' and consequential considerations – the 'least harm' principle (see Chapter 2). While this is unarguably a vitally important position to take when the overriding issue is the safety of children, it is rarely uncomplicated by the absence of other competing considerations, such as the following:

- The child's view might be that they do not need or want protection.
- The interests of parents may be seen to be in conflict with the needs of their children, and from the worker's viewpoint, may be in conflict with the 'best interests of children'.
- The interests of parents may conflict with those of other stakeholders, such as agency policy, the availability of resources or demands for efficiency, and the rights of others.
- There may be conflict between the practitioner's duty of care, which involves both helping and social control functions and their commitment to the rights of parents and communities.
- Cultural ways of parenting may be in conflict with the societal expectations.
- There may be conflicting views between families, communities and statutory authorities about the most appropriate and effective ways of ensuring children's safety.
- Practitioners, whose focus is the welfare and safety of a child or children, may be in conflict with colleagues whose focus is the welfare of a parent or other caregiver, or indeed a community of caregivers.

There are clearly multiple competing interests in working ethically with children and families. At heart, practising ethically in child protection involves making sound moral judgments, a combination of rights and duties, and making judgments about the best interests of children. Given the nature of ethics (see Chapters 2 and 3), and the nature of ethical decision-making frameworks outlined above, reflective questions are offered at the end of this chapter as a guide in developing an ethical decision-making framework for child protection.

Conceptual framework

Three conceptual elements form the basis of the DECIDE model, first described by Thompson *et al.* (2006), and refined over the years through use in research and teaching ethics to human service students (Hegge, 2012; Harries *et al.*, 2007). These are:

1 Competing ethical principles;
2 Unequal power relationships; and
3 Complex stakeholder responsibilities.

Competing ethical principles

There are at least three competing primary ethical principles central to all decision making and always in tension with one another (Thompson *et al.*, 2006). It is important to note that the order in which these principles are presented does not imply or suggest a hierarchy; rather, their prioritisation is in the hands of the decision maker. These concepts, dating back to the early work of Beauchamp and Childress (2001), have been nuanced over the years, and include:

- *Beneficence* (often referred to as duty of care) constitutes the duty to do good and minimise harm; its mirror principle is *non-maleficence* – to do no harm;
- *Justice* involves protecting the weak and defending the rights of those who cannot defend themselves, treating people fairly and equitably, and avoiding discrimination; and
- *Respect* means the duty to treat people as ends in themselves and never as means to your own ends; it means valuing the rights, autonomy and dignity of all people and, in so doing, being truthful and honest with them.

Beneficence

Beneficence refers to the moral obligation to act so as to benefit others. It also involves defending the rights of those who cannot defend themselves. One of the most enduring criticisms of the use of this principle in professional activity, particularly in medicine and nursing, is it generates paternalism, that is, it limits the autonomy of people and reduces their ability to take charge of their own lives. In its application to the work of caring for and protecting children, it means having a duty of care towards them, that is, a duty to reduce harm and remove conditions that cause harm (Beauchamp and Childress, 2001). This responsibility sits comfortably with an understanding of childhood and vulnerability. Virtually everyone would agree that adults have a duty to care for and protect children. We have already noted in the contemporary risk-aversive child protection environment, the primary activity associated with the duty of care to children revolves around assessing risk or predicting the likelihood of harm. This is absolutely in keeping with the duty to protect children from harm. Observing harm and saving children from its effects is one matter but using the principle of beneficence in predicting risk of harm to protect children is a more fraught and highly speculative endeavour. Prediction of risk is, by every definition, a most inexact science and yet it has won almost universal favour as the guiding structure for defining the duty of care to children and for allocating resources. As Kemshall (2002) forcefully asserts, risk has replaced need as a determinant of the duty to provide a service.

Justice

Justice, or, put as simply as possible, the quest for universal fairness, promotion of the common good and avoidance of discrimination, is another principle to which most people would commit – and yet it too is, as Beauchamp and Childress (2001) say, 'elusive' when we try to 'capture its diverse conceptions' (p. 225) and attempt to explain it within the various contexts in which it might be applied. Most people believe in fairness and social justice. But what does this principle mean in decision-making practice? At the most basic level, it is interpreted to mean practitioners should treat people as having equal rights; at another level, it means people should not be treated as a means to someone else's ends. Yet, at another level, it suggests practitioners must recognise and ameliorate, wherever possible, the disadvantages experienced by people due to discrimination and inequality in terms of poverty, race, disability, sexual orientation and so on. One of the many questions is how equality for individuals is defined when conditions vary and absolute equality is unachievable.

In child protection practice, justice is increasingly a concept in the headlights, yet in some ways is defined by its absence! Child protection services are known to concentrate on disadvantaged groups, particularly Indigenous people, those with a disability, single parents, people from minority and low-income groups, and people with mental health problems and physical disabilities (see Chapters 6 and 8). Serious questions are being asked about how, in the name of social justice, society recognises and addresses bias and inequality. Hudson (2008) believes 'justice is under threat in the risk society' (p. 203). Those who are seen to be the source of the risk are considered less worthy and labelled 'bad' or 'dangerous' (see Chapters 5 and 13). In considering risks to children in a risk society, the individuals who are held primarily responsible are the biological parents. Indeed, Urek (2005) argues, it is the 'bad mother' who is primarily named and shamed. A preoccupation with the procedures of risk assessment threatens to ignore issues of justice and the duty of practitioners in a moral community to value the humanity and dignity of all people, not just that of the child.

Respect

Respect in Kantian terms means recognising the unconditional value and worth of every person. It is a fundamental principle in the codes of ethics of all human service professions. Respect is more broadly used to mean the valuing of the rights of people to their own autonomy. There are, of course, limits to the exercise of autonomy, for example, when someone's rights are interfering with the rights of others – a significant issue in child protection concerns. Valuing each individual, respecting their rights and working towards maintaining their dignity and autonomy suggests associated duties of truthfulness, confidentiality and the seeking of informed consent before intervening in their lives. Again, all these are well-acknowledged values in human service provision. Yet their consideration is always context driven. Attendance to these multiple duties requires practitioners who can grasp the complexity of the context in which rights and duties coalesce, and discern and name their priority duties, while recognising their decision making will require the recognition and balancing of sometimes competing ethical principles.

Respect and justice are two principles that can, and must, be held in tension with duty in all ethical decision-making processes in human services. Yet, these principles are often overlooked as the requisite preoccupation of statutory workers and the legal advisory system merge around the seemingly exclusive priority given to the 'best interests' of the child. In this instance, the threat to the ethical decision-making process is that of excluding the fundamental respect owed to parents: human beings who are themselves in trouble (Sennett, 2003).

Unequal power relationships

It is now an accepted truism that all relationships mediate, and are mediated by, power, and that some people and groups have more power than others. Also, people's power varies in different situations. Due to the understanding that professionals have expert knowledge and associated positional authority deriving from their expertise, they are generally recognised as having more power and authority than their clients. Accepting this premise, it would follow that practitioners have a duty to pay attention to the need for respect, justice and fairness in all their work. Hence, they need to pay particular attention to the workings of power and the potential for power imbalances in their relationships with their clients.

Professionals in child protection typically work with populations of people who are structurally disadvantaged and would, by any definition, be seen to be marginalised in terms of their access to power. This has been acknowledged by many scholars, particularly those writing about anti-oppressive practice (Clifford and Burke, 2009). Many are Indigenous or from culturally and linguistically diverse communities. Many are single parents or have a mental health, intellectual, addiction or other health problem, and they are almost always faced with an added disadvantage of having limited access to financial, legal and social support services. When parents and children meet with child protection workers, or any practitioner who is an 'agent of the state', they are confronted with the additional force of formal statutory power.

Research into the experiences of families with experience of the child protection systems repeatedly attest their feelings of powerlessness (Dumbrill, 2003, 2006, 2010; Harries, 2008; Hinton, 2013). Families talk of being confronted with a powerful bureaucracy about which they understand very little, if anything; they talk of having no access to assistance. Amid the powerlessness they feel, they experience a coercive environment and the threat that their children might be removed if they fail to conform to expectations; and they talk of their perception of the worker's power and their feelings of despair associated with their helplessness (Dumbrill, 2003, 2006, 2010). Chapters 7 and 13 expand on this recurring theme.

McConnell and Llewellyn (2005) argue most persuasively that, in not recognising their own power and the inherent powerlessness of these families, professionals are subscribing to the 'de-politicisation of social inequality' (p. 554). In two recent research reports, Bywaters (2015), along with his colleagues (2014), exposed the social determinants of poverty and deprivation underpinning child protection data, and appealed for a re-theorising of child protection and family welfare in terms of a social inequalities discourse. The inattention to inequality in the lives of children and families coming to the attention of child protection agencies is linked to the dominant individualistic neoliberal discourses that underpin policies and practices (see Chapters 5 and 6).

Of course, recognition of structural disadvantage does not reduce the need to simultaneously recognise the relative powerlessness of children. All children have limited power and those who come to the attention of child protection and family welfare agencies are inevitably definable by their vulnerability in the face of the power of others. To acknowledge the vulnerability of the child does not require an either/or choice, but a need to recognise the indeterminacy of power imbalances and to pay attention to this (Tew, 2006). Helpfully, Tew (2006) proposed a multidimensional matrix of protective, cooperative, oppressive or collusive power that might assist workers to pay attention to the different ways in which they might use their power, and avoid any tendency to further disempower relatively powerless service users. In summary, decision-making processes must take contextual variables that mediate power imbalances, such as poverty, addiction or mental illness, into account.

Complex stakeholder relationships

As observed to this point, two prerequisites for ethical decision making in child protection are the identification of ethical principles and the addressing of power relationships. The third element is recognition of the diversity of people who have a stake in the outcome of the decision, and an analysis of any ethical duties owing to each of them. Historically, child protection practice was presented simplistically as the application of the duty of care in a dyadic relationship between abused children and the practitioners who rescued them from abusive parents (Scott and O'Neil, 2003). The dominant child protection assessment model focused mainly on determining the suitability of parents, generally the mother (Sinclair, 2005; Swift, 1995; Urek, 2005). On this basis, decisions were made as to whether or not a child had been maltreated or was 'at risk' of harm. In this child protection model, children assessed to be in need of protection were safeguarded by professionals who had the duty to protect them from harm.

Even in more holistic contemporary child protection models, the primary stakeholder is the child whose well-being and safety is an overriding concern. Without jeopardising the undisputed and primary duty to the vulnerable child or children, the analysis of who else is owed a duty is central to the factual review of the situation and problem at hand. This is not an easy task but is an important one as it demands an appreciation of the physical, human and social context within which any decision is made. Unarguably, parents and siblings and other family are also stakeholders. Although the harmful or neglectful actions of people may be the reason for reporting the child, they remain people to whom a duty of respect is owed. The practitioner, while protecting the child, does have a duty of care to all stakeholders, including parents, siblings, grandparents and perhaps significant others in the extended family. Some have referred to these stakeholders as 'unheard clients' (Dale, 2004; Kapp and Vela, 2004). It is increasingly clear that these stakeholders want and expect their concerns and needs to be heard (see Chapter 7).

While the child's interests are paramount, parents too need help and support, and deserve respect. Research shows that few parents feel respected in child protection encounters (Freymond and Cameron, 2006; Holland and Scourfield, 2004; Thomson and Thorpe, 2004). While paying primary attention to the protection of the child, there is no morally acceptable argument for practitioners to dismiss the needs of the child's biological parents to whom, no matter what the circumstances, the child is likely to be attached.

Additionally, there are stakeholders in the organisational context. It is impossible to understand the practitioners' work without appreciating the duties owed in the context of that work. Significant in this context is the obligation to comply with the range of duties and responsibilities owed to the employing organisation (see Chapter 9). Practitioners have an ethical duty to comply with the legal and policy mandates of their employing organisation, as well as ethical duties to their managers and colleagues (see the case example in Chapter 11). Additionally, there is a range of people who have a stake in the outcome of child protection and family welfare decisions. No doubt, among these, are the media and the public who have a stake in system outcomes and preventing tragedies (see Chapter 6).

Because of its complexity, child protection and family welfare practitioners involved in assessing risk to children and ensuring their well-being have to conceptualise and articulate the decision-making task comprehensively. Without doubt, the seriousness and sensitivity of the decision-making task has always been uppermost in the minds and concerns of these practitioners. However, recent scholarship about poor system outcomes and a growing articulation of stakeholder rights, including those of children, families and, importantly, adults who have experienced being in care as children, have added a new dimension to practitioner concerns.

Preoccupation with what is unarguably a relatively singular deontological approach focused entirely on duty to a child may well have obscured the significance of stakeholder interests. It is no longer sufficient to say that one only has a duty of care to a vulnerable child. It is also vital to take evidence of outcomes into consideration. Adopting some components of a more teleological approach requires practitioners to pay attention to reports of devastating consequences of some child protection practices worldwide, among these the removal of minority and Indigenous children from families and communities, abuse in care, forced adoption and child migrants in detention. Many of these negative outcomes were identified in a Eurochild (2010) review profiling children in care in Europe and the aftermath of that care. It seems imperative that any assessment of the risk of harm should specifically include an examination of the longer term outcomes, as well as the immediate and pressing issue of safety.

The DECIDE framework

As outlined in Chapter 1, the DECIDE model pays attention to the complexity of decision making we have described, particularly the situational context – both the internal (understanding and intuition) and the external (matters such as race, poverty and illness). It assists in what Platt and Turney (2014) call 'sense-making strategies' (p. 1) that capitalise on relationship-centred and relational practice, and the capacity for reflection and reflexivity on the part of decision makers (see Chapters 8 and 11). Though represented as a staged process for the purposes of description, it is not linear in practice because, at every stage, practitioners are invited to make their own interpretation and reflect on internal and external factors, as well as on facts, principles and anticipated outcomes. We describe its application in Chapter 12 and provide case examples in the last two sections of the book. It comprises six stages:

- Define the problem;
- Ethical review;
- Consider options;
- Investigate outcomes;
- Decide on action; and
- Evaluate the results.

Define the problem

Before expressly defining the ethical problem to be solved (and there may be a number), the facts of the situation need to be ascertained and the questions to be asked outlined. What are the facts that have a particular bearing on the situation and what ethical issue/s demand a decision? Some of the 'facts' may include disputed events, organisational and cultural perspectives, personal anxiety or political pressures. In identifying the facts, the people involved and those who have a stake in the decision are more easily identified. Name these stakeholders. Defining the problem is almost always the most difficult part of this process and often a number of problems can be named before the priority one is established. It is useful to compare notes with colleagues at this stage to be alert to the different ways problems may be perceived.

Ethical review

Identify which ethical principles are relevant to this problem or decision, and reflect on which of the principles have priority for particular stakeholders. In all child protection matters, the dominant stakeholder is the child or children, and to them a dominant duty of care is owed. However, the parents are inevitably stakeholders and, particularly if young, ill, vulnerable or otherwise disabled, will require a duty of care on the part of those in authority. The matter of context and, in particular, power relationships, is critical here. Identifying the structural factors influencing the problem assists in understanding the relevant social justice matters and in balancing the twin duties of justice and care. All people are owed respect. The process of identifying dual, and sometimes complex, responsibilities and balancing competing principles and duties is always difficult. However, practitioners who have used an ethical framework for their decision making will already be used to such discernment.

Consider options

With the ethical question at the forefront, and as practitioners name the principles and duties owed to various stakeholders, it is possible to identify fairly quickly the options available and the practicality of the choices therein. Brainstorming the choices from the various stakeholders' perspectives, and determining how they accommodate important principles and duties, will lead to options that are easily excluded or otherwise listed as real options. The chosen option must recognise legal and procedural constraints, while not using these as the sole determinant of action. The question is what are the most reasonable, ethical and practical choices available? It is important to brainstorm all the possible ways to deal with the problem and to spend time focusing on the most sensible and practical options, as well as those that intuitively feel to be the best.

Investigate outcomes

In listing options – perhaps around three – consider the likely outcomes for each. Some considerations might include: will anyone be harmed and, if so, how can that harm be minimised and what are the highly charged concerns framing this decision and how are they influencing my choice? Identify the likely ethical outcomes, costs and benefits of each option? Check each of the options against the three principles of beneficence (duty), justice and respect for persons and review that outcome to see which is the most ethically acceptable or, at worst, least harmful.

Decide on action

It is important now to decide on a clear plan of action – one that has a clear objective and plainly articulates the reason for the decision, and the balancing of principles and priorities required in the process. Indeed, at this point, it is important to remember there are no absolutely 'right' answers, only answers and plans that are well-reasoned and somehow recognise and accommodate the emotional tensions in the decision making (Gray and Gibbons, 2007).

Evaluate the results

In the busy world of frontline practice, this endpoint of decision making is often left out or is addressed at a much later stage when the best or the worst of outcomes are sometimes incidentally raised. Reflexive and reflective practice is used at as early a stage as possible to learn about what has worked well or otherwise, and to learn from successes and mistakes and discern the part the practitioner has played in generating positive outcomes. Evidence of outcomes is often slow in coming and, in the area of protecting children, is particularly fraught because of the potential dissonance between short- (immediate safety) and long-term (life chances) outcomes being addressed in recent literature.

Conclusion

People working to safeguard children and ensure their safety and well-being generally work in a space characterised by dilemmas. Herein they face uncertainty and anxiety, where the requirement for reflection is shadowed by the fear of risk to a vulnerable child, and the additional fear of making a decision that fails the child and leads to public exposure. Gray and Gibbons (2007) have usefully referred to this space as a dialogical and relational one requiring practitioners to 'go beyond formulaic responses' and 'reflect on their values and commitments, as well as intuitions and emotions' and 'incorporate situational and intuitive understanding' (p. 223).

It is clear that ethical decision making is a craft not easily acquired and for which there are no rulebooks providing simple procedures (Pawlukewicz and Ondrus, 2013). The DECIDE model explicitly acknowledges this space and assists in addressing the emotional elements present in as rational a way as possible. As well as balancing different principles, managing complex relationships, respecting people's rights and assessing the risks involved, the need to anticipate longer term outcomes for children, their families and communities is a component of the framework. Conceptualising ethical decision making in child protection and family welfare within a framework that pays attention to context and outcomes offers an important opportunity to provide a balance to dominant rule-based deontological models. The inclusion of concepts from virtue-based prudential ethics enables principles of respect, justice and beneficence to be incorporated in the decision-making process. In addition, matters of power, always present when vulnerable people confront statutory services, are acknowledged and named as such.

It is important to note that this model provides substantial challenges for policy makers, managers and legislators, as well as practitioners. To place all responsibility for change in the hands of frontline practitioners only is untenable. Practitioners must work within the constraints set by legislation, policies and managerial procedures, and within a pervasive awareness of public and media scrutiny that leaves them feeling vulnerable to exposure.

We now turn to Part 2, in which we critically examine the context of child protection practice and explore the underpinning ideologies and discourses that drive contemporary practice, knowing that a prerequisite for good practice in protecting children are 'top level' policies that are not 'remedial and punitive' but are 'proactive, preventive and supportive' (Durrant, 2006, p. 14).

Reflective questions

1   What principles can best guide practitioners who work in rule-governed environments, where there are risks involved (deontological)?
2   What do professional codes tell practitioners about how to balance competing rights and interests and the many rules and procedures to be followed (deontological)?
3   What long- and short-term outcomes for children and families can testify to the utility of decision-making processes (teleological)?
4   What are the skills, characteristics and attributes required of workers who have to make decisions in these highly fraught areas (virtue)?
5   How can decision makers demonstrate respect for all parties (deontological) and value and build relationships with them (care ethics)?
6   How can social factors like class, gender, culture, religion, ethnicity, mental illness and disability be considered in decision making (rights and virtue)?

Part 2

The context of child protection practice

Chapter 5 Competing perspectives on child protection and family welfare

This chapter explores the dominant perspectives that have shaped contemporary Western approaches to protecting children. These perspectives have emerged from uneasy battles between top-down and bottom-up concerns to reproduce or destabilise power relations across the lines of gender, generation, class and ethnicity. Contemporary dominant perspectives appear to cohere around child rescue, children's rights and social investment. These operate within specific welfare and organisational settlements characterised by a neoliberal logic and new public management (NPM).

Oppositional alternative or emerging perspectives often centre on concerns to support families in the context of structural inequalities, legacies of dispossession and racism, and the recognition of the importance of rights. Strengths-based practice approaches and those emphasising individual capacity development and resource mobilisation within communities are increasingly promoted by those seeking to engage with the complexities of contemporary contexts and counter individualistic policies and practices focused on risk and deficit linked to older traditions.

Emergence of child protection perspectives

From the law of the father to children's rights

Fox Harding (1997) outlined four value perspectives that have influenced child care policy and practice historically:

1 laissez-faire and patriarchy;
2 state paternalism and child protection;
3 the modern defence of the birth family and parents' rights; and
4 children's rights and child liberation.

Laissez-faire and patriarchy

At the heart of the laissez-faire perspective lie mistrust of the state and an acute awareness of the dangers of its powers. Domestic and family life, in particular, is seen as the realm of the private and should be left alone. From this perspective, the family is the one institution that has continued throughout history and still continues to challenge the state. The emphasis on the desirable separateness of the family from the power of the state appears to mean, in effect, that power in the family should lie where it is allowed to fall (Fox Harding, 1997, p. 11). This perspective has been influential historically, but while antipathy to the intrusion of state power into the realm of the private continues today, a concern with the needs and rights of children is widely understood to trump such antipathies.

In the late nineteenth century, first-wave feminists played a crucial role in challenging patriarchal power relations within families, drawing attention to the injustices experienced by both women and children (Gordon, 1989). Feminism, in that period, located itself as part of a modernisation project, seeking to use the state to support women and children in power struggles with men. Subsequent waves of feminism from the 1960s onwards initially exhibited a more suspicious view of the state, but over time feminists in many countries have been advocates of state intervention in many areas, such as domestic abuse and family violence. As we explore further in Chapter 13, the insertion of domestic abuse into a child protection paradigm has had both welcome and problematic consequences.

State paternalism and child protection

State paternalism and child protection is the term Fox Harding (1997) uses for the school of thought favouring extensive state intervention to protect children from poor parental care. Where parental care is inadequate, finding the child a new permanent home is favoured. The rights and liberties of parents are given low priority; the child is paramount. This perspective has in some countries, such as England, merged with some elements of a child-focused perspective.

Modern defence of the birth family and parents' rights

The modern defence of the birth family and parents' rights emphasises the importance of birth or biological families to children and parents, and posits these should be kept together where possible. The role of the state should be neither paternalist nor *laissez-faire* but supportive of families, providing the services they need to stay together and thrive. This perspective emphasises the importance of class, poverty and deprivation in explaining much of what occurs, and points to the evidence that those children who are removed from their families of origin are overwhelmingly located in economically disadvantaged communities.

Children's rights and child liberation

The fourth perspective identified by Fox Harding (1997) is that of children's rights and child liberation. This emphasises the importance of the child's own viewpoint and wishes, seeing the child as a separate entity with rights to autonomy and freedom. While the language of liberation has largely disappeared today, the importance of children's rights has been emphasised particularly, although not exclusively, within a *child-focused* orientation.

Other classifications have emerged from comparative research into different countries. Gilbert (1997) conducted a study of social policies and professional practices in nine countries – the USA, Canada, England, Sweden, Finland, Denmark, Belgium, the Netherlands and Germany – and found variations between countries were linked to whether they used a *child protection* or *family service orientation*. These two orientations were distinguished along four dimensions, as follows: problem frame; preliminary intervention; state/parent relationship; and out-of-home placements. To summarise, in *child protection systems*, abuse was conceived as something that demanded the protection of children from harm from family members. Preliminary interventions operated as a mechanism for investigating this abuse. Professionals acted in an adversarial way and out-of-home placements were often the result of court orders. By contrast, in countries characterised by a *family service orientation*, child abuse was seen as related to conflict or dysfunction within the family arising from social and psychological difficulties. A therapeutic response was offered by professionals who tended to work in a spirit of partnership with parents and children. Out-of-home placements were often the result of voluntary agreements.

Further comparative work followed linking different orientations to differing welfare state types as explored further below. When Gilbert returned with others (2011) to re-examine the same countries, plus one extra, they noted a transnational *child-focused* orientation. This orientation concentrates on the child as an individual with an independent relation to the state. It is not restricted to narrow concerns about harm and abuse; rather, the object of concern is the child's overall development and well-being. This is evident in many of the policies and programmes that target children as important means to advance the welfare state and levels of state expenditure. These programmes seek to go beyond protecting children from risk to promoting children's welfare. With a child-focused orientation, the state takes on a growing role for itself in terms of providing a wide range of early intervention and prevention services. This role represents the state's paternalistic interests in children's needs and well-being. By addressing the child as a separate entity in the family, the state promotes policies that lead to *defamilialisation*, as it reduces parents' responsibilities for their children in some ways, while expanding them and regulating them in others.

Dominant perspectives

From this discussion of the emerging discourse on child protection, three dominant perspectives have emerged:

1   a child protection orientation (see Chapter 6);
2   a family service orientation; and
3   a child-focused orientation.

Given the contemporary focus on the last, it is to this we now turn our attention.

UN Convention on the Rights of the Child

The child-focused orientation, as used in contemporary practice, is undergirded by the emphasis on the child's rights. Although it borrows elements from both the child protection and family service orientations, Gilbert *et al.* (2011) suggest that this child-focused orientation is qualitatively different in character and is shaped by two major, somewhat contrasting, lines of influence that do not always sit easily together; the growing priority attached to *individualisation* and ideas related to the *social investment state*.

Individualisation is linked to the democratisation of childhood so that actual children are able to call upon discourses that support their rights to be heard, have a view and be recognised as individuals. The clearest manifestation of this is the UNCRC. As Melton (2010a) notes, this fits within international human rights law and a global consensus about what it means to be human. Hence, this covenant provides a broadly applicable vision about the obligations that accrue to democratic governments, and to all adults as actual or potential voters – as a product of respect for humanity. Melton (2010a) argues that human rights law invites discussion about minimal norms of action consistent with respect for persons, stimulates innovation in ensuring such basic protections and, thus, demands personal and collective consideration of the ingredients in a culture of respect.

Melton (2010a) notes also that even though human rights law generally regulates the conduct of governments, not individual people, it is the province of all. He quotes US human rights advocate Eleanor Roosevelt who, when addressing the UN General Assembly, described where human rights begin: 'In small places, close to home – so close and so small they cannot be seen on any maps of the world. Yet they are the world of the individual person; the neighbourhood he lives in, the school or college he attends; the factory, farm, or office where he works' (p. 162). Ms Roosevelt eloquently explained: 'Such are the places where every man, woman, and child seeks equal justice, equal opportunity, equal dignity without discrimination. Unless these rights have meaning there, they have little meaning anywhere' (Melton, 2010a, p. 162). Ultimately, the core idea in international human rights law is universality. If human dignity is to be protected, then the humanity of every person must be recognised and respected.

The UNCRC, adopted by the UN General Assembly in 1989, begins with an affirmation of the inherent dignity, and the equal and inalienable rights, of all members of the human family without distinction of any kind. Children's rights are interwoven and inseparable from those of their parents and family, and community, with cultural connection essential. The rationale for family related rights acknowledges the family and community as a necessary foundation of values and socialisation. Family and relationships are central to this as they are fundamental to nurturance, identity, purpose, fulfilment and safekeeping.

Given the foundation of human rights law in Western moral philosophy, ongoing concerns have been raised about its applicability across differing cultural contexts, and whether rights are truly universal or instead dependent on culture (Connolly and Ward, 2008; Melton, 2010a). Tension has also existed between civil liberties and social entitlements; a tension that is, according to many, including Melton (2010a), grounded in a false dichotomy, as is the supposed conflict between rights and responsibilities. Melton argues that respect for personal dignity implies social responsibility to safeguard intimacy. Individual rights lack meaning without social relatedness; relationships are unsatisfying without mutual respect. Accordingly, personal autonomy is maximised in the context of community; social cohesion is most likely when rights talk is taken seriously. In a compatible argument, Featherstone *et al.* (2014b) advance the importance of understanding children as well as adults as *selves in relationships* and the notion of *relational autonomy*; this combines a concern for the individual's autonomy rights with an understanding of all family members as situated and engaged in relationships that are dynamic and multidimensional (see also Chapter 12).

Social investment discourses

The contemporary child-focused orientation is tension ridden, as together with reflecting the focus on children as subjects whose well-being in the here and now matters, social policy concerns are represented in social investment discourses that position children as objects who will secure the future. Over the last decades, these discourses have been reshaping social policy developments in relation to children in ways that extend beyond concerns with maltreatment or neglect. They emerge from anxieties associated with rapid economic, technological and social changes. In particular, in a globalised world, all national economies are increasingly exposed to expanded economic competition, prompting political parties occupying differing positions on the left/right spectrum to re-think and re-structure their welfare settlements.

According to Giddens (1998), responding to globalisation required a move away from the postwar welfare state towards a social investment state. This requires 'investment in *human capital*, wherever possible, rather than the direct provision of economic maintenance' (Giddens, 1998, p. 117). While the old welfare state sought to protect people from the vagaries and inevitable risks posed by the market, a social investment state seeks to facilitate the integration of people into the market. Thus people's security comes not from the role played by the state, but from their capacity to re-skill themselves. The state spends not to enable individuals to exist in the here and now, but to ensure the spending has a future payoff:

> The notion is that such investments will be more suited to the labour markets of global capitalism, in which job security is rare, and flexibility is highly valued. For its part, social policy should be 'productivist' and investment oriented rather than distributive and consumption oriented. The emphasis in social policy should shift from consumption and income maintenance programs to those that invest in people and enhance their capacity to participate in the productive economy.
>
> (Jenson and Saint-Martin, 2001, p. 5)

This is a future-oriented and child-focused project; state spending should be carefully directed to supporting and educating children, *especially in their early years,* because they hold the promise of the future. Early spending will insure against future risks, such as those of criminality, poor health and unemployability. An instrumental approach to parents emerges in social investment approaches; they are constructed primarily as a means to ensuring children's welfare rather than as subjects in their own right. Thus their own needs, desires and hopes are not accorded legitimacy. A key responsibility of all parents is to engage in paid work in order to support themselves and their children, and also to provide the right environment for their children to grow up in. They are also expected to take responsibility for their children's engagement with school and desistance from crime. Parents, especially those on precarious work contracts and with few social and economic resources, can find themselves caught between different and often contradictory sets of expectations.

In England, in the last decade, *safeguarding* became the term used to signal a broader, more ambitious remit for children's services than that encompassed in *child protection*. Safeguarding not only encompassed the need to pay attention to harms to children not usually considered, such as bullying or traffic accidents, but was also located within a broader project concerned with tackling social exclusion. The term 'family support', used since the Children Act 1989, and the subject of considerable debate throughout the 1990s, was subsumed within a broader language of intervention and prevention. However, several child deaths and the attendant media exposure (in particular, that of Victoria Climbié) continued to ensure that the risks to children of being harmed by their parents or carers retained very strong purchase in the public discourse. In practice, this meant that activities associated with 'child protection' remained central to the duties of social workers.

With a change of government this has intensified in recent years through a very explicit commitment to rolling back the state citing the need for austerity as a cover. Social investment has morphed into child protection/rescue in this context. It is argued that the conditions for today's developments in England emerged under the Blair government; catch them early, focus on children, treat parents either instrumentally or render them invisible, and identify and treat the feckless and risky. While there was money being spent on support programmes, the consequences were not quite so obvious. However, under 'austerity', matters are rather different. The focus on early intervention has been sharpened, incorporating elements of social investment and moral underclass discourses (Gray, 2014; Lister, 2006). It incorporates an unforgiving approach to time and to parents – improve quickly within the set time limits!

As Kirton (2013) notes, the intensified focus on adoption and permanency planning that is evident in England and in other countries, such as the USA and Australia, but notably absent in others, fits well with a neoliberal emphasis, offering a largely privatised solution to the consequences of social problems. Indeed, it is the epitome of individualised responses premised upon construction of children as unfettered individuals, rather than as relational beings with profoundly vital connections to kith and kin, culture, neighbourhood and community.

The child-focused perspective, therefore, takes different forms in different national welfare contexts and can encompass shifts either in the direction of family support or child protection. Moreover, as Gilbert *et al.* (2011) note, there is considerable fluidity because changes of government can significantly, and rapidly, alter matters. Policies can be influenced by specific events, particularly child deaths or tragic cases of maltreatment. Butler and Drakeford (2005), for example, have argued that certain deaths become 'scandals' and accelerate a particular policy shift because they are used by governments to bring about changes that were desired but may not have been feasible, for whatever reason, to implement.

The social investment approach is a future-oriented perspective that considers children as worthy investments because of their potential in the future (see Featherstone, 2004; Lister, 2006). By contrast, the rationale for policies and practices that perceive children as individuals in the *here and now* concerns the quality of children's childhood. Overall, despite the tensions between them, the child-focused orientation puts children's rights above parents' rights and emphasises parents' obligations as caregivers. As we explore further, for example in Chapters 13 and 14, this is ethically problematic at a range of levels, not least in the way parents (especially mothers) are blamed for endangering their children in situations where they have very little control (for example, in the contexts of domestic abuse or where they are caught between the demands of work, welfare systems and child protection systems) (Gray, 2014). The perspectives explored above have also been considered within an understanding of differing welfare regimes, many of which, however, have become subject to the imperatives of neoliberalism and the eclipse of the language of *needs* by that of *risk*.

Neoliberal and public management discourses

Esping-Andersen's (1990) oft-cited distinction between three broad 'ideal-types' of welfare regimes has provided a historical starting point for those considering context.

He distinguished between: *neoliberal regimes* which seek to minimise the role of the state and promote market solutions; *social-democratic welfare regimes* that are redistributive and in which the state assumes the greatest part of responsibility for welfare; and *conservative or corporatist regimes* in countries which fuse compulsory social insurance with traditions emphasising social assistance rather than welfare rights. Policy approaches are, of course, ever shifting and within and across countries it is possible to discern pendulum shifts in relation to the balance to be struck, for example, between the responsibilities considered appropriate by the state or individual parents. Over several decades, however, there has been an inescapable shift towards neoliberalism and new public management across diverse welfare regimes. Although we recognise the term neoliberal is not a satisfactory one, as it is reductive, lumps together too many things, sacrifices attention to internal complexities and lacks in geo-historical specificity, we agree with Hall (2011) that there are enough common features to warrant using it:

> Neoliberalism is in the first instance a theory of political economic practices that proposes that human well-being can best be advanced by liberating individual entrepreneurial freedoms and skills within an institutional framework characterized by strong private property rights, free markets, and free trade. The role of the state is to create and preserve an institutional framework appropriate to such practices.
>
> (Harvey, 2005, p. 2)

Across a range of countries, deregulation, privatisation and withdrawal of the state from many areas of social provision became common, transcending welfare regime typologies and encompassing post-Soviet era states through to social democracies, such as Sweden and New Zealand. As Culpitt (1999) notes, under neoliberalism social policy successfully eclipsed the former moral imperatives of mutual obligation that sustained political support for welfare states. A new rhetoric of governance argued for the lessening of risk, not the meeting of need.

This is vitally important as a myriad of people and issues became known only through the language of risk. Indeed, Kemshall (2002) noted that social work shifted from a preoccupation with need to one of risk, and Webb (2006) argued that need and risk became conflated with social work taking on a role in risk regulation and expert mediation for problematic populations and vulnerable people. Webb (2006) noted an ambivalence here, which was manifest through instrumental rationality in terms of calculating and regulatory practices, and substantive rationality in securing personal identity through dialogic and expressive face work. Thus in child protection work this has been evident in the expansion of practices that seem designed to facilitate audit rather than meaningful relationships as explored further below. Within a neoliberal logic:

> The disadvantaged individual has come to be seen as potentially and ideally an active agent in the fabrication of their own existence. Those 'excluded' from the benefits of a life of choice and self-fulfilment are no longer merely the passive support of a set of social determinations: they are people whose self-responsibility and self-fulfilling aspirations have been deformed by the dependency culture, whose efforts at self-advancement have been frustrated for so long that

they suffer from 'learned helplessness', whose self-esteem has been destroyed. And it thus follows, that they are to be assisted not through the ministrations of solicitous experts proffering support and benefit cheques, but through their engagement in a whole array of programmes for their ethical reconstruction as active citizens.

(Rose, cited in Culpitt, 1999, p. 39)

Thus those who are poor are active agents in their own poverty and, moreover, their poverty becomes transformed into an indicator of risk to themselves or others. Parents are deemed responsible for their children's poverty because of their poor choices (Parton, 2014), and poverty is recast as a personal deficit rooted in perceived individual failings and moral turpitude (Ridge, 2013). The relationship between poverty and forms of maltreatment, such as neglect, becomes obscured in such a context as does the corrosive and negative impact of shame and stigma on people living in relative poverty (see Featherstone *et al.*, 2014b). A vital accompaniment to the rolling back of the state's responsibilities has been an intensive focus on reorganising how services are delivered.

New public management and an audit culture

The introduction of many of the disciplines of the private sector into welfare services since the 1980s has served a range of very diverse political purposes. For example, Parton (2014) notes that a Conservative administration in the 1990s made a significant shift towards giving managers the right to manage, with the implementation of a variety of regulatory and audit systems known as new public management (NPM). These aimed to produce accountability to the taxpayer and the government on the one hand, and the customer and the user on the other. Over time, NPM has taken on differing forms in different countries. In the area of child protection in some countries, such as England, it has been a central tool in a deadly engagement between those who do not trust the public sector and seek to control it, and a media hungry for the next scandal.

Featherstone *et al.* (2014b, p. 79) argue that many of the child protection 'reforms' were predicated on a set of erroneous assumptions:

- people need extrinsic motivation to do a good job;
- strong top-down management is the key to quality and performance;
- standardisation of processes and explicit targets drive quality;
- technologies, including ICTs, are integral to this reform agenda;
- errors are a result of professionals failing to share or record information; and
- managing institutional risk is the policy priority.

The reforms are based on a pessimistic view of human motivation, a view that is at odds with what research on human performance in complex domains suggests (Wastell, 2011). Moreover, it is premised on a serious misunderstanding of the motivations of those who enter public service. Command and control approaches assume the need for extrinsic motivation, whereas research suggests that self-set goals are more effective in motivating people. If goals and targets are set and performance is measured against them, then metaphorically speaking, 'leaders' who do 'well' are often those 'teaching to the test' rather than those engaging with how the test is understood and experienced.

Such developments have privileged confidence measures over those designed to foster trust. Smith (2001) makes an important distinction between confidence and trust. *Confidence* refers to the general sense of safety and reliability that we invest in systems – having certain expectations in relation to professional roles and the regulatory frameworks governing these systems. However, a focus on these must not be at the expense of *trust* which serves as a guide to interpersonal relationships where the outcome cannot be guaranteed and, indeed, where the possibilities of disappointment and regret are ever present. If activities such as social work and child protection work are to bring about positive outcomes in people's lives, then trust is essential. Many of those who need services will have experienced situations where their trust was betrayed very profoundly. This might lead to the conclusion that it is better to concentrate on developing systems based upon rights and entitlements. Rights are a vital underpinning for children's services, but rights are exercised relationally in interpersonal encounters, whereas services (including those based upon rights) are mediated by people (Smith, 2001).

Research evidence suggests that *how* a service is delivered really matters in terms of whether people continue to access it. For example, young people constantly give feedback on the importance of how they are talked to by workers and whether they feel such workers care about them (Robb, Featherstone, Ruxton and Ward, forthcoming). Thus, while it is important to measure how many children and young people attend the meetings that are held to discuss their care, it is just as important, if not more so, to devise meaningful measures that assess their real level of participation and how they feel about the quality of meetings.

In order for risk to be assessed and change to happen, service users need to tell the truth (Smith, 2001). While this may not always be possible, it is quite unlikely to happen if practitioners are not able to build up relationships that are compassionate and truthful in return (see Chapter 14). Service users value and respond to those who are honest and can deliver the bad, as well as the good news, in a respectful manner. Integral to the building of relationships is that workers have enough time to assess what is happening, to reflect on differing versions of events, to weigh up conflicting sets of evidence, and to elicit truthful accounts. This kind of work cannot be done by harried workers running from one case to another without proper space for consideration. Good-quality supervision is essential (Munro, 2011). The research on human cognition suggests everyone is prone to cognitive error, particularly when tired and emotionally overwhelmed. Supervision should offer a space to reflect, challenge judgments made, and to process the emotions that arise when dealing with painful and distressing situations.

Trust and confidence are related but not the same, and systems that focus only upon confidence building can destroy the possibilities for developing the kind of trusting relationships upon which child protection practice rests. It is widely recognised that it is vital for child protection and family welfare services to grasp opportunities to embrace principles of system design which aim at building trust and supporting the frontline professional's tasks, including providing reflective supervision, and guarding against the seductive proxies for quality that timescales and targets produce. These create new arenas for blame and tend to spawn more of themselves in response (Featherstone *et al.*, 2014b).

Alternative perspectives

Human capabilities approach

Alternative oppositional and emerging perspectives in different jurisdictions often centre on developing policy and practice models that support families in the context of structural inequalities, provide advocacy around parental rights breaches, and recognise and ameliorate the pain of cumulative losses in the context of colonisation and racism. The difficulties of raising children safely in the context of poverty and structural inequalities were central to Fox Harding's (1997) third perspective: the modern defence of the birth family and parents' rights. Historically, writers such as Parton (1985, 1991) have stressed the role of poverty and deprivation in making the safe care of children difficult to achieve, and the role of practice and policy in attending to issues arising from material deprivation, poor housing and so on; a perspective marginalised within a neoliberal logic emphasising individual responsibility and risk. For example, in research that explored how poverty related to child maltreatment, Hooper *et al.* (2007) found in discussion with professionals, that poverty often slipped out of sight as they focused on drug or alcohol problems, and on individual attitudes, values and priorities. They concluded:

> A limited conception of poverty, lack of resources to address it, and lack of attention to the impacts of trauma, addiction and lifelong disadvantage on the choices that people experience themselves as having may contribute to overemphasising agency at the expense of structural inequality.
>
> (Hooper *et al.*, 2007, p. 97)

However, the perspective has not disappeared and, since the economic crisis of 2008, there seems to be increased interest in revisiting it. Gupta, Featherstone and White (2014) explore how the human capabilities approach can inform critical analysis of child protection policy, with particular reference to poverty, parenting and maltreatment, and provide an alternative conceptual framework for practice that challenges the dominance of neoliberal ideology in ways consistent with the promotion of human rights and social justice (Reisch and Jani, 2012). The human capabilities approach was originally developed by Nobel Prize-winning economist Amartya Sen (1999) and philosopher Martha Nussbaum (2000), who revivified neo-Aristotelian virtue ethics (Gray, 2011). They developed aspects of Aristotelian thinking relating to human flourishing and the kind of conditions in society needed to allow human capabilities to develop. In other words, they addressed the question of what social conditions were needed for people to develop their full human potential (see Chapter 3). This approach is now widely used in a range of disciplines and policy domains and provided the framework for the Human Development Index embraced in development aid discourse (Carpenter, 2009; Gray 2010c). Not only does it offer a multidimensional definition of poverty, but also a way to measure the extent to which societies are meeting the conditions needed to create human well-being. This framework went on to inform the Millennium Development Goals (MDGs) to end poverty by 2015. For our purposes here, its multidimensional framework enables the incorporation of individual and social factors into our analyses of social policy and its impact at various levels.

Rather than a precise theory, the human capabilities approach has been used as a flexible, multipurpose framework to assess human well-being; evaluate social arrangements; and develop policies and practices to effect social change, such as the MDGs mentioned above. It challenged orthodox neoclassical economics and neoliberal ideologies that focused on economic growth and *per capita* income and offered an alternative to resource- and income-based approaches to evaluating human welfare. Instead, it focuses directly on the quality of life that individuals are actually able to achieve, and proposes that we consider *not* just resources but, rather, the valued things people are able to do, or to be, as a result of having them – the *capabilities* they command. It recognises that, due to structural inequalities, people are not equally placed to realise their human capabilities and tackling these is central to its theory of social justice (Carpenter, 2009). Poverty is regarded as a *capability deprivator* because it interferes with a person's ability to make valued choices and to participate fully in society (Sen, 1999). Thus poverty is not just about material resources, it also leads to the deprivation of basic human capabilities. Echoing Maslow's hierarchy of needs, Sen (1999) has argued these can vary:

> from such elementary physical ones as being well nourished, being adequately clothed and sheltered, avoiding preventable morbidity, and so forth, to more complex social achievements such as taking part in the life of the community, being able to appear in public without shame, and so on.
>
> (Sen, 1999, p. 15)

The direct negative impact of poverty on children's development has been well documented. Children who grow up in poverty are at greater risk of a wide range of adverse outcomes affecting their physical and mental health, educational attainment and victimisation by crime, as well as criminalisation for antisocial or offending behaviour (Bradshaw, 2011; Hooper *et al.*, 2007). Cooper and Stewart (2013) found that children in lower income families have worse cognitive, social-behavioural and health outcomes in part *because they are poorer,* not just because low income is correlated with other household and parental characteristics. Gupta *et al.* (2014) argue that, when considering the relationship between poverty, parenting and maltreatment, it is essential not to adopt a binary approach that on the one hand pathologises poor parents (the 'if Ms X next door can parent adequately on benefits why can't you' approach), and on the other reduces the problem of maltreatment to one solely of material poverty. The former perspective is currently dominant, with the prevailing discourse constructing both poverty and poor parenting as resulting from individual failings (as occurs in social investment discourse – see Gray, 2014). A more nuanced and multifactorial analysis is necessary.

The human capabilities approach offers a framework that stresses the importance of multidimensional assessments of poverty, which requires analysis of the interaction of individual, relational and social factors on a person's capabilities and functioning. This is consistent with growing research on parenting and poverty. Poverty impacts differentially on individual families, with particularly serious consequences for more vulnerable individuals, for those who are less resilient, or who lack informal and formal sources of support (Ghate and Hazel, 2002; Quinton, 2004). Hooper *et al.* (2007) found that 'stress, unless buffered by sufficient social support and/or mitigated by other sources of resilience, is likely to be significant in the increased risk of some forms of maltreatment among parents living in poverty' (p. 105). They found that parents' own experiences of violence and abuse had ongoing impacts on their lives and were compounded by poverty. As with the human capabilities approach, they suggest an individualistic focus is inadequate and recommend a more holistic approach so practitioners have a fuller appreciation of the many ways poverty impacts on family life. Hooper *et al.* (2007) acknowledge that recognition and respect are fundamental human needs often denied to marginalised and oppressed groups, and that the 'spoiled' identities associated with poverty and other life experiences could lead to social isolation and 'othering' processes.

While the human capabilities approach is well developed in other disciplines, it remains relatively unknown in the child protection and family welfare literature. It has been applied to thinking about children's rights, however, by Nussbaum and Dixon (2012). They argue that, while the twentieth century saw the near universal recognition of children's rights as human rights, the conceptual basis for this remains largely under theorised. They draw on the insights of the human capabilities approach to provide a fuller theoretical justification based upon recognition of children as human beings with dignity. This is a vital underpinning for the analyses of those who seek to counter a largely individualistic understanding of children's rights by emphasising the importance of understanding all of us, children included, as relational beings (Featherstone *et al.*, 2014b; Melton, 2010a). Thus our connections with each other at the deepest levels must be recognised and supported and not ruptured without the most careful thought about the implications and consequences (see Chapter 12).

Neighbourhood-based approaches

These understandings underpin calls to re-imagine or reform child protection and to move it away from an individualist risk-saturated lens in order to engage with families' everyday realities of seeking to survive and thrive in challenging material and emotional circumstances (Featherstone *et al.*, 2014b; Lonne *et al.*, 2009). These calls emphasise the importance of practitioners re-engaging with communities from which many have become distanced, and with more collective neighbourhood-based models of practice, working with and within communities. Such calls are longstanding and are echoed across many countries. The edited collection by Melton *et al.* (2002) offers compelling examples of neighbourhood-based protective programmes exploring efficacy alongside articulating a flexible and responsive strengths-based, practice model (see Chapter 6) (see also Gray, 2011).

In exploring the potential for strengths-based approaches, the potential that already exists in specific communities is highlighted. In this vein, an ethnographic study in Wales by Holland *et al.* (2011) explored how notions of children as a risk, as well as at risk, were enacted within a specific locale; what perceived geographies of safety/ risk there were in a neighbourhood; and neighbourhood experiences and perceptions of formal and community safeguarding agencies. As these researchers noted, there is much empirical evidence relating to the prevalence of informal care of children in neighbourhoods across social classes, and there is substantial evidence of care within family networks (Morris and Featherstone, 2010). During the fieldwork, Holland *et al.* (2011) became interested in 'community parenting', which they defined as the informal, everyday, shared culture of looking out for, or looking after, children within the immediate neighbourhood:

In Caegoch we noticed several features of activities we labelled community parenting. Parents and other residents said they would 'look out' for other people's children on the estate and trust that others would look out for their children. Therefore they were happy to allow their children to play out on the understanding that someone would intervene if their child was distressed or engaged in behaviour they shouldn't. Adults in Caegoch were thus perceived as willing to intervene to care for, or regulate other people's children.

(Holland *et al.*, 2011, p. 7)

The parents also shared information about risk with one another. This culture of community parenting was aided by social and spatial aspects of the estate, such as the close proximity of family and kinship networks, and the layout of housing and gardens that allowed for easy visibility of children playing in the street. There was, of course, a downside, namely, that the collective culture could be seen as exclusionary to outsiders or to those who became labelled as outsiders following disagreements.

As the researchers note, it is important to recognise the real social and economic problems in Caegoch, strongly exacerbated by high levels of poverty. However, many analyses can overlook the positive aspects of life in such communities. Moreover, we would suggest contemporary individualist models of practice do not include a concern with harnessing such aspects to support families to flourish. This has not always been the case however. Jack and Gill (2010) offer a number of practice examples from the past in order to counter what they consider are essentially individually oriented and reactive approaches by practitioners to safeguarding children and young people. One example was the Canklow Estate project in Rotherham in the north of England, which involved a model of work known as *patch* endorsed by the Barclay Report (1982) that operated on the premise that:

[an individual] will usually have developed relationships varying from the very intimate to the very distant: he will be in sympathy with some and at odds with others ... He is part of many networks of relationships whose focus is a local area ... whatever his position in, or attitude to the networks, if he falls on hard time, becomes handicapped or is confronted by acute personal crisis, he will be vitally affected by the extent to which networks can be a resource to him by way of information, practical help, understanding or friendliness. It is these local networks and collective responses that constitute ... community.

(Barclay, 1982, p. xiii)

Patch workers in the Canklow Estate project adopted a community development approach that aimed to reduce the pressures on local parents and their children by enhancing the range of activities and informal social supports available to them. A five-year project evaluation found there had been significant reductions in the numbers of children in care or of supervision orders, and that numbers on the child protection register had fallen to almost zero. The workers helped to increase the levels of informal activities and social supports, but also reduced mistrust between parents and workers so that help seeking occurred earlier.

Other projects explored by Jack and Gill (2010) included the Henley project in Coventry. This began by taking a broad view of the factors affecting children's health and safety and aimed to develop a community which was informed and thoughtful about child protection, emphasising that high levels of poverty, unemployment, traffic and crime provided the context in which most safeguarding concerns and childhood accidents had to be understood. It developed neighbourhood-based family support, community action with young people, and positive action to build on the strengths of families and communities.

An interesting feature of the research by Holland *et al.* (2011) was their exploration of the overlapping spheres of safeguarding in Caegoch. The informal sphere concerned the residents of the community; the semi-formal sphere included the local community development project and a family and early years project run by a large voluntary organisation; the formal sphere was the statutory safeguarding sector such as social workers and so on. They explored qualitative accounts of formal relationships between these spheres, including referrals and informal aspects such as attitudes, beliefs and experiences. There was considerable overlap between the spheres with residents volunteering or working in the community or statutory sector, and projects in the community sphere being funded to perform safeguarding services. Availability and approachability were important in facilitating positive relationships between the spheres. These had spatial, temporal and biographical features: Proximity, flexibility around time, trust in people who were known, local and had been through difficult times themselves, and who had approachable personal manners and flexibility in terms of scope of services. Thus practical and emotional help could be accessed and was available. These enabling features were often apparent in the informal sphere (between neighbours for example), and were also particularly associated with the community safeguarding sphere but much more rarely associated with the formal sphere (particularly children's services).

A particularly inspiring example of the potential of parents and communities can be found in the challenging context of the residual, protection focused child welfare service of New York City. Tobis (2013) describes a process by which mothers whose children had been removed into foster care were transformed by self-mobilisation and community action from 'pariahs' into 'partners'. It is a story of how individual parents, mostly black and Latino, living in extreme poverty and having overcome domestic abuse and addictions, fought to become stakeholders, and thus transformed the system, reducing the numbers of children in foster care from 50,000 in the early 1990s to 14,000 in 2012.

They supported parents' rights to advocacy and parents as advocates and such initiatives are found in many countries, often supported by small voluntary organisations and charities operating with short-term, highly precarious funding (see Tobis, 2013, for an excellent account of the vagaries of funding for advocacy). Some organisations concern themselves with the needs of specific groups of parents, for example those with learning disabilities, who are disproportionately represented among those who lose their children (Featherstone *et al.*, 2011). These groups face considerable challenges, including from a child-focused orientation that can construct parents as means towards the facilitation of children's welfare, rather than ends in themselves and central to children's lifelong identities. 'Rights' talk on the part of parents is often not supported in a climate which stresses parents' legal and moral responsibilities towards children and demonises those who become caught up in child protection systems (Tobis, 2013).

Recognising and repairing multiple losses

Nowadays it has become imperative to engage with the complexities attached to place and community, and be wary of seeking to re-imagine forms of practice that are inattentive to the consequences of shifts in identities and meanings. In a late modern world, where tradition no longer defines the individual, and people are constantly required to re-create their roles, *attachment to place* can encompass both the 'real' and the imagined and be both fixed and fluid. The experience of migration and, in particular, of forced migration is of considerable importance here. Loss is constitutive of many identities: the loss of one's own place; history; the loss of a sense of the achievements of one's group or class; and the loss of valued role models and icons (Frost and Hoggett, 2008). Loss is completely central to the experiences of Aboriginal and Indigenous peoples; loss of land, history, culture, connection and children. The removal of children has had long lasting intergenerational effects (Berland *et al.*, 2011). As we see in Chapter 13, for example, fathers have lacked a history of being fathered themselves, as well as meaningful social roles to support their identities as fathers and men.

Alongside such histories of loss and displacement, Aboriginal and Indigenous peoples have highlighted the ongoing, grossly disproportionate numbers of children in child protection and family welfare systems (Blackstock *et al.*, 2004). This is, it is argued, only partly explained by their significant economic, social and health disadvantage:

> Across these nations, *institutionalized racism* and *colonization* have also led to a range of destructive practices such as assimilation, child removal and widespread adoption into white families, and oppression via schooling regimes that entailed enforced residential ... and had profound effects on people's collective and individual identities.
>
> (Lonne *et al.*, 2009, p. 22)

A range of practice developments to challenge continuing oppressive practices has emerged from within communities themselves and from allies. Perhaps the most significant example of such developments has been the family group conference (FGC), which offers possibilities for voice to be exercised by all family members. The origins of FGCs lie in Māori traditions developed in Aotearoa-New Zealand as a response to widespread concerns from within the Māori community about the disproportionately high numbers of their children being removed from their families, and a sense that 'traditional' decision-making and problem-solving approaches were not being used to engage more positively with children's difficulties. The approach now appears to have been exported successfully to a range of different contexts, such as the UK, USA, South Africa, Canada and Scandinavia. Its potential in relation to developing and supporting inclusive models of family (rather than normative and restrictive notions based upon a particular model) has been highlighted (Featherstone, 2004) and, in Chapter 13, we explore its potential for engaging fathers and men more generally, often a gap in more mainstream approaches.

The signs of safety approach to child protection casework was developed in Western Australia by Andrew Turnell and Steve Edwards in collaboration with child protection workers and has been used across many jurisdictions in the USA, Canada, UK,

Sweden, Finland, Holland, Aotearoa-New Zealand and Japan (Turnell and Edwards, 1999). The impetus to create the signs of Safety approach arose from dissatisfaction with most of the existing models and theory regarding child protection practice, especially when used with Aboriginal families. The approach seeks to build partnerships with parents and children in situations of suspected or substantiated child abuse. It is a strengths-based, safety-oriented approach to child protection work, expanding the investigation of risk to encompass strengths and *signs of safety* that can be built upon to stabilise and strengthen the child's and family's situation. A format for undertaking comprehensive risk assessment – assessing for both danger and strengths/safety – is incorporated within the signs of safety assessment protocol. The approach is designed to be used from commencement through to case closure and to assist practitioners at all stages of the child protection process, whatever the setting. It is grounded in action research practice and use of appreciative inquiry, and draws upon practitioners' experience and wisdom, using a basic framework to explore: what are we worried about? What's working well? And what needs to happen?

Conclusion

Overall, competing perspectives have always been evident in this area of welfare and have usually encompassed different views on balancing family support and child protection and, therefore, the responsibilities of the state and parent. A child-focused orientation emphasising children's rights and social investment seems to be in the ascendancy across many countries. However, it can morph into a narrow child protection rescue approach in particular contexts where neoliberal concerns to roll back state responsibilities for support for families are dominant. An array of alternative oppositional perspectives are to be found emphasising that we are all, children included, relational beings. These stress the importance of developing systems that do not further oppress the most marginalised in our societies by depriving families of the means to care safely. Child protection processes need to be highly attuned to ensuring such processes act to heal and repair, rather than intimidate and rupture precious identities and bonds.

Reflective questions

1   How have social constructions of children, families and childhood changed?
2   How do you perceive and understand children and childhood?
3   What are the key features of the UN Convention on the Rights of the Child and how can these be a foundation for ethical practice?
4   Is it helpful to conceive of children as having rights but their parents as having responsibilities?
5   How can we best promote children's relational identities?
6   What are the barriers to promoting neighbourhood-based support services?
7   What would be the advantages and disadvantages of parents who have been through the child protection system acting as advocates for other parents?

Chapter 6   System mandates, policy, theory and practice

Following on from the discussion on the emergence of child protection discourses in Chapter 5, in this chapter, we explore how, over time, altered social constructions of children, parents and families have led to changed responses to the state concerning governance of the family (Fox Harding, 1996; Parton, 2006b). Enduring issues confronting child protection are explored and major theories for practice in this area are described.

Emergence of protective systems

Literary coverage of child maltreatment reveals changing social constructions and understandings of protecting children over time. Two fictional characters help exemplify this. Mark Twain's Huckleberry Finn was neglected and endured regular beatings from his alcoholic father, relying on his wits and others' generosity to get by. Charles Dickens chronicled the impoverished social conditions and cruelty Oliver Twist and numerous poor children experienced at the hands of adults and family members. Individualised rather than institutionalised responses to these injustices were the norm in Victorian times.

Ferguson (2004) posited that the development of Western child protection policy and practice occurred in the late nineteenth century through civil society initiatives, such as England's National Society for the Prevention of Cruelty to Children (NSPCC) setting in train a charity model that spread to the developing world through colonisation. External interventions to bring poor families into line were motivated by charitable intentions of 'doing good' to those in need. Gradually, however, with pressure from the voluntary sector for, and the emergence of, state welfare services, the government began to expand its jurisdiction to protect children 'in need of care'. For the most part, services were highly individualised with families managed on a case-by-case basis. During the course of the last century, 'developmental waves' expanded professional interventions following recognition of the 'battered baby syndrome' (Kempe et al., 1985), which led to child-saving approaches (D. Scott, 2006). Along with the advent of the UNCRC in 1989, notions of the child as a psychological being and bearer of human rights gathered momentum (Melton, 2010a) (see Chapter 5). At the same time, during the 1980s, the discourse of risk emerged along with increasingly conservative social policies. Evolving family-state relationships led to the emergence of the 'preventative surveillance state', with increased and earlier intervention sitting alongside greater regulatory authority and governance of the family. Parton (2006b) claimed these developments threatened the civil liberties and human rights of children and parents alike. These changes affected the value position of, and ethical frameworks used by, practitioners in exercising their power and statutory authority – from paternalistic values of protecting children to rational approaches to assessing risk and justify intervention.

Child protection systems within nation states around the world developed differently with 'social configurations rooted in specific [national and local] visions for children, families, communities and societies' (Cameron and Freymond, 2006, p. 3). Generally, however, three broad system models developed over the 1970 and 1980s, each of which entailed different permutations of state and professional power, although, to some extent, every jurisdiction had elements of each. They were statutory child protection, family services and informal community care (Cameron and Freymond, 2006).

1   *Child protection* approaches delineated the boundaries between the private and public spheres of responsibility in which the public sphere entailed legally authorised investigations and interventions by statutory agents and agencies into the private lives of families in cases of suspected child abuse and neglect, with private community-based services offering limited support for families.
2   *Family support services* restricted state intervention, instead promoting voluntary state-subsidised family support services, generally provided by community organisations, often faith-based agencies.
3   *Community care,* rendered through informal familial, social and cultural networks, provided assistance to vulnerable families.

In effect, the type and level of service received hinged on the particular jurisdiction's dominant discourse about: (i) the necessary extent of state intervention into the family; (ii) the degree of preference for voluntary involvement; and (iii) perceptions of problem severity. Hence, child protection and family welfare systems displayed a variable mix of the following elements:

1   In most systems, families involved in reported cases of serious abuse and neglect invariably came to the attention of the *statutory child protection* system, undergirded by legislation authorising child protection officers to exercise coercive state authority to protect vulnerable 'at-risk' children from significant harm.
2   Within *family services* dominated systems, the orientation focused on safeguarding the general well-being, development and social functioning of children through education and accessible social support to families when needed.
3   *Community care* approaches strongly promoted available family support through local and culturally bound relationships and connections.

While aspects of all these approaches still remain in contemporary protective systems, as discussed in Chapter 5, there is now a much more concentrated focus on early intervention and prevention (Gilbert *et al.*, 2011). This is increasingly based on the economic discourse of social investment, which emphasises early childhood education and development, whereby investing in young children's well-being will produce active citizens who would contribute to society in constructive ways (Gray, 2014) (see Chapter 5). Major changes in approaches have often followed critical events in child protection practice, not least high-profile scandals involving the deaths of children (Lonne and Parton, 2014). Given that child protection entails a system of social surveillance that invites citizens to report children at risk of harm to the statutory authorities, with protective investigations to follow, such failures were bound to call practitioners to account for their actions and lead to service transformation.

Contemporary protective systems: key stakeholders and diverse models

In all protective systems, the child is the primary stakeholder, although within the citizen-oriented, community-care model, the primary stakeholders are children, parents and families. Service providers in community-based services may be closer to their service users than their statutory counterparts and there is evidence to suggest that they are better perceived, approached more for help and less distrusted than statutory agencies (Holland *et al.*, 2011; Queensland University of Technology and Social Research Centre, 2013). And a very recent research report in Australia made the 'disturbing finding' of major tensions between community workers and statutory workers that had, among other features, major 'adverse consequences for families' (Hamilton and Braithwaite, 2014, p. ii). Secondary stakeholders include the broader community, comprising diverse cultural and Indigenous groups (see Chapter 7).

Within the statutory child protection model, professional managers and practitioners construct norms of effective and ethical child protection practice, and significant power differentials pertain, with families, parents and children having relatively little power. Powerful politicians and government agents determine child protection policy, which broadly involves health, welfare and education authorities, the police and judiciary, and other community services. This powerful system is usually subjected to rigid review and accountability mechanisms, including public inquiries.

Community campaigners, agency personnel, academics, researchers and professional bodies also seek to influence child protection policy (McCosker *et al.*, 2014), while the media facilitates debates about contentious issues, and sometimes initiates reform campaigns (Lonne and Parton, 2014). Indeed, in some countries, such as England, there have been ongoing discussions about the role of the media and 'the politics of outrage' in response to particular child deaths (Parton, 2014). For example, Ray Jones (2014) conducted a particularly incisive analysis of the role of the media in England in the wake of the death of Peter Connelly. Fear of media exposure sometimes occurs (Lonne and Parton, 2014). Further, the risk-aversive practice apparent in some systems (see for example Queensland Child Protection Commission of Inquiry, 2013a, 2013b), partly results from the acute sensitivity of key child protection organisational stakeholders to negative public opinion and media coverage.

Tensions are ever present in the dynamic relations between governments and community stakeholders: 'their roles, responsibilities, agendas and motivations differ and may be complementary or opposed. Rivalries, jealousies, synergetic alliances, competitive relationships, and boundary and role disputes abound' (Lonne and Parton, 2014, p. 824). While diverse stakeholders are united on the social obligation to protect children from harm, they can disagree on the best means to this end. As well as differing on what the desired community standards are, there are constant debates on what constitutes ethical, just and effective practice, and the accountability processes to ensure procedural fairness. External scrutiny is a crucial check on how statutory agents and private agencies use their power and authority with vulnerable people and, as Lonne and Parton (2014) note, has exposed bad practices. Contemporary examples are evident in Australia's Royal Commission into Institutional Responses to Child Sexual Abuse, which is exposing injustices perpetrated by state and church-based institutions.

Enduring issues surrounding child protection

Overrepresentation

While child abuse and neglect occurs within all sociocultural groups and across all societies, a number of groups are overrepresented within particular child protection systems. There is consistent evidence of a statistically significant link with deprivation (Ben-Arieh, 2015; Bywaters, 2015; Bywaters *et al.*, 2014). Generally, parents with intellectual and mental health disabilities, single female parents, migrants and people of colour are overrepresented in Western child protection systems (Bilson *et al.*, 2013; Child Trends, 2012; Daniel *et al.*, 2010; Gilbert *et al.*, 2011; Gillespie *et al.*, 2010; Jonson-Reid *et al.*, 2013; Kaplan, 2013; LaLiberte and Lightfoot, 2013; MacLaurin *et al.*, 2005; McConnell, 2013; Pelton, 2014; Saunders *et al.*, 1993; Scott, 2014; Tilbury, 2009). Disability discrimination is evident (Kaplan, 2013; LaLiberte and Lightfoot, 2013). Race and cultural relativism are also at play (Lonne, 2015; Maitra, 2005).

Overrepresentation of Indigenous children is a legacy of colonisation, intergenerational trauma and compounded poverty and disadvantage. For example, Australian Indigenous children are overrepresented relative to the non-Indigenous population; whereas Indigenous people constitute only 2.5 per cent of the population they are eight times more likely than non-Indigenous children to have a substantiated notification (45.3 per 1,000 children compared with 5.7), and ten times more likely to be under a protective order and in out-of-home care (57.1 per 1,000 children compared with 5.4) (AIHW, 2014). The Australian Institute of Health and Welfare (AIHW, 2013) identified a relationship between Indigenous overrepresentation and 'perceptions arising from cultural differences in child-rearing practices' (p.16). In some parts of Canada, more than half of the children in care are Aboriginal (MacLaurin *et al.*, 2005; Strega and Carriere, 2009).

Poverty-associated neglect is often the largest category of substantiated maltreatment (Dubowitz, 2013a; Lonne, 2015; Pelton, 2014). For example, 78.3 per cent of substantiated cases in the USA in 2012 involved neglect (US Department of Health and Human Services, 2014). In England, Bywaters and colleagues identified an unmistakeable association between a range of inequality indicators and increased involvement in the child protection system, particularly for neglect (Bywaters, 2015; Bywaters *et al.*, 2014). There is similar evidence in Israel (Ben-Arieh, 2015) and the USA (Pelton, 2014). Recent Australian data revealed that 42 per cent of children who were the subject of substantiated maltreatment were from the lowest socioeconomic status areas, with Indigenous children 'far more likely to be from areas of the lowest socioeconomic status – 59% compared to 38% for non-Indigenous children' (AIHW, 2014, p. 23).

However, several interrelated factors contribute to the overrepresentation of certain groups, including social, economic and health inequalities, race, culture, and physical and mental disabilities. In addition to these social factors, policies like mandatory reporting, discussed further below, also play a part. Most child protection approaches focus on investigating individual cases and largely ignore the underlying social and structural factors exacerbating child neglect.

The overrepresentation of particular groups has social implications, because the large-scale removal of children from their cultural connections has intergenerational impacts, as seen in the Stolen Generations of Australia, where children forcibly removed from their families experienced significant emotional and psychological trauma resulting from their loss of identity, spirituality and relational connections (HREOC, 1997). Successive child removals, along with associated practices, such as holding individuals responsible and blaming and stigmatising them for their social disadvantage, have exacerbated these problems. As a result, subsequent generations have experienced historical trauma, disrupted familial and cultural connections, profound mental and emotional health difficulties, and poor parenting skills (Berland *et al.*, 2011).

This is a complex problem that seems to defy solution. At root lie widely divergent cultural values surrounding family and community existence. Minority groups are forced to conform to dominant values and expectations and their overrepresentation signifies the difficulties associated with adapting to Western norms (Gray *et al.*, 2008). Hence Gray *et al.* (2008) argued that seeking culturally relevant solutions to social problems was an ethical imperative (see also Gray *et al.*, 2014).

Mandatory reporting

As noted earlier, the advent of *mandatory reporting* (MR) has often followed tragedies and systemic inquiries. We refer here to three types of MR: legislatively authorised, policy-based and contractually required reporting. This controversial policy obliges child protection practitioners, and other professionals working with children, to report cases of suspected child abuse and neglect, thereby ensuring that statutory authorities are informed and can take early investigative and protective action (Mathews, 2012; Mathews and Bross, 2015; Mathews and Kenny, 2008). Since child abuse and neglect are often concealed, MR urges citizens to report cases to the authorities rather than become personally involved (Melton, 2005); this overcomes legal and ethical barriers to reporters releasing confidential information (Mathews, 2012). MR entails a compulsion to report designated matters irrespective of the consequences. While some jurisdictions do not have a legislative basis to MR, nearly all have inter-organisational policies, procedures and service-delivery contracts that require staff to pass on information about children at risk to appropriate authorities. However, these are implemented in diverse ways, with various definitions, thresholds, specified reporters, protocols and information systems, and requirements in place; reporting may not result in investigation and interviews with the child and family, but does mean a risk assessment of the available information is undertaken and recorded by authorities.

To its proponents, MR is a necessary system to ensure children are not left unprotected and their situation neglected by authorities (Mathews and Kenny, 2008). However, for others, MR is deeply problematic because it appears to target particular groups (as discussed above), who become reluctant to seek help fearing their children will be removed (Harries and Clare, 2002). Lonne (2015), when examining MR for serious neglect, identifies:

> A serious flaw of mandatory reporting regimes, however, is that to a large degree their effectiveness relies upon robust inter-agency collaboration, system integration, role clarity, clear policy and procedure, regular cross-agency training, and mindful management to ensure that the whole system shares responsibility for the welfare

> of children and providing assistance to struggling families. There is little evidence of this being evident in most jurisdictions ... there are numerous unintended consequences and critical system failures that require us to rethink the merits of basing our approaches primarily on social surveillance and mandatory reporting of neglect situations rather than providing more accessible help and less blaming and stigmatizing through a public health approach that addresses social structural factors.
>
> (Lonne, 2015, p. 268)

Depending on the specific jurisdictional MR requirements, failure to report constitutes a potential breach of the law and organisational directions, as well as an ethical transgression for professionals working with children, especially if harm results. It is a vexed issue due to the complexities within professional confidentiality (Clark, 2006b) and can threaten therapeutic relationships with families and children (Steinberg *et al.*, 1997). The very act of being reported and investigated can be devastating for families, leaving them suspicious and mistrustful of those trying to help them. While the duty to report is designed to protect at-risk children, it has also led to an ever-widening net of surveillance and consequent significant increases in the demand for child protection services (Lonne *et al.*, 2009). There can be huge disparities between child protection systems and family services models in the overall proportions of reports coming from mandated reporters compared with service users' self-reports (Kojan and Lonne, 2012). It has led some to proffer 'differential response' and the public health – early intervention and prevention – model as a way of diverting less serious cases away from the statutory system (Gray, 2014; Kapland and Merkel-Holguin, 2008; Kyte *et al.*, 2013).

Differential response

In the 1990s, concerns about child protection investigations unnecessarily capturing children and families in need of preventive rather than statutory intervention led to the development of *differential response*, sometimes known as 'alternative responses' and 'dual pathways'. It typically entails early screening, assessment and referral processes to help families access needed support and divert them from the investigation pathway. As with MR, there is a wide diversity of approaches to differential response with variable definitions, thresholds, processes and requirements. For example, in Australia, the community-based sector is centrally involved but this is less the case in the USA (Lonne *et al.*, 2015). Cash-strapped child protection services tend to give priority to the riskier, more serious cases, and differential responses address unmet need through diverting children and families to alternative assessment and service processes (Kapland and Merkel-Holguin, 2008; Kyte *et al.*, 2013). To be fully effective, differential response systems require robust integration of the statutory child protection and community-based service systems.

These services seek to foster family cooperation through increased engagement in holistic strengths-based assessments and interventions, and there is mounting evidence of their relational and outcomes effectiveness, particularly from service users' perspectives (Fuller *et al.*, 2013, 2014, 2015; Kapland and Merkel-Holguin, 2008; Kyte *et al.*, 2013; Loman and Siegel, 2015; Lonne *et al.*, 2015; Merkel-Holguin *et al.*, 2015). Recent evidence also shows enhanced service-user help seeking, service accessibility and community engagement in differential response systems (Cameron and Freymond, 2014), decreased risk assessments (Winokur *et al.*, 2015) and reduced re-reports, investigation and substantiation rates (Harries *et al.*, 2015; Janczewski, 2015; Loman and Siegel, 2014). However, some researchers argue that more robust evaluation of these processes and their outcomes is required and that resources are unnecessarily being diverted away from child protection, thereby placing children and families at greater risk (Hughes *et al.*, 2013).

How child protection practitioners relate to service users is an important ethical and moral consideration. Whether involved in investigative or alternative pathways, practitioners need to be respectful, courteous, open, and fair in all their dealings with them and particularly with those who are powerless and vulnerable. This requires acting with moral purpose and integrity, using power and authority wisely and active reflexivity, all of which are fundamental to relationship-centred practice (see Chapters 10 and 11).

Out-of-home care

Child protection and family welfare systems require a well-functioning out-of-home care capacity if they are to achieve their mandate; they must provide a standard of care better than what was provided within the child's family so that children are not only safe, but their well-being is improved. Yet these systems have been plagued by poor outcomes, such as gross failures in institutional and foster care, and especially in residential care (Berland *et al.*, 2011; Brown *et al.*, 2007; Cummins *et al.*, 2012; Eurochild, 2010; Parliament of Australia Senate Community Affairs Committee, 2004; Pecora *et al.*, 2007; Queensland Child Protection Commission of Inquiry, 2013a). The abuses of children in care that have been identified have highlighted the terrible impacts on many children who have experienced out-of-home and, particularly, institutional care around the world (Commission to Inquire into Child Abuse, 2009). This includes sexual abuse by carers, including clergy (see, for example, the Australian Royal Commission into Institutional Responses to Child Sexual Abuse at www.childabuseroyalcommission.gov.au).

Out-of-home care can involve considerable risks for children, not least from the high rates of placement breakdown and turnover, which have sometimes lifelong attendant impacts upon children's psychological and emotional health and well-being (Osborn *et al.*, 2008; Pecora *et al.*, 2007; Sinclair *et al.*, 2007; Withington *et al.*, 2013; Wulczyn *et al.*, 2003). This is not to deny the positive benefits experienced by many children in care (Munro, 2011) but, rather, to make the point that out-of-home care systems are not automatically benign; their history bears out an unhappy legacy for many children (see, for example, Parliament of Australia Senate Community Affairs Committee, 2004; see also Chapter 7, this volume).

Further, these are very expensive care systems for governments to operate and sustain. For example, Australia spent AUD2.1 billion in 2012–2013 on the out-of-home care system for children and young people, which was 64.3 per cent of the total child protection system costs (Steering Committee for the Review of Government Service Provision, 2013). The recent Queensland, Australia, judicial inquiry, as part of its terms of reference, examined the fiscal sustainability of the child protection system because the increasing numbers and rates of children per 1,000 child population in out-of-home care were even greater than those for Australia, which had doubled in the previous decade (AIHW, 2014; Queensland Child Protection Commission of Inquiry, 2013b). These rapidly increasing numbers of Australian children in out-of-home care

are largely driven by the increasing overrepresentation of Indigenous children, discussed above, despite specific policies to reduce this, such as the Child Placement Principle which requires Indigenous children to be placed in culturally safe placements with Aboriginal or Torres Strait Islander families (AIHW, 2014; Queensland Child Protection Commission of Inquiry, 2013b). Similar issues are being experienced in some Canadian provinces, such as Alberta.

Permanency planning

Given these system outcomes, it is not surprising that policy makers look closely at measures to reduce service demands and decrease the numbers of children in out-of-home care. *Permanency planning* is a policy that has periodically gained momentum around the world, only to stall when its shortcomings become evident. Essentially, it seeks to prevent the problems stemming from placement instability by setting often arbitrary time limits on parents to satisfactorily address the reasons the child has come into care, or have their child placed into permanent care either through a long-term guardianship order or forced adoption.

As explored further below, neuroscience is being misused, in our view, to promote a 'now or never' removal practice involving permanent severing of the legal ties between parents and children (Wastell and White, 2012). There are many difficulties with this approach, not the least of which are that frequently there are insufficient support services available to meet the families' needs, or parental care issues result from problems that are not easily addressed within the 12–24 month rehabilitation period permanency planning policies typically demand. Issues of identity, emotional and relational connection, and associated health problems are pushed aside in the endeavour to provide long-term placement stability, with the expectation that the child's health and well-being will thus be assured. But there are no guarantees in this regard, ethical issues abound, and the policy is highly contested. A key point here is that the establishment of new legal guardianship does not mean that there are no ongoing emotional connection issues for those involved – usually the opposite is the case, with these matters of identity and intergenerational linkages remaining unresolved and deeply troublesome over the long term, particularly for children.

Forced adoption

Issues of identity and intergenerational connections are to the fore when considering *forced adoption,* also known as adoption without consent. This entails the permanent cessation of parental guardianship rights through a legally enforced severance of the birth parent–child relationship, and the placement of the child with another family via adoption that, in turn, constructs a new legal parent–child relationship. A recent Australian inquiry highlighted the tragic legacy for multiple stakeholders that resulted from well-intentioned forced adoption policies in the twentieth century (Parliament of Australia Senate Community Affairs Committee, 2012). A major study of stakeholder viewpoints was undertaken by the Australian Institute of Family Studies to provide an evidential base for the inquiry (Kenny *et al.*, 2012). It is sobering reading as it chronicles the lifelong impacts on children, siblings, adoptive parents, relinquishing parents and families. Importantly, this policy and practice was developed in a period where single mothers were publicly shamed and given no welfare support, and the actions taken to remove children from their mothers were described as often being 'the source of ongoing trauma for them' (Kenny *et al.*, 2013, p. 37). Another example is the Magdalene Laundries in Ireland. The policy was:

> considered by society as a suitable 'solution' for a young unwed mother who was expected to 'soon forget' (unfortunately for many this was not the case). It also provided married 'respectable' infertile couples with an opportunity to have a child to raise as their own ... the range of people involved suggests the potential for wide-ranging impacts ... and that past adoption practices were at times illegal, unethical, immoral, had the potential to do damage, and often did.
>
> (Kenny *et al.*, 2013, p. 37)

Currently adoption is promoted in countries such as England as part of policies that ensure children are removed from neglectful parents in a timely manner. It is argued that timeliness is of the utmost importance so they are not left with irreparable damage either neurologically or socially (see Wastell and White, 2012). Birth parent consent is not required and it is not possible to reverse an adoption order once made. This might be seen as a bizarre extension of the early intervention and prevention social investment discourse (Gray, 2014).

Integrated multi-agency responses

Integrated multi-agency responses, such as 'whole-of-government' approaches or *joined up* services, have long been part of the overall policy thrust in most child protection and family welfare systems. However, many inquiries have found that poor interagency responses and relationships abound (Cummins *et al.*, 2012; Queensland Child Protection Commission of Inquiry 2013b). Ross (2009) identifies 'cross-cutting' issues for multifaceted organisational arrangements:

> coordinating any two complex systems is a challenge. Government departments are specialised – they focus on one set of services – and they employ large numbers of people ... competition and culture clashes prevent collaboration between any two agencies, and incorporating additional agencies adds exponentially to the obstacles such efforts encounter. The byproduct of a decentralized government, these challenges often lead to bewildering laws, regulations, policies and court decisions that further complicate developing cross-cutting solutions.
>
> (Ross, 2009, p. 3)

Nonetheless, governments have generally uncritically accepted the idea of 'joined up' or networked multi-agency responses to child and family welfare services, whereas social critics have highlighted the negative implications of the increased social surveillance such approaches entail when agencies are forced to share confidential information about service users (Parton, 2006b; Wrennall, 2010). As discussed in Chapter 14, sharing information about clients is a risky business.

Joined-up services rest on the idea that *coordination* and *collaboration* between services leads to improved outcomes for children and families, because they result in more efficient, holistic assessments that collect consistent information across cases. They provide, it is argued, accessible and timely supports, lead to greater clarity of roles and responsibilities, and avoid wastage and duplication. Standardised assessment and assistance processes, along with information sharing, it is claimed, also lead to greater service equity. However, there is little empirical evidence demonstrating that collaboration achieves such outcomes for vulnerable and at-risk families, especially where service users' problems lie between respective agency domains, such as homelessness and poverty (see Cross *et al.*, 2009; McDonald and Rosier, 2011a, 2011b; Morris, 2008).

Contemporary health and human services systems are often complex, 'siloed', fragmented, competitive, and difficult to navigate and integrate (McDonald, 2006; McDonald *et al.*, 2003; Morris, 2008). Child-focused systems also face many difficulties in linking with adult-oriented services, and building awareness of children's issues. To address this, significant resources, high-level leadership support and prioritised networking at all levels are required (Cummins *et al.*, 2012; McDougall and Gibson, 2014; Winkworth and White, 2010). Further, there is evidence that increased service coordination can decrease service quality due to decreased individual accountability for care (Glisson and Hemmelgarn, 1998).

Collaboration can be viewed as a continuum that differentiates cooperation, coordination and collaboration, with agencies having variable interdependence, risk, rewards, commitment and contribution (ARACY, 2009a), while Winkworth and White (2010) assert that it may be conceptualised as a tiered problem-solving approach. McDonald and Rosier (2011a) identified collaboration's key characteristics as dense, interdependent connections; frequent communication; tactical information sharing; pooled, collective resources; negotiated shared goals; and shared power between organisations. There can be significant tensions between achieving such arrangements and the competition and rivalry between stakeholders noted earlier. While there is a range of interagency activities that exemplifies collaborative practice, the involvement of children and parents may be unclear, yet has the potential to 'be part of a strategy to increase community capacity, social capital and community empowerment' (McDonald and Rosier, 2011a, p. 4). Community members can play critical roles providing informal support within community-based agency networks for improving child and family well-being, particularly when inequality is prevalent (Featherstone *et al.*, 2014b; Holland, 2014; Holland *et al.*, 2011; Jack, 2004; Kimborough-Melton and Campbell, 2008; Landau, 2011; McDonell and Melton, 2008; McLeigh, 2013; Melton 2010b, 2014).

To be effective, collaboration needs to be well-conceived, planned for and embedded into everyday business; but it also needs a shared vision and goals, a legislative and policy remit, role and responsibility clarity, unreserved executive and management backing, standard operating procedures, resourcing of the time and energy for the regular meetings required to build and maintain trust and cooperation, and support at all tiers within organisations (Ross, 2009; Winkworth and White, 2010). Furthermore, coordination is practitioner-centric and requires sound relational practice for the dialogue and negotiations that underpin it. Yet, within complex systems and competitive and sometimes conflicted interagency environments, is collaboration truly achievable? Are its supposed benefits worth the effort? Does it merely consume resources and divert attention from addressing families' needs? Without rigorous research it is hard to evaluate this. For most practitioners, however, collaboration remains an organisational directive they are duty bound to follow, albeit one with ethical implications, particularly surrounding the exchange of information (see Chapters 9 and 14). Hence, it needs to be an embedded part of agencies' and practitioners' ethical frameworks for practice.

Media impact

As outlined in Chapter 5, the impacts of media coverage upon child protection systems should not be underestimated. The media is a powerful shaper of public perceptions of social problems and what should be done about them. Print media tend to focus on criminal cases involving sexual and physical abuse, even though neglect and emotional abuse are far more prevalent (Lonne and Gillespie, 2014). Media coverage through whatever medium is often critical, targeting individuals – naming and shaming parents and 'perpetrators' – and overlooks social and structural factors at play (Lonne and Gillespie, 2014). But it can also inform the public by grappling with complex, nuanced policy issues, such as MR, thereby facilitating policy reform though public debate (Gillespie *et al.*, 2014; McCosker *et al.*, 2014).

Media reporting has contributed to the progressive politicisation of child protection (Parton, 2014) and shaped unhelpfully blaming public discourses on maltreating parents and the communities in which they live (see Chapter 5). Practitioners are also not immune from such vilification (Lonne and Parton, 2014). Despite laws generally protecting the identity of children and the confidentiality of service delivery, child protection cases can become high profile and impact significantly on practitioner morale when scandals are exposed. Fear of public vilification can result in practitioners and agencies becoming 'even more sensitive to public criticisms, and evermore likely not to release information into the public domain' (Lonne and Parton, 2014, p. 832). Media coverage impacts on organisational cultures, which are key determinants of ethical practice (see Chapter 9).

Influential theoretical frameworks

An ethical framework must be embedded in practice at all levels: individual, organisational and frontline practice. Also required is an in-depth understanding of families across eras, and over the life cycle, and the ways in which culture, political change and social forces influence them (Gardiner *et al.*, 1998; Lindsay and Dempsey, 2012; White and Wu, 2014). Practitioners need theoretical frameworks to guide their understandings of maltreatment and practice, and to be able to critically examine the many factors at play.

Many jurisdictions have developed *assessment frameworks* like those used in the UK in previous decades, such as the Children's Assessment Framework triangle, which shows the domains of the child's developmental needs, the parental capacity and the family and environment. It arose from work commissioned by the UK government including *Child Protection: Messages from Research* (UK Department of Health, 1995). *Every Child Matters* (HM Government, 2004) promoted the Common Assessment Framework designed to operate as an early intervention tool to be used by any lead professionals involved with the child. These tools derived from ecological systems theory (see Jack, 2012; Payne, 2014). They condense a myriad influences upon families and children into simple depictions that provide a framework for understanding the factors contributing to children's well-being and safety.

While useful in some respects, they involve particular social constructions of children, families and childhood that arise within predominant neoliberal political contexts, which entail broader roles for the state, such as greater technologically based social surveillance (Featherstone *et al.*, 2014b; Parton, 2006b; Wrennall, 2010). Their primary orientation is deficit-based and individualises the causes of maltreatment while minimising influential social and structural factors, thereby downplaying the importance of relational and community supports critical to resourcing family coping. They also enable the framing of practice through technologically based tools that scientise the assessment process and minimise the relational aspects of caring (Featherstone *et al.*, 2014b; Pithouse *et al.*, 2011).

Where these frameworks reinforce child protection's incident-based investigative orientation and emphasis on risk, they tend to bypass an understanding of families' life journeys, relationships and communities in holistic, long-term ways that recognise the need for people's identity, culture and connection to be sustained (White and Wu, 2014). The pervasive and intergenerational impacts of gross inequality due to race, class, gender, disability and other social differences are minimised, while they uncritically embrace neoliberal ideology because they emphasise individual responsibility and risk within normative assumptions applicable to the dominant discourses (see Chapter 5).

Nonetheless, all frameworks still require theories to explain children's development, the life cycle, how we connect with others through relationships, the influence upon cognition, emotions and behaviour of culture, gender, race and class, how different groups relate and communities function, and how people change. Here we will succinctly describe some of the more influential theories, with further learning encouraged.

Systems theories

Ecological systems theory was developed by Bronfenbrenner (1979, 1986) to explain human development and uses ecology's foundational conceptions of the microsystem, mesosystem, mexosystem and macrosystem to describe person-environment relations and interactions (O'Donoghue and Maidment, 2005). It explains complex human behaviour, recognising that social structures and institutions shape people's culture, beliefs and values, and the narratives they use to understand life (see Chapter 8). This theory makes 'clear the need to see people and their environments within their historical and cultural contexts, in relationship to one another, and as continually influencing one another' (Kilpatrick and Holland, 2009, p. 16). Systemic interdependencies are highlighted, with change being a continual and dynamic process of adaptation to feedback and altered circumstances. Correctly applying this theory requires practitioners to methodically identify the myriad factors at play in complex cases and their respective levels of influence.

Systems theory, and family systems theory, was formulated with concepts such as structure, boundaries, roles, alliances, rules, power, processes, feedback, change, and equilibrium being core (Payne, 2014; Walsh, 2010). Outsiders can become potentially powerful systems change agents. When used in conjunction with Germain and Gitterman's (1980) *life model*, it is a powerful conceptualisation of the developmental pathway for families explaining life stressors, coping and transition, with relatedness emphasised. Family systems theory has particular relevance for child protection because it enables the underlying causes and processes eventuating in maltreatment to be identified and understood at the relational and interactional levels, within their cultural, gendered and social contexts. While it can aid understanding, it does not provide 'model' interventions, instead requiring practitioners to creatively develop unique approaches for case situations.

Attachment theory

Bowlby's *attachment theory* helps us to conceptualise the formation of relationships between parents/carers and children, and to understand the impacts of bonding, separation and disrupted attachments upon children's cognitive, emotional and relational development (Howe, 2011; Watson, 2005). Psychosocial development, it is asserted, is shaped by the four types of attachment: secure; insecure ambivalent; insecure avoidant; and disorganised and controlling (Howe, 2009). These result from different types of parenting that can themselves be related to their own childhood maltreatment (Watson, 2005). While awareness of attachment theory facilitates the assessment of family relationships, dynamics and signs of maltreatment, and understanding of parents/carers' background, needs and aspirations, it needs to be borne in mind that there is a limited supportive evidence base. Moreover, there has been criticism of its assumptions of universality, and cultural relativism in its application with Indigenous children and cultures (Neckoway *et al.*, 2003).

The focus on early intervention, as well as removal, is shored up by the use of attachment theories that have a deterministic emphasis on the importance of the early years and support 'now or never' (Munro, 2011) arguments (see Featherstone *et al.*, 2014b). As mentioned above, early intervention and removal is also bolstered by a particularly potent neuroscientific argument, which has been widely critiqued from within neuroscience itself (Bruer, 1999; Uttal, 2011; Wastell and White, 2012). The original neuroscience literature shows that the infant brain has quite remarkable resilience and plasticity when exposed to ordinary patterns of 'chaotic' neglect, usually seen in the population referred to children's social care. Indeed, if changes to the brain were the criterion for removal from parents, very few children would be removed (Wastell and White, 2012).

Strengths-based approaches

Strengths-based approaches have been increasingly adopted in child protection in an attempt to improve service-user engagement and redress its deficit-based assessment framework, which is arguably fundamental to the investigation of risk (see Chapter 5). Saleebey (2009) has written extensively on the strengths perspective, a relationally oriented practice, with its key principles being:

- every individual, group, family and community possesses strengths;
- while maltreatment and trauma may be injurious, they can also be sources of challenge and opportunity;
- it is important to not assume the levels of growth and change in others;
- collaborating with service users is the best approach;
- every situation has many resources available; and
- caring, caretaking and context are central.

(Saleebey, 2009, pp. 15–19)

In practice it provides a basis for entering the world of families, forming partnerships, being context sensitive and working with them to develop alternative narratives about the struggles they face (Munford and Sanders, 2005). Gray (2011) argued that with its underpinnings in Aristotelianism, humanistic individualism and communitarianism, strengths-based practice is at risk of co-optation within dominant neoliberal ideologies emphasising individualistic service responses. Its overly optimistic and uncritical understandings of community development, social capital and the subjective well-being movement accompany an overall emphasis upon individual, family and community responsibility for finding solutions and a simultaneous downplaying of government responsibility to address social and structural inequalities. Gray has queried whether its claims of success have a supportive empirical evidence base, as well as whether the equality in the client–worker relationship that strengths-based approaches rely on was actually possible within contemporary managerialised service-delivery systems – a point of direct relevance in child protection.

Strengths-based *solution-focused models* of practice are perhaps most often used in child protection (Oliver and Charles, 2015). Examples include *signs of safety* and solution-based casework (Christensen *et al.*, 1999; Turnell and Edwards, 1999) (see Chapter 5). These models provide a structure, process and relationship-based principles for service-user engagement, assessment and intervention, and emphasise the relational aspects of the helping process that have been increasingly stressed within child protection and social care more broadly (Ruch *et al.*, 2010). They are consistent with many aspects of systems and psychodynamic theory that emphasise complexity, use of self and reflective practice (see Chapter 11).

However, questions remain about whether strengths-based approaches are truly possible within the deficits-based orientation of child protection. The most commonly cited Saleebey (2009) – 'Kansas' – model and its variants rest heavily on collaboration, which is not always possible in child protection work (Folgheraiter, 2004; Folgheraiter and Raineri, 2012; Oliver and Charles, 2015). As Featherstone and Gupta (2014) argue, in a societal context of widespread inequality, not enough attention has been paid to the implications for relationships of mutuality between service users and practitioners. Oliver and Charles's Canadian study found:

> the common conflation of strengths-based and solution-focused approaches ignores important differences in the conceptualization of practitioner authority and leaves practitioners attempting to implement versions of strengths-based practice that do not fit statutory child protection work. Only when practitioners choose solution-focused models that support their use of mandated authority is consistent implementation a reasonable expectation.
>
> (Oliver and Charles, 2015, p. 1)

More optimistically, the *signs of safety* model holds promise as it has been specifically designed for child protection work (Oliver and Charles, 2015).

Anti-oppressive approaches

Anti-oppressive, anti-discriminatory and *feminist* perspectives have particular relevance for child protection work because of overrepresentation issues (Strega and Carriere, 2009). These conceptual frameworks use a multifaceted social lens shaped by critical and structural theory; principles of social difference; power and powerlessness; linking the personal with the political; incorporating socio-political and historical contexts; and emphasising the importance of reflection and reflexivity for practitioners (Burke and Harrison, 2009; Dumbrill, 2003, 2006, 2010; Orme, 2009; Payne, 2014). The linkages to structural factors, poverty, human rights and social justice principles are crucial because they enable broader systemic analysis rather than just individualising the causes of maltreatment and inequality (Mullaly, 2007). In our view, sound ethical practice must entail critical analysis of injustice and its social structural causes so that we can empathise and work with people who experience lifelong discrimination and oppression (see Chapters 5 and 14).

Conclusion

In this chapter, we have critically examined how dominant discourses have shaped social mandates and models of child protection, the ethical issues surrounding these, and the theoretical frameworks underpinning practice approaches. While many practice theories are used in child protection work, such as psychodynamic perspectives and crisis intervention, a major flaw in some practice frameworks – and models of child protection – is the narrow conceptualisation of community, which is often limited to seeing family, neighbours and others merely as 'reporters' (Melton, 2005), and community-based organisations as the primary providers of supportive services (see Chapter 5). Significant benefits can flow from a far broader conceptualisation of community members' roles in protecting children and helping struggling families through informal supports (Holland, 2014; Holland et al., 2011; Jack, 2004; Jack and Gill, 2010; Kimborough-Melton and Campbell, 2008; Landau, 2011; Melton, 2010a; Melton et al., 2002; McLeigh, 2013). In Chapters 10 and 11, we show how, by recognising and using the informal community web of care, we open up opportunities for prevention strategies within everyday family, neighbourhood, cultural and community networks, as well as secondary and tertiary supports that are accessible, acceptable and do not necessarily stigmatise. In Chapter 7 we take up service users' perspectives of child protection and examine the emerging evidence concerning the poor outcomes children and parents, and many staff experience.

Reflective questions

1 What are the emerging and dominant policy trends in child protection?
2 Who are the key stakeholders in the protection of children and how well do their interests align and differ?
3 How do mandatory reporting and differential response fit within the dominant child protection discourses?
4 What are the ethical issues in overrepresentation of particular groups?
5 How might social surveillance in child protection affect the nature of your practice relationships with service users and practitioners in other agencies?
6 What are the key theories for child protection practice and how might you embed your ethical framework within them?
7 How can a critical socio-structural framework assist you to understand injustice and work with the diversity of service users and their life experiences?

Chapter 7   Service-user and other perspectives

This chapter examines the diverse perspectives of child protection service users, with a particular focus on the general exclusion of the voices of children and parents from practice-related decision-making processes and policy forums, and the impacts of new stakeholder organisations, particularly those representing past service users and advocacy groups. *Service users* is a term used to describe the people who use health and other care services. In the context of this book, it means those who are reported to, or who are otherwise involved with, child protection and family welfare services. The term *service user* emerged in the 1980s to describe a 'movement' in mental health services wherein people previously called patients and later, consumers, started to define themselves as more than passive recipients of paternalistic services. By adopting this nomenclature, it was suggested that people for whom services were developed had a right to 'involvement in their services', 'to be able to give voice to their own experiences' and, in doing this, to be able to influence services to improve quality and outcomes (Wallcraft *et al.*, 2009, p. 8).

It is noteworthy that, as with child protection, many service users in mental health do not willingly use these services and, instead, are often mandated to do so. This means their engagement as service users is not always consensual, power differentials are accentuated and rights are easily, albeit unintentionally, compromised (Rooney, 2013). Therefore, this term was a progressive one for its time carrying with it a contested but clear message about the need to rectify power imbalances between service providers and service users by fostering empowerment and participation for vulnerable people.

Generally, service users in mental health are identified as those people living with mental illness or serious mental health problems. Their families and carers are considered to be separate stakeholders, albeit with a clear and important role in influencing services. There is little doubt the contribution of service users and families and carers in mental health worldwide is highly advanced, and this has had a significant impact at every level of policy, practice and research. The same cannot be said for child protection where, as Ivec (2013) notes, 'consumer-led initiatives are in their infancy' (p. 13). Indeed, as is evident, the language of *client* and *consumer*, rather than service user, continues to be used in child protection in many countries.

Service-user perspectives and voices

Children and their parents are the primary recipients of child protection services; they are typically identified as the key service users (Buckley *et al.*, 2008; Dumbrill and Lo,

2007). An understandable public perspective might be that, as a service user, a child is a passive recipient of these protective services, and is affected by them to the extent he or she is assessed and then guaranteed safety and a nurturing environment in which to grow and mature. Parents, on the other hand, are likely to be perceived by the public as compulsory service users, especially when reported to the statutory service as having 'failed' the child, in which case they are suitably chastised, learn their lessons and so maintain care of their child or, in more extreme circumstances, fail to change their behaviour and lose such care. These perspectives are also likely to have been those of the early architects of services aimed at protecting children from the harms perpetrated by their parents, or by the failure of their parent(s) to protect them from harm (Bessant, 2013; Dickey, 1986) (see Chapter 5).

It is salutary to note, as does Pelton (2011), that it was only in the 1990s that serious research attention was given to the views of child protection service users. He notes that, until this time, most of the little research undertaken, studied children and parents as 'objects' rather than paying attention to their 'subjective realities'. One of the key principles of the UNCRC, as expressed in Article 12, asserts that the views of children and young people should be taken into account, wherever possible, in decisions that affect their future well-being. This has undoubtedly stimulated an increase in research about the participation of children and young people, and their experiences of child protection interventions and services. Much of this research has been undertaken by organisations set up worldwide to represent the voice of children as citizens and service users, such as variously named offices of children's commissioners, guardians or ombudsmen.

Children and young people's voices

What does this research tell us about the views of children and young people? It is acknowledged that research involving children has methodological and ethical challenges. However, the significant amount of research conducted over the last decade or so, despite these difficulties, shows considerable dissatisfaction among children who are, or who have been, subjected to the care and child protection systems (Carroll-Lind et al., 2006; Sanders and Mace 2006; Westcott and Davies 1996; Woolfson et al., 2009). Although positive outcomes are reported and it is important to acknowledge these, many children often find the processes intimidating and feel overlooked, impotent, ignored and uninformed about proceedings, and ill-prepared for what happens to them. The evocative words of a manager in a statutory care service who spent almost all his life in the care of the state captures the importance of listening to children and young people:

> Over this journey through the care system there were a number of transformative moments that if the system had stopped long enough and really listened to what I and other people were trying to say, things may have been very different. The problem was that I was part of a care system focused on having total control over the lives of children in care. That control meant that what they thought was best for me was going to happen. This led to a battle for control that I now feel that both the Department and I lost.
>
> (King, 2014, p. 1)

Adults such as Michael King, who experienced out-of-home care, and who have had both positive and not-so-positive experiences, are contributing as part of an increasingly interdisciplinary cohort urging changes that enable the voice of children at risk or in care to be heard during decision-making processes that involve them and in policy making that amends the system.

Generally, the now substantial body of research evidence confirms children and young people want to be involved in decisions affecting their lives and attests the 'ethical, practical and therapeutic legal reasons for doing so' (Montserrat, 2014, p. 688). This research evidence speaks to the efficacy of actively engaging children and young people in decision making (Bilson, 2007; Dalrymple, 2005) and most legislation worldwide now confers this right on children. Despite the research evidence, the empowering legislation and the strong voice of children about their wish to be involved, there appear to be obstacles and perhaps resistance to fully engaging young people in child protection decisions. (Vis *et al.*, 2012). There are at least two reasons for this.

First, there appears to be some continuing adult resistance to engaging the voice of children and young people. Leeson (2007) researching the experiences of young people in care, found the problem was not in the interest or capability of young people but the problems lay with adults' 'ability and preparedness to involve young people in decisions about their own lives' (p. 268). This restriction of child engagement comes from a range of workers and leads inevitably to a reliance on adult voices in the affairs of children. Bruce (2014) expresses his concern about the now considerable evidence showing that 'children are not being adequately included in child protection work' (p. 516).

Second, practitioners are caught in multiple binds, among which are the different ways in which decision making is defined, roles allocated and the 'complexity of what actually happens in practice' (Hudson, 2008, p. 3). Among the other imperatives, it is undoubtedly hard to calibrate the voice of the child among the other demands and the risks involved. Given practitioners are responsible for implementing legislation on child involvement, practice standards and protocols need to make this possible (Munro, 2011).

Parents' voices

Swift's (1995) ground breaking *Manufacturing Bad Mothers* focused on the way in which mothers were vilified in child neglect discourse, when poverty was the underlying cause. Pelton (2011) highlights the ongoing risk of attributing culpability to mothers, and the untenable stance of focusing on the personality of the mother alone rather than paying attention to the situational factors of the family. Structural causes rather than individual or familial failing should be the targets of change (Bywaters, 2015; Featherstone *et al.*, 2014b; Marmot, 2005). Those who have listened to parents' voices on their engagement with the child protection services over the years reveal their overwhelming experience of hopelessness, fear, blame and shame (Buckley *et al.*, 2011a; Cleaver and Freeman, 1995; Dumbrill, 2003, 2006, 2010; Hansen and Ainsworth, 2007; Spratt and Callan, 2004). This research attests the imbalances of power between parents and statutory authorities, parental experiences of powerlessness and futility and the potential harm to children when the importance of familial bonds is ignored (see Chapters 8 and 12). More optimistically, Pelton

(2011) observes that, while services tended to focus on risk assessment and interventions to change the behaviour of parents, 'the studies converged upon an important fact': what parents generally found most helpful was practical help and 'concrete supports' (Pelton, 2011, p. 482).

There has been increasing attention to the experiences of parents and their rights in relation to child protection investigations and interventions (Hinton, 2013; Pelton, 2011). These have led to the development of an increasing number of advocacy and support services for parents (see, for example, the Family Inclusion Network: http://familyinclusionnetwork.com). Importantly, recent researchers have been helpful in identifying what parents have found positive and useful in their contact with child protection authorities (see Chapter 12). In summarising their research findings, Ghaffar, Manby and Race (2012) highlight the positive experiences of some parents and the potential for positive outcomes noting the importance of 'systematically harnessing parents' views and advice, not least to secure improvements in assessment processes and case conference settings' (p. 93). In a similar vein, Kapp and Vela (2004, p. 205) noted:

> The predictors of overall satisfaction (of parents) suggest that if solid social work skills (i.e. respect for client values, making expectations clear, preparing clients for meetings, asking clients about problems and services, including them in decisions, and respecting their culture) are practiced, it is likely that the parents will have a satisfactory experience.

Other stakeholder voices

Besides service users, other *stakeholders* have an interest in the processes and outcomes of child protection decisions (see Chapter 6). These stakeholders might include neighbours, teachers, family friends and, indeed, the media and broader public. Almost always, children and their families live in some form of connection within geographic, racial and cultural communities or communities of interest be they schools, churches, sports groups or employment organisations. Inevitably, many people have an investment or stake in the outcomes of child protection decisions, since children themselves have a connection with a wide variety of communities and networks (see Chapters 5 and 11).

The predominant focus on parents and children conceals a much more complex service-user collage. Very young children are 'passive recipients' and it is hard to conceptualise them as service users, while older children and young people vary greatly in their capacity to have a voice as service users. Parents are individuals and their involvement is often disparate and also variable and, as Featherstone *et al.* (2014b) comment, parents are often seen through a simplified prism of success or failure rather than through 'an understanding of the subtle shading of (their) relational life' (p. 114). As outlined in Chapter 13, mothers appear to have greater involvement than do fathers (Brodie *et al.*, 2014; Featherstone, 2010; Scourfield, 2006), and single mothers as a demographic group are highly represented in child protection data internationally (Allan, 2004). However, in the broader collage, grandparents are increasingly involved in child care and child protection matters (Murphy *et al.*, 2008; Worrall, 2005) and extended families, particularly in countries with minority Indigenous populations, are necessarily involved in child protection interventions (Roberts, 2002).

Beyond that, other groups, such as foster carers and kinship networks have a direct interest in outcomes for children and families. All of these groups might be seen as service users in a broad sense.

Foster and kinship carers' voices

Debates about how to provide care for children who are removed from parental care are far-reaching and increasingly preoccupied with considering the risks and benefits of alternative care arrangements in environments in which numbers of children are increasing, care options are limited and many poor long-term outcomes of care are being confronted. A large number of reports worldwide include extensive service user feedback from foster carers, kinship carers as well as parents and young people, and attest the contemporary understanding that the out-of-home based care for children is in crisis (Fostering Network, 2011; Harber and Oakley, 2012; Jarmon *et al.*, 2000; Osborn and Bromfield, 2007; Thomson and Thorpe, 2004). Evidentially these crises are multifactorial but include questions about efficacy and outcomes and the nature of ethical practice when decisions have to be made quickly, short-term safety and long-term well-being are in tension and power imbalances are experienced between all of the players – children, workers and foster carers or kinship carers.

The ethical aspects of the tensions involved are captured intrepidly by Little (2010) and responded to coherently by Sinclair (2010) in an article titled, 'Looked after children: Can existing services ever succeed?'. Little provides four arguments against the continuation of current models of substitute care for children. All arguments provide excellent starting points for questions about the ethics of such care and each, by their nature, invite service user perspectives. The four points made by Little (2010, pp. 3–6) are: care services are not ethical; state care belongs to another historical context; the selection of children for care is haphazard; and, the evidence base for state care is weak. Sinclair's response engages with the importance of this contemporary, ongoing and confronting debate and, as he says, in the absence of a convincing 'blueprint for what we should put in place' invites ongoing dialogue about how to improve care outcomes. There is no doubt that the experiences of foster carers is essential in this debate particularly as along with their unrelenting contribution to children in need they have voiced their concerns over many years about important matters such as lack of consultation, powerlessness in the face of statutory agency and poor partnership arrangements with practitioners (McHugh and Pell, 2013).

Formal placement of children in kinship care, as opposed to the dominant form of child welfare care in Western societies of foster care or 'placement with strangers', has increased dramatically in recent years. These newer care arrangements have been accompanied by ongoing debates at all levels of policy, legislation and practice, about government versus family responsibilities for children and young people in such care and their carers (Nandy *et al.*, 2011). The complexities of service user perspectives of the care system are highlighted well in a number of recent research reports about children's and families' experiences of kinship care as opposed to foster care (Burgess *et al.*, 2010) and they summarise with a challenge relevant for all decision makers in child protection and particularly relevant in terms of relationally based ethical decision making:

The service system needs to work with the difficult issues of family contact and relationships, rather than moving quickly to ordering regular, controlled contact arrangements, or attempting to forbid contacts unless absolutely necessary. Within safe limits, young people may sometimes need to explore what will work for them. This requires support workers to have the skills to deal with the complexity of family relationships where there has been abuse and neglect.

(p. 32)

There are also advocacy organisations representing the interests of children and young people in the care system. For example, CREATE in Australia, and the American Children's Advocacy centres aim to empower children and young people to have a say in their own lives, particularly when they are involved in the care system. In Australia, the Care Leavers Australia Network (CLAN) and the Alliance for Forgotten Australians (AFA) among others, have testified to the horrific experiences of adults who were removed from their families as children and spent a significant amount of time in state care. These increasingly influential organisations, bringing together individuals and groups of adults who were once in care, comprise 'prior service users' with valuable information to contribute on the impact of care in children's lives. Many of these people refuse to use the term 'care system' and see themselves as 'survivors of care'.

These and other stakeholder communities have made a significant impact on child protection policy and practice through public inquiries highlighting abysmal service outcomes (Parliament of Australia Senate Community Affairs Committee, 2004). Additionally, there are now a significant number of biographies, such as the powerful work of Penglase (2005), *Orphans of the Living*, attesting the need to engage children and young people more directly in child protection assessment and care provisions. There are also group histories, such as Roberts' (2002) *Shattered Bonds: The Color of Child Welfare* and the *Bringing them Home* report in Australia (HREOC, 1997) on the ongoing crisis in the disproportionate representation of Indigenous and black children in the care system (Busch *et al.*, 2008) (see Chapter 6).

Further, recent inquiries have highlighted the experiences of service users and stakeholders affected by past adoption policies and practices, particularly those subjected to 'forced adoption' (see Chapter 6). A recent Australian inquiry captured the permanence of the tragic outcomes for many women: 'a mother whose child has been stolen does not only remember in her mind, she remembers with every fibre of her being' (Parliament of Australia Senate Community Affairs Committee, 2012, p. 29). Beyond the direct impacts on women and children, the 'wide-ranging ... ripple effect of adoption' is felt by the mother's family, siblings, fathers, and adoptive parents and their families (Higgins, 2011, p. 64). While these experiences are not always negative for all involved, the testimonials speak to matters of real significance in ethical decision making – a coercive environment in which mothers' choices were limited and attributed shame left them powerless (Freymond, 2003).

Many have highlighted the ongoing grief and trauma and 'untold damage' associated with these 'past practices' and, importantly, the sociological context shaping the 'views of broader society' around 'illegitimacy, infertility and impoverishment' (Higgins, 2011, p. 64) that framed these adoption practices. Decision making in past adoption practices is under scrutiny around the world, and a growing body of research suggests coercion, poverty, restricted options and related factors continue to shape some contemporary adoption practices, particularly intercountry adoption (Smolin and Smolin, 2012). The highly contested push to 'permanency planning' that has been a policy response to research about risks associated with discontinuity in foster care and the neurological *sequalae* of trauma is seeing a return to accusations by various service users and stakeholders that this is simply a new form of forced adoption (see Chapter 6).

Given the ongoing problems in child protection, several 'communities of interest' have emerged to express their concerns about the negative impact of child protection practices and services. These, increasingly national organisations are exerting a strong transformative influence and include organisations such as the US National Coalition for Child Protection Reform (NCCPR) and the Family Advocacy Movement. Their stakeholders, representing associations of service users and professionals, are attempting to alter the politics and morality of child protection. Among them a large number are focused on the racial and deprivation geography of child protection (Roberts, 2008) and its nexus with the systematic disadvantage associated with inequalities, poverty and illness (Bywaters, 2015, p. 4).

Practitioners as stakeholders

As already indicated, practitioners, academics and policy makers along with others across a spectrum of disciplines have been active in suggesting, generating and advocating for changes in child protection practice and decision making. Some of the associations in which they have been and are involved are named in earlier sections of this chapter. Not the least of these campaigners and activists are practitioners who work or have worked in this hugely challenging (and rewarding) arena of child protection and who have themselves experienced the organisational difficulties that lead to a sense of anxiety, fear and risk, none of which auger well for considered decision making (see Chapter 9). The multiple challenges involved in managing the complex organisational context of child protection leads to agencies undergoing almost constant organisational change, which entails its own uncertainties and anxieties. Additionally, these challenges lead to significant problems, such as high levels of work stress, inadequate staff supervision, constant staff turnover and recruitment problems (Claiborne *et al.*, 2011; Collins, 2008; Lonne *et al.*, 2012). The media often portray these systems as being constantly in crisis (McCosker *et al.*, 2014) and, as Lonne and Parton (2014) highlight, staff in turn feel and react to the public blaming that follows when tragedies or scandals occur:

> The fear and anxiety that is engendered for child protection workers and related health, education, and police staff promotes risk-averse practice and a slavish adherence to policies and procedures, often ignoring the specific familial and community circumstances that exist. Good practice subsequently becomes 'I have followed the rules', rather than 'I have done the proper thing in this particular situation'. Protective systems are fundamentally human and relational, and the impact of these sorts of punitive and blaming portrayals upon staff attitudes and behaviour should not be under-estimated. Even though very few actual staff 'casualties' result from this sort of media-driven public vilification, other staff watch and listen, take note of the punitive process, and act accordingly.
>
> (Lonne and Parton, 2014, p. 832)

Risk-aversive practice generally emerges under conditions of such stress, with result-ant over-reliance on policy and procedure, including defensive, self-protective work cultures. Risk-averse environments have been found to affect case-related decision making by altering the ways practitioners undertake assessments and define abuse thresholds (Queensland Child Protection Commission of Inquiry, 2013b). Further, research indicates that personal and organisational cultural variations in practitioner definitions, thresholds and assessments, and differences in how agencies and jurisdic-tions make determinations about these (Harris, 2011; Horwath, 2007; Maitra, 2005; Platt and Turney, 2014; Steen and Duran, 2014). These factors lead to variable case-related decision making and increase pressure for more consistent evidence-based practice. They also lead to demands for change. And there are a large number of practitioners who, along with academics and others and despite the difficulties and risks in doing so, provide ongoing evidence of the need for change.

Implications for practitioners and ethical practice

So why this lengthy account of viewpoints from the range of people who are service users or significant stakeholders in child protection? And how does it relate to the matter of ethics and ethical decision making? The examination of child protec-tion and family welfare services from the viewpoint of different service users and multiple stakeholders invites us to think much more comprehensively about what is important in decision making in child protection, including about race and dis-advantage. As Featherstone *et al.* (2014b) observe, service users and many other stakeholders tell us that the families who are investigated, and the children who are removed 'are overwhelmingly economically and socially disadvantaged' (p. 4). This presents as a significant political, ethical and moral matter relating to our duty as a community and as child protection practitioners to families trying to parent in soci-eties in which economic, social and racial inequalities are profoundly present and define the vulnerability of populations. Associated with poverty and disadvantage is vulnerability and always the intimidating companion of powerlessness. And that powerlessness is ever accentuated in the presence, or threatened presence, of state agents and practitioners carrying the weight of that authority. Nowhere is this more pronounced than in the power and authority of the state to intervene in the family and remove children! We return to the management of power in Chapters 9 and 12, where the matter is dealt with in more detail in terms of how it is applied in an inte-grated decision-making framework.

For practitioners, who are also stakeholders in the outcomes of child protection decisions, various failures in the safeguarding of children has led to endless inquir-ies that impact on individuals in particular and the workforce in general (Lonne and Parton, 2014). Most significantly, a 'focus on the media is important because of the power the media have to help transform the private into the public, but at the same time, to undermine trust, reputation, and legitimacy of the professionals working in the field' (p. 822). The performance of any worker is affected by a large range of external and internal factors. Externally, organisational demands and stresses, media focus and political attention generally lead to fear and uncertainty. The result of inquiries and media-mediated public responses to these has no doubt dramatically increased the work stress, staff turnover and anxiety of practitioners. Devaney (2004) noted this was producing a crisis in statutory child welfare departments, where 'there is a chronic shortage of staff wishing to work with children and families ... departments are operating with high vacancy rates' (p. 30). This has resulted in *toxic work environments,* for some, as the fear of public vilification amid impossible work pressures has led to increased anxiety and a culture of risk management (Kemshall, 2002; Stalker, 2010; Webb, 2006).

Alongside this, an increasing number of websites vilify the child protection workforce (e.g. www.lukesarmy.com) and invite opprobrium to those who 'steal children'. The creation of complex audit systems creates an additional environment of surveillance for practitioners (Munro, 2004). Practitioners who feel under siege, and who are experiencing intense anxiety, are also working under severe time constraints often mediated by organisational and legal priorities (Waterhouse and McGhee, 2009) (see Chapter 9). In these situations it is inevitable that problems may be defined in personal ways and some decision making distorted. This is exemplified in the findings of the research undertaken by Beckett *et al.* (2007) in which they sought the views of child welfare practitioners having to make decisions under pressure. These practitioners talked about the 'bias towards safety where failure can lead to public disgrace' (p. 61), and the implications of this, among other factors, to frame problems and decision making in certain ways.

While the historical and contemporary individual and community realities of child protection practices are being highlighted as seriously problematic, practitioners are experiencing varying degrees of helplessness associated with ever-increasing pressures to safeguard growing numbers of children. As noted by Ungar (2004), the irony may well be that 'a deeper sensitivity to the marginalization experienced by disempowered and at-risk populations' has not been credibly translated 'into an appreciation of the implications of this interpretation for the practitioner themselves' (p. 489). There is little doubt that child protection and family welfare practitioners can be trapped in the same way that impoverished and disadvantaged parents, families and communities are, in unintentionally damaging worlds 'not of their own making' (Pelton, 2011, p. 485). Ungar (2004) urged practitioners to understand the implications of this and the associated need to understand new potential paradigms, discourses and power, and acknowledge the need to share resources to become 'architects of something different' (p. 495).

In their comprehensive recent research, Gladstone *et al.* (2012) acknowledged the centrality of relationship and engagement in child protection practice and noted the role of power in mediating this engagement. They summarised with words that speak to the significance of ethics in practice: 'A challenge for the child welfare system is to not only express a philosophy that promotes engagement between clients and workers but [also] to establish an environment where this can come about' (p. 117).

Alongside an acknowledgment of the role of power, the ethical point of reference should be the imperative to respect all services users, appreciate the context provided by other stakeholders and attend to contextual matters of justice for all involved. These imperatives derive from the principle to respect all people and to avoid discrimination and harm. Doing so does not detract from the centrality of the child in decision making about safety but acknowledges the child is deeply connected in profound and permanent ways to others – to family, friends and community. The 'best interests' of the child cannot be separated from his or her connections to the family of origin – connections that, if severed, have the potential to seriously harm people to whom the child may well be attached, regardless of what they have done to invite the attention of statutory authorities. Arguably, to the extent that one harms the birth family of a child, one also potentially harms the child. In the words of an early report urging reforms to child protection:

> It is extremely difficult to take a swing at 'bad mothers' without the blow landing on their children. Therefore if we really believe all the rhetoric about the needs of the children coming first, we must put those needs before anything – even our anger at their parents.
>
> (Wexler, 2003, p. 48)

Conclusion

The experiences of service users and other stakeholders are vitally important to include in ethical practice and policy development. Yet reports from across the globe suggest all these important stakeholders often feel excluded and that the dominant discourses of child protection, with the attendant emphasis on risk and the immediate protection of children, have left them feeling voiceless and impotent to contribute to improving practice and policies. They consistently say there are serious impediments to their participation in practice-related processes and decision making in ethically important matters. Perhaps more importantly, service-delivery outcomes poorly meet their needs, and it is to a closer examination of this that we now turn.

Reflective questions

1 How might children, young people and parents participate more fully in decision-making processes and how can the practitioner facilitate this?
2 To what extent do organisational constraints stand in the way of such engagement?
3 What feedback loops might be put in place to ensure that the voice of service users informs ethical practice?
4 How might service-user powerlessness be addressed within child protection practice?
5 How might the demanding practice and organisational environments for child protection practitioners be altered to reduce stress and promote their capacity for effective and ethical practice?

Chapter 8   Needs and circumstances of service users

Some parents do harm to their children in intentional and desperately harmful ways. We hope these families are reported to statutory authorities. However, the majority of parents and children reach the attention of child protection authorities because they, like all families, need help. Raising children has many challenges, and there are numerous pressure points at particular developmental milestones, such as a new baby entering the family, children going to a new school and adolescents leaving home. When dealing with these stressful periods, people find needed support from family, friends and neighbours – the *web of care* provided by *informal sources of community care* (Melton, 2010b, 2014) (see Chapter 5). However, access to support is crucial but not always available when required to those who need it. For most families, most of the time, there is little reason for the formal involvement of child protection authorities, and contact rarely happens. But the situation is quite different for people from particular groups that are overrepresented in the child protection and family welfare system, such as the socially marginalised, alumni of the care system, single parents (mostly women), Indigenous people, refugees, people of colour, and those from socially excluded ethnicities, especially where families are experiencing issues associated with divorce, alcohol and drug misuse, domestic and family violence, disabilities or health conditions, poverty and mental ill-health.

Pathways to contact include an ongoing relationship with the statutory authorities, mandatory reporting, self-referral or professional referral (see Chapter 6). Causes for contact might include a one-off incident of harm or potential harm to a child (accidental or intentional), a series of harmful events (which might be minor but are perceived as cumulative or increasing in risk) and chronically poor parenting seen as warranting outside intervention. As we shall see in Chapter 11, the pathway and cause for contact can significantly influence service users' experience of statutory and other service involvement, and how they are treated is pivotal to the ethical practice of practitioners and agencies.

High and complex needs

Most child protection and family welfare service users have multifaceted needs that test a parent's, or family's coping and resilience, and their ability to weather harsh times often depends on service accessibility. Further, service users often have multiple needs simultaneously. Yet, many disadvantaged communities lack resources, *capabilities* and *social capital* and have depleted levels of connectedness and trust (Bywaters *et al.*, 2014). People in these communities are already struggling to make ends meet and may simply not be in a position to provide assistance. Help may not be at hand.

Even families in wealthier communities may not have access to the assistance they need as limited resources may be directed elsewhere. Further, high service demands for child protection have led to the prioritisation of urgent or crisis cases and targeted services. In situations assessed as low risk – usually when statutory involvement is deemed unnecessary – practitioners can find themselves referring families with high needs to community agencies, perhaps through differential response arrangements (see Chapter 6). This can result in 'churning', where high-need families undergo repeated investigations as they go from agency to agency seeking, but not receiving, the help they need due to limited resources (Cummins *et al.*, 2012; Wood Inquiry, 2008). To add to this, service-delivery systems are frequently fragmented, making it difficult for people to access resources within complex structures, processes and eligibility requirements. Hence, the frequent calls for 'joined-up' services with shared protocols, policies and data collection systems, despite problems associated with the ever-widening social surveillance of marginalised groups (Wrennall, 2010) (see Chapter 6).

As already discussed in Chapter 6, most jurisdictions have mandatory reporting requirements of one form or another, which have led to increased stigmatisation and contributed to families' reluctance to request services for fear of statutory involvement resulting in the removal of their children (Lonne, 2015). Within this context, the ethics of relational practice between service users and practitioners is crucial in building and maintaining the trust necessary for effective and humane interventions (see Chapter 11).

Families may themselves contribute to their inability to access available resources, either knowingly or unwittingly. For example, highly mobile families are often unaware of how to find resources in their new communities, and some parents are wary of others' motives and have trouble engaging in reciprocal relationships. We expand on this later but, in short, their past experiences of familial, kin and friendship relationships can contribute to distrust, ambivalence, and an inability to manage emotions and hostility, particularly for people who have been emotionally abused and neglected (Crittenden, 1999; Howe *et al.*, 2000). Having learned to be guarded about the *attachments* they form, they may find it very difficult to build sustainable relationships, thereby hindering their ability to access help.

We briefly examine areas of need often associated with a higher incidence of child maltreatment, although we note that association does not equate with causation. Our purpose in exploring these areas is to increase the awareness of the plight of people whose lives entail these sorts of problems, but also the need for understanding and empathy so that we can avoid stereotyping and prejudice, and promote ethical and humane practice.

Alcohol and drug misuse

Child abuse and neglect is often linked to *parental substance misuse*, which can be a catalyst for people physically and sexually harming children, and also for neglect situations (Gilbert *et al.*, 2009a, 2009b). Yet, alcohol use is a prominent part of the cultural milieu of many societies. While adults are generally viewed as responsible and free to make choices around alcohol consumption, despite the severe consequences for family life, especially domestic violence, illicit drug use is viewed differently. The public discourse around misuse, however, is predominantly a blaming one. Most adults behave responsibly or are able to address addiction issues themselves through personal control or self-help groups. Others need the help of health and welfare professionals and more prolonged treatment for their addictions. Many struggle to regain their equilibrium and relapses are commonly part of the process. Child protection workers frequently encounter cases of maltreatment involving parental alcohol and drug use and therefore need to know and understand the research around *substance misuse treatments*. They have to make difficult decisions about the best interests of children in these circumstances and must operate from an informed rather than a biased standpoint. How practitioners perceive and relate to people engaged in substance misuse is an important factor in the prospects for ethical and effective protective interventions.

Domestic abuse

Domestic and family violence are major problems in society, mostly affecting women who are abused by their intimate partners (see Chapter 13). This directly impacts on children who witness ongoing violence in the home and those who are themselves physically harmed in these circumstances. While women are most at risk of serious *domestic violence*, including homicide, men also suffer physical and emotional abuse from women and some couples are mutually violent (Office for National Statistics, 2014). Domestic violence is frequently linked to alcohol and drug misuse. While the links with poverty and deprivation are complex, the lack of economic and social resources impacts in a range of ways on causation and consequence. The social construction of gendered identities has particularly pernicious impacts upon economically and socially disadvantaged men and women (Rivett, 2010). *Domestic abuse* is a key issue in child protection as seen in policy and legislation regulating the sector and, as we explore in Chapters 6 and 13, there are a range of ethical issues associated with societal attitudes toward women and men, the construction of gendered roles and the protection of children (Featherstone *et al.*, 2014b). For example, is the suffering of women effaced or indeed even intensified by practices and procedures that focus in an instrumental way on the needs of children? (See discussion on early intervention in Chapter 5.)

Poor parenting experiences and intergenerational trauma

There is a higher likelihood of abuse and neglect occurring in those families where a parent has also experienced childhood maltreatment. Though the long-term impacts are diverse and variable, *intergenerational trauma* is especially seen in Indigenous communities alongside the effects of colonisation (see Dubowitz, 2013a; Gilbert *et al.*, 2009a, 2012; Lonne, 2015). Developmental theories emphasise the long-term impacts of unhealthy childhood attachments, child removal and adoption (see Chapter 6). Many children removed from their parents find it difficult to form healthy adult relationships and sound *emotional attachments* with their children (Crittenden, 1999; Howe *et al.*, 2000; Tanner and Turney, 2003). Hence, failures in parent–child attachment often repeat across generations and result in fractured relationships (Reder and Duncan, 2001). This is especially seen in Indigenous communities where people have experienced the debilitating impacts of colonisation and its long-lasting impacts on individuals, families, kinship connections and communities (Berland *et al.*, 2011; Sinha *et al.*, 2011). *Cumulative harm* results in new generations experiencing the fallout from the historical trauma, pain, misery and desperation of their forebears. This partly explains the overrepresentation of Indigenous children in the child protection system, but, as Wilkinson and Pickett (2009) show, it also reflects the insidious impacts of health and social inequalities on particular groups in society, especially those with a colonial history.

Disability

Disability is often linked to child maltreatment as disabled children are particularly vulnerable to violence and abuse. While most people with disabilities are highly capable parents who form loving and caring bonds with their children, there is an overrepresentation of parents with intellectual or mental health disabilities in the child protection system. This has been attributed to *systemic discrimination* as parents with a *disability* frequently find themselves subject to others' stereotypes and prejudices (LaLiberte and Lightfoot, 2013; McConnell, 2013). Hence, child protection practitioners need to be ever mindful of social constructions of disability and their discriminatory impacts, especially on risk assessments and child protection interventions.

Unemployment and poverty

There is 'strong evidence linking [child] neglect to poverty' (Dubowitz, 2007, p. 605) and race (Carter and Myers, 2007; Jonson-Reid *et al.*, 2013). The recent analysis by Bywaters *et al.* (2014) of inequality and maltreatment data in England highlighted the important links between area-level deprivation and child protection interventions and the requirement to understand how poverty played out in the lives of children in impoverished communities (see Chapter 5). Looking more broadly, however, higher rates of maltreatment in disadvantaged communities may be associated with the increased surveillance activity as well as other factors. Communities with high levels of *poverty* tend to have lower levels of social capital and trust, and a decreased capacity to aid those who struggle. Unemployment compounds these problems. Particular groups, such as single mothers, young people and specific ethnicities with lower levels of education, are more vulnerable than others to social marginalisation with the flow-on effects of low-quality housing and poor physical and mental health.

Wilkinson and Pickett (2009) found strong connections between *social and economic inequality* and other negative economic, social and health indicators:

> Inequality ... is a powerful social divider, perhaps because we all tend to use differences in living standards as markers of status differences ... Our position in the social hierarchy affects who we see as part of the in-group and who as out-group – us and them – so affecting our ability to identify with and empathize with other people.
> (Wilkinson and Pickett, 2009, p. 51)

Their work highlighted the pervasive impact of social and health inequalities and their relationship to quality of life, not just for the poor but for all people, particularly those in poor physical and mental health. They argued that societies that were more homogeneous and equal tended to be stronger. The societies that were most unequal had greater social problems and there was less trust between its members, as well as higher levels of anxiety arising from the shame experienced by those who perceived societal reactions to them as derogatory. How people in poverty were portrayed and perceived impacts upon the discourses used to shape child protection interventions, and therefore were vital to address in developing ethical practice (Featherstone *et al.*, 2014b).

Mental health

Poor parental *mental health* is prominently associated with statutory child protection involvement (Kaplan, 2013). Mental ill-health often has a strong impact on people's ability to parent, not least due to a reduced capacity to earn a consistent income. Thus, poverty and disadvantage compounds the impact of mental illness. Nevertheless, with effective treatment and integrated supports many parents living with mental illness are able to care for their children. Mental health, however, is often poorly understood and people who are mentally ill frequently encounter stereotypes, prejudices and unfounded fear. Child protection practitioners can also be prone to these attitudes, potentially resulting in ongoing stigma and discrimination. Embedding ethics into professional and organisational practice frameworks can go some way to preventing this.

Ethnicity and race

Indigenous peoples, people of colour and marginalised ethnic groups are overrepresented in child protection data around the globe, with cultural relativism at play (AIHW, 2013; Bilson *et al.*, 2013; Blackstock *et al.*, 2004; Child Trends, 2012; Gilbert *et al.*, 2011; Sinha *et al.*, 2011). Hence, ethnicity, race and culture are strong determinants of child abuse and neglect (Gilbert *et al.*, 2011; Reading *et al.*, 2009). Yet there are wide variations in definitions of what does or does not constitute an incident of child abuse and neglect (Dubowitz 2013b; Jonson-Reid *et al.*, 2013). Lonne (2015) highlights that:

> Overrepresentation by reporting and intervention systems should not be viewed as arbitrary. Rather, these are patterns associated with poverty, marginalization and race and we find that groups with these characteristics find themselves targeted within our reporting systems ... Moreover, not only are these social structural dimensions not taken account of and corrected within our mandatory reporting systems, they are reinforced by it.
>
> (Lonne, 2015, p. 250)

The part that *ethnicity and race* play within social systems is complex but is associated with the higher levels of inequality experienced and an increased probability of being reported to statutory authorities (Bilson *et al.*, 2013; Bywaters, 2015; Harries and Clare, 2002) (see also Chapter 13).

Services and programmes to address high and complex needs

Circumstances for families with high and complex needs can present serious obstacles to garnering emotional and practical support, particularly when service systems are fragmented. When families have high and complex needs, they require a variety of supports and services, and these are best delivered within an *integrated framework* rather than a piecemeal patchwork of disconnected service responses (see Chapter 6). Further, programmes need to be delivered in ways that meet the diverse needs of the individuals and communities involved, attending to cultural and other requirements (Arney and Scott, 2013). We now briefly examine the sorts of services relevant for struggling parents, although it is noted that there is not a strong evidence base for identifying precise programme and service responses for specific family needs and maltreatment behaviours – what works, for whom and when (Kirkman and Melrose, 2014).

Broadly speaking, the following sorts of services are beneficial for family members in addressing the underlying issues contributing to abuse and neglect, although it should be noted that the *aetiology* and *sequelae* of neglect are often different to abuse and therefore require different interventions and treatment (Lonne, 2015). There are numerous sources that assist in guiding support and treatment interventions (see Arney and Scott, 2013; Gilbert *et al.*, 2009a). Families need practical support, such as assistance with food and household necessities, home management and affordable housing, particularly where poverty is present. Emotional supports, including self-help interventions, facilitate the sometimes lengthy journey that people need to undertake to address longstanding matters. Psychological guidance and counselling may assist in addressing behavioural, cognitive and emotional problems. Similarly, relationship and family counselling that focuses on unsatisfactory emotional engagements and problematic relational interactions can be very helpful.

Therapeutic treatments that address disability, alcohol and substance misuse, and mental and physical ill-health are often a high need for families as they are strongly associated with the issues hindering coping. Because of the associations with poverty, education, skills training and support that helps people to gain suitable employment and thereby address problems arising from low income are required. When families are struggling to cope, respite care and alternative accommodation arrangements can provide necessary space for family members to withdraw temporarily from intense relationships while their protective and personal needs are addressed. We have outlined in Chapter 5 the evidence base showing that community work and social development strategies can be fundamental to building capabilities, trust and the community connections essential for increased support and resilience.

Children's needs

Children have a range of needs and these alter across the developmental stages with, for example, increased need for independence. While a generalised dependence upon adults, particularly their parents, is present, this is nonetheless quite variable across cultures and contexts, and beliefs and attitudes about childhood and child rearing. This said, the domains of children's needs relate broadly to:

- Physical – shelter, food, nutrition and appropriate clothing for the physical, climatic and social environment.
- Supervision and safety – ensuring their surroundings do not present unacceptable threats to their health and safety.
- Health and well-being – their physiological being and welfare, security and physical activities.

- Educational – accessing age-appropriate schooling and training.
- Psychological – cognition, emotional responses and mental hygiene related to their developmental progression to adulthood.
- Emotional and relational – their needs for nurturance, affection, attachment and belonging met within consistent caring relationships within the family.
- Cultural – behaviours, mores, beliefs and practices in keeping with those held broadly within their community of connection.
- Spiritual and moral guidance – values-based and religious instruction.
- Identity – their essential character and sense of self, with personal, familial, cultural and community aspects that define their being in relation to others.

While there is a great deal of debate about the relativity or universality of children's needs (Redshaw, 2012), constructions of childhood and definitions of child abuse and neglect are generally socially, culturally and community contingent (Parton, 2006b). Within this complex context, making determinations about child maltreatment is as much a moral activity as a technical-rational one, and involves both *the head and the heart* (Horwath, 2007). Practitioners not only need to know the facts and knowledge-based aspects of children's needs and maltreatment, and particular sociocultural thresholds for determining harm and appropriate interventions, they also need to be mindful of the range of organisational, legal, professional and personal influences relating to the care and protection of children (Lonne, 2015).

Impact of child maltreatment

Recent meta-analyses of *prevalence studies* of child abuse and neglect have demonstrated its pervasive and significant impacts on children and families (Gilbert *et al.*, 2009a, 2009b; Radford *et al.*, 2011; Stoltenborgh *et al.*, 2013). Maltreatment can occur in the various relationships and contexts of the child's life, but most often occurs in the family and is due to parental and sibling behaviour. More widely, peers engage in bullying and aggressive behaviour. However, child protection issues, more often than not, centre on the child's family.

Social science research highlights the critical link between social and structural factors, such as gender, social class, race and inequality, and child maltreatment. Nevertheless, child abuse and neglect result from a messy interplay of events and risks, and determining what needs to be done presents a veritable ethical minefield. Deciphering impacts and determining consequences is not an exact science (Gilbert *et al.*, 2009b; Stoltenborgh *et al.*, 2013) and individual circumstances and *resilience* are important factors to consider. There is a huge variation in the noticeable consequences of maltreatment. Some incidents of maltreatment have imperceptible impacts while others are clearly observable.

Given the complex interrelated *sequelae* affecting multiple aspects of maltreated people's lives, effective support and treatment are more accessible when delivered via integrated coordinated service networks. A *web of care*, involving a mix of informal, semi-formal and formal help, is required to deal with the multiple impacts of child abuse and neglect, including:

- Physical injuries and disablement that hinders or prevents everyday activities and may involve long-term medical and other interventions.

- Emotional and psychological trauma leading to serious mental health issues, including anxiety disorders, PTSD, depression and substance misuse.
- Disrupted and fractured family relationships leading to the abuse of power and trust that characterises sexual and physical abuse, and an absence of affection, empathy and caring that emotional abuse and neglect entails, including transference to other intimate relationships.
- An inability to function independently and financially support oneself in adulthood as a consequence for some maltreated children, who require ongoing support from formal social services (see Gilbert *et al.*, 2009b).

Child maltreatment can have a long-lasting impact on people's identities and life narratives, many of whom carry stories of trauma, and a loss of faith and trust in others and the joys that life can bring. Aspirations are filtered through imprisoning, often judgmental, self-narratives such as:

- 'I am a bad person and incapable of being loved'.
- 'I will always be imprisoned by the events and circumstances of my abuse as a child'.
- 'People always look after themselves and are untrustworthy'.
- 'I cannot depend on others because they will let me down'.
- 'I always seem to pick up the bad people as friends'.
- 'People like me will never get ahead no matter what'.
- 'I always seem to stuff things up'.
- 'You have to fight hard to stop others from treating you badly – don't trust them'.
- 'My life is just never-ending episodes of being abandoned by others'.

Narratives can also be located within maltreated people's geographical and relational locations such as:

- 'Most people round here don't have happy endings'.
- 'None of my family have done any good so they say "you won't do any good either"'.
- 'I'd like to be a decent mum but that's unlikely to happen in this place. Too many bad things always happen'.

These narratives epitomise many service users' feelings of failure, helplessness and hopelessness. They are often reinforced by social stereotypes and prejudices that influence how services respond. Narrative therapy offers an approach that assists people to critically review their self-defeating life stories and reconstruct new empowering ones (see Brown and Augusta-Scott, 2007). By developing alternative life narratives, outdated understandings are replaced with powerful messages of surviving past events and thriving on life's opportunities. A narrative approach is particularly useful when working with parents who have had their children removed, with the consequent impacts on their emotions, roles and self-identity. It offers practitioners a perspective from which to understand and interpret abusive and neglectful relationships and their consequences non-judgmentally. Importantly, this enables practitioners to be inspirational *agents of hope* and to care for people who carry a pervading sense of their fragmented and damaged lives (Featherstone *et al.*, 2014b).

Implication for practice

Rampant neoliberal ideology and attendant inequality, privatisation and individualisation impacts heavily upon our child protection systems and leads to the overrepresentation of certain groups (see Chapters 5 and 6). Rapid social, economic and technological changes heighten many people's anxieties and fears about a world that seems more alienating and less trusting and connected (Melton, 2010a). Increasing inequality separates us from one another, fosters distrust and social angst, undermines the community's capacity for social care, and results in greater social division (Wilkinson and Pickett, 2009). Unsurprisingly, child protection interventions reflect broader social and structural inequalities (AIHW, 2013; Bywaters, 2015). In this context, there are three issues of which practitioners need to be acutely aware as they assess the need to intervene. The first is awareness of what service users want, the second is awareness of difference and othering, and the third is the need for reflective and reflexive practice.

Knowing what service users want

It helps if practitioners are aware of what service users want. Indeed, as shown in Chapter 12, this is essential to relational practice. While evidence of service efficacy is patchy and non-specific (Kirkman and Melrose, 2014), there is emerging empirical work on service users' views of services. In 2011–2012, a major Australian study of three cohorts of parents/carers – child protection ($n = 289$), family services ($n = 293$) and out-of-home care ($n = 391$) – found statistically significant differences between the child protection and family service groups regarding perceived improvements in their parenting skills. The proportion of the family services group responding positively (84.8 per cent) was nearly twice that of the child protection cohort. Similar differences were found in perceived improvements in their child's well-being and health. Participants from both groups who responded positively identified particular areas of improvement including being able to meet their child's needs, communicate with them and manage their behaviour, and improve the child's mental health, health, safety, confidence and relationships with others (QUT and SRC, 2013).

Logistic regression analyses showed that parents/carers from both groups, who positively viewed workers' responses to requests for assistance, were four times more likely than others to perceive an improvement in their parenting skills. When the worker had contacted them as often as was needed, there was a twofold increase in their perceived improved parenting skills, and when they had the opportunity to express their views about the service, and felt welcome in the agency, there was a threefold increase (QUT and SRC, 2013). While, overall, participants agreed that the services were useful all or some of the time, a far higher proportion of the voluntary family services participants reported that the worker provided information about the sorts of services they needed and contacted them regularly. Responses regarding access to agency records and feedback and complaint mechanisms showed similar between-group differences, but 25 per cent of the child protection participants believed the information they provided to the department had been used inappropriately and this distressed them. Many studies of differential response services have also involved service-user feedback and have found similar results concerning the relational aspects of practice (see Chapters 6 and 11).

The Buckley *et al.* (2011b) study of 67 Irish service users, including young people, found that good client-worker relationships could offset power differentials. They valued courtesy, respect and skilled, accountable and transparent practice. An Australian study similarly found that socially excluded and isolated sole parents of young children felt judged and surveilled by social care agencies, but valued assistance in everyday, non-stigmatising environments (Winkworth *et al.*, 2010). Such consumer research highlights the centrality of having ethical relationships embedded within practice.

Difference and 'othering'

Attribution theory explains how we usually deal with differences between us. It explains how we are prone to attribute the ambiguous behaviours of those from other groups as hostile, using erroneous assumptions, stereotypes, biases and prejudices to describe how others think and behave – essentially, we judge them differently. We often see ourselves as the *in-group* and others as the *out-group*. We tend to over-emphasise situational and underemphasise dispositional explanations for our own behaviour, thereby placing less responsibility on ourselves. When judging others' actions, we tend to emphasise dispositional explanations and personal responsibility, while downplaying broader situational determinants. Overrating individual motivations and factors for maltreatment and undervaluing or ignoring influential social, structural and other situational factors can lead to assessment errors, and therefore has implications for ethical practice.

Othering is a sociological term for this tendency to think in terms of in- and out-groups. It refers to our tendency to differentiate and exclude 'others' who hold fundamentally different values, and whose cultures and behaviours we perceive as threatening. This leads to *social discrimination* – sexism and racism – and can involve the subjugation of those who do not 'fit in'. Politicians often 'other' particular groups deemed responsible for unacceptable social problems and events; child maltreatment is a good example with 'child abusers' (often parents) viewed pejoratively and experiencing stigma, and paedophiles being vilified (Lonne and Gillespie, 2014). The community workers who were interviewed in Hamilton and Braithwaite's (2014) research talked of the 'courtesy stigma' (p. 58) they experienced as the stigma associated with families for whom they were advocating was transferred to them. We are all prone to use assumptions, stereotypes, biases and prejudices when explaining how others think and behave, and this makes it imperative for child protection practitioners to have ethics central in their practice framework, and to use a reflective and reflexive approach to practice.

Reflexive and reflective practice

Reflective and reflexive practice, explored further in Chapter 13, is a sound approach for dealing with this fraught aspect of practice, given child abuse and neglect are socially constructed phenomena, and prone to blame, prejudice, discrimination and othering. It is a good tool for understanding better how we are relating with parents, young people and children who are being treated badly and stigmatised at multiple levels (Fook and Gardiner, 2012). Reflective practice requires that we remain acutely aware of the diverse and complex factors at play in working with highly vulnerable people in child protection situations that are replete with ethical issues, tensions and dilemmas, and competing ethical rules and principles. Likewise, reflexive practice focuses on our own history, background, gender, culture, class, ethnicity and values as powerful factors that shape our beliefs and attitudes about, as well as our emotional responses to, child abuse and neglect. This awareness makes us cognisant of the factors shaping our own interpretations and reactions. Reflexive practice is an introspective approach, where we subject our own values, biases, assumptions and emotions to critical analysis within the context of our personal, professional, social, cultural and organisational allegiances. It works well within a relational ethical approach (as discussed in Chapters 9–14). However, before addressing this, in the following chapter we examine ethical practice within the child protection environment, with a particular focus on regulatory measures, including the law, policies and procedures used in everyday practice.

Conclusion

In this chapter, we explored the high and complex needs of service users who are most affected by social and health inequalities. As shown in earlier chapters, harsh neoliberal social policies result in exclusionary targeting and service cuts most affecting those reliant on welfare support. Within these systems, single parents, people with disabilities and people living with mental illness, as well as Indigenous people affected by intergenerational trauma, are especially vulnerable and experience the long-term impacts of policy changes and service cuts. In this context, we have argued, practitioners need to be acutely aware of what service users want and need, of the dangers of difference and *othering* and the need for reflexive and reflective practice.

Reflective questions

1 What do you see as the causes and impacts of inequality?
2 What experiences have you had that shape your understandings of the high and complex needs of service users?
3 How do you tend to respond when engaging with people who have fundamentally different viewpoints than you about child rearing?
4 What sorts of personal and background factors have influenced your decision to practise in child protection?
5 How do you feel about child abuse and neglect and the harm this causes children?
6 How might this influence the ways you practise and your relationships with service users and colleagues?
7 What are the areas of working in child protection that are most challenging for you?

Part 3

Professional ethics and ethical child protection and family welfare practice

Chapter 9   **Ethics, organisations and the law**

We outlined in Chapter 6 the many stakeholders and agendas present in the contested socially constructed arena of child protection. Given this dynamic interplay, it is little wonder significant rivalries, tensions and hostilities can exist and interfere with the overall goal of protecting vulnerable children and supporting struggling families. As already noted, within this context, practising ethically needs to be central to sound child protection practice because the work:

- is dominated by the exercise of power and authority;
- involves decision making that has material impacts on service users' lives;
- comprises individuals and communities that are highly vulnerable; and
- has the potential to be stigmatising and damaging.

Ethical decision making is influenced by the organisational context, which in turn is bound by legislative and policy requirements, in light of which duties are interpreted. An *integrated framework* for child protection decision making uses professional knowledge and skills and relational practice, and a sound ethical framework, including key principles to address case-specific factors (see Chapters 10, 11 and 12). In order to make ethically appropriate decisions, practitioners must consider these diverse influences and use a decision-making process that incorporates the potential consequences for all who have a stake in the decisions reached, not least the child, their parents and family (see Chapter 7). The DECIDE model discussed in Chapter 12 facilitates this and positions ethics centrally in decision making rather than as an 'add on' to 'normal' practice.

As outlined in Chapters 5 and 6, child protection legislative, policy and organisational environments often individualise responsibility, particularly for parents, and downplay social and structural factors, including economic, cultural and social inequalities. Additionally, in light of the poor outcomes and community concern outlined in Chapters 6 and 7, the child protection organisational environment is frequently characterised by ongoing, significant institutional reform. Associated with this is the pressure for more openness, transparency and accountability of public institutions. These demands occur within a turbulent media and community environment that is often deeply distrustful of governments and their attempts to prevent information release, particularly when there is a hint of scandal.

These systemic push and pull factors mean that practitioners are ever mindful of, and sensitive to, the continually changing landscape of legislation, policy and practice.

Yet, to practise ethically, practitioners need to be constantly aware of the uncertain and contested nature of their daily work. It is to this daily work environment we now turn, first by examining the legislative and policy context, and then some specifics of the organisational environment.

Legislative and legal context

Criminal and protective civil legislation is perhaps the primary requirement affecting child protection practice and, unsurprisingly, it is shaped by local jurisdictional cultures, beliefs and priorities, within an overall hierarchical power structure which dictates that *adjudication* of disputes is undertaken according to law and justice principles. As outlined in Chapter 5, legislation is driven by community and government attitudes about governance of the family as well by broader neoliberal approaches to working with marginalised groups in society, such as harsh measures to reduce 'welfarism'.

The broad protective models outlined in Chapter 5 all contain elements of forensic investigative responses to child abuse and neglect. Dominant forensic models associated with powerful sociolegal discourses frequently compete with preferred models of family support found in community-based voluntary services and informal approaches to care (Fernandez, 2014). The salient point is that all protective models require some state capacity for legislatively authorised state intervention into families, but their scope and level varies. Within child protection models, the major legislatively driven service is one that involves receiving notifications of suspected maltreatment, investigating whether harm or risk of harm has occurred and intervening compulsorily, including the use of protective orders and out-of-home care.

Forensic child protection is linked closely to the criminal and civil protective systems, with delineated roles for police and protective practitioners, often along with interagency agreements to ensure multilevel collaborations and the sharing of relevant information. A diverse array of legislative definitions, configurations and arrangements occur worldwide and it is beyond the scope of this chapter to cover these details (see Bala *et al.*, 2004; Bromfield and Higgins, 2005; Dubowitz, 2013b; Mathews and Kenny, 2008; NSPCC, 2012; US Department of Health and Human Services, 2014). However, common child protection features include:

- definitions of child, child abuse and neglect, and the thresholds and principles for state intervention;
- authorisation of statutory officers to investigate defined matters and intervene in suspected maltreatment situations to protect children at risk of harm;
- identification of responsibilities of associated practitioners and agencies to provide services or undertake particular duties, such as mandatory reporting;
- categorisation of protective orders, including the transfer of guardianship and placement of the child with authorised caregivers, such as foster parents, kinship carers and residential carers;
- systems and procedures for providing services to children and their families, such as case management and family meetings; and
- designation of decision-making bodies, often judicial and external to the child protection authority, to review matters and adjudicate findings and guardianship, and make protective orders.

Internationally, there is marked variation in legislation and processes relating to mandatory reporting requirements and, in many jurisdictions, such as the UK, there is no such legislation (Mathews and Kenny, 2008). However, most countries do have policy and contractual arrangements with government and non-government agencies requiring them to report incidents of children at risk of harm to the statutory child protection authority. As discussed in Chapter 6, ethical issues abound for practitioners who are legislatively or organisationally mandated to report. Some practitioners refuse to comply with it because they believe it is detrimental to children and families, and the net effect is damage to their service-user relationships with no guarantee that the child protection authority will subsequently intervene to render protective assistance (Harries and Clare, 2002; Steinberg *et al.*, 1997).

Ensuring legislation to protect children and support their families and communities is implemented is the shared responsibility of all practitioners and agencies. Practitioners have an essential duty to uphold the law, but this can be difficult when they believe that applying the legislation would be oppressive or harmful and, therefore, unethical. Professional practice is not without complications, tensions and conflicts, particularly ethical ones when workers have to make judgments about how to intervene most effectively and they are constrained by aspects of the law (Kennedy *et al.*, 2013).

The law is open to interpretation; it is seldom black and white, but characterised by various shades of grey and, as such, requires judicious consideration. While it is unethical not to have a good working knowledge of the law, by the same token, uncritically following the law, particularly in discriminatory or oppressive ways that reinforce inequalities, threatens ethical practice. In such situations, practitioners have a duty to alert their supervisors and managers within the organisation to their concerns so as to negotiate an acceptable resolution. Importantly, discretion is always required in the work of street-level bureaucrats. Practitioners must weigh up all the relevant information available to them when considering how they might best exercise their legal responsibilities; this is fundamental to integrated practice (Kennedy *et al.*, 2013). Judiciously applying the law involves incorporating not just case-related facts and information, but also legal definitions and interpretations, the tenets of *procedural fairness* (sometimes called *natural justice* or *due process*), organisational policy, procedural and practice requirements, and ethical considerations. Given the differing expectations of the law and ethics, practitioners need to know the laws, policies and ethical principles. As Dickson (2009) warns:

> There is an assumption among many professionals that if one acts ethically then one is also acting legally, or conversely, if one is acting legally then one is acting ethically. While this is often the case, it is not always so.
>
> (Dickson, 2009, p. 266)

Dickson (2009) identified a number of significant areas where legal–ethical conflicts arose in child protection work. First, its social control aspects might conflict with ethical duties surrounding informed consent, confidentiality and privacy. Second, reporting child abuse, especially where mandatory reporting requirements were in force, created a range of ethical conflicts (as already discussed in Chapter 6). Third, compulsory investigations and searches of property could be an invasion of privacy, especially where reports were not substantiated. Fourth, the removal of children always carries ethical implications, even in voluntary removals, concerning the information – or lack of it – and therefore whether parents and children are properly informed about the intervention and the short- and long-term implications. Families may not subsequently receive the services they need. Out-of-home care is prone to placement breakdown that impacts on children. Finally, practitioners perceived as being coercive, misleading, deceitful, or breaching confidentiality by misusing information gained through their discussions with service users and other practitioners and agencies, are not only in breach of ethics but also the law. Dickson (2009) concluded that practitioners required training in legal and ethical matters and such potential conflicts; agencies should provide access to legal advice and ensure their policies are both legally and ethically justifiable. Practitioners well versed in the legal and ethical requirements of their work are able to exercise discretion and make prudent judgments. Without an associated capacity to critique the law, and ethical considerations in its application, legal training initiatives may unwittingly reinforce the inherent legalism of dominant sociolegal and managerialist organisational cultures (see Chapters 5 and 6).

Courts and review processes

Judicial and accountability forums, such as external case review panels, have a critical role in overseeing the exercise of statutory power. In all jurisdictions there are either adversarial or inquisitorial models for courts to determine child protection matters. Additionally, alternative dispute resolution processes may be used (Kennedy *et al.*, 2013). These are usually much more affordable for service users, many of whom may not have the available resources to meet the considerable expenses involved in legal representation and court proceedings. Whatever the mechanisms in place, it is clear that in all jurisdictions, legislative and legal frameworks determine procedures for the hearing of matters, the evaluation of evidence and the adjudication of disputes. There has been little research into the efficacy of the various legal processes worldwide but an Australian judicial inquiry identified that, within ongoing system reform environments, there can be significant dispute concerning the role of the court and its jurisdiction over case-related decision making (Cummins *et al.*, 2012). Additionally, it is evident from research that complexity increases in situations when broader family law intersects with child protection legislation (Kennedy *et al.*, 2013).

In these legislative arenas, fundamental disagreements often occur around the application of principles of justice and fairness, the actions of professionals and the need to protect vulnerable children. Available evidence can be ambiguous, is often based on professional assumptions and assessments, and service users can be hostile toward the intervention. Notwithstanding that the 'best interests of the child' principle is central, a clash of institutional logics can occur between the courts and legal system and child protection authorities. The law is based on a particular rational judicial approach to problem solving that is quite different to more holistic human services approaches.

Legal processes:

- are rights based and rule driven;
- eschew emotionality for rationalism;
- are directed by *justice and legal principles*;
- are underpinned by particular notions of how to properly and defensibly use *discretion* in authorised decision-making processes (*administrative law*);

- entail legalistic interpretations of the admissibility and veracity of evidence; and
- focus on the *legality of actions* in law and not necessarily whether they are the *right thing* to do ethically.

Human services approaches are:

- driven by *humanistic concerns;*
- rational though not strictly rule driven;
- *relationally based* and in touch with the emotional landscape;
- non-judgmental, often entertaining diverse viewpoints; and
- creative in meeting people's needs and negotiating settlements, rather than adjudicating them.

It is little wonder then that many child protection workers feel out of their depth when immersed in legal processes and proceedings – but so too do service users, usually more so, and there are lifelong implications for them. Within such situations, practitioners might be called to give evidence and explain their assessments. Besides being stressful for all concerned, legal proceedings entail the examination of different versions of events, alternative perspectives and areas of disputation. Practitioners have a duty to gather the best available evidence and to present this in an impartial manner before the court (see Chapter 10). There is much at stake for all parties. It is right and proper, given the significant issues present, that a high threshold is set concerning involuntary state intervention and removal of guardianship, with its attendant short- and long-term consequences for children and their families. Practitioners must give sworn testimony in a professional and impartial way; this is not easy when these matters are highly emotive and have dramatic consequences. When practitioners are highly committed to children's safety and well-being, temptations can arise concerning whether to slant their evidence to ensure 'the right outcome'; this is a clear risk to ethical practice and just outcomes.

In order to increase rigour in assessments and reduce ambiguity in evidence, a 'scientific' approach such as that adopted in *decision-making technologies* (DMTs) has increasingly been used in care assessments for case-related decision making and presentation to courts. It is proper that the veracity of evidence be tested in courts, however, the utility and value of these tools remains contested, as outlined below. They may have been erroneously used, or incorrect assumptions may have been made; they are in no way foolproof.

It is not unusual for child protection authorities to be able to have quality legal representation and the capacity to bring the full resources of the state to bear in court proceedings. It is not necessarily a 'level playing field' and legal processes can further accentuate service users' sense of powerlessness and injustice. Hence, in this decision-making environment, adhering to the principles and processes of procedural fairness (or due process) provides a check and balance on the use of power, and helps to safeguard ethical practice (Kennedy *et al.*, 2013). Procedural fairness requires timely decision-making processes that are:

- consistent with the employing organisation's legislative remit, and formal policies and procedures;
- transparent, fair and unbiased;

- inclusive of all those affected or who have a stake in the outcomes;
- based on a complete and reliable information gathering inquiry (*a duty to inquire*), with the results shared, where possible, so that all parties are properly informed;
- fully documented, with explanation and justification of any actions taken; and
- able to uphold the rights of all parties, including provision of advice about appeal processes.

Universally applying procedural fairness helps meet practitioners' duty of care to all stakeholders. Because service users are often socially marginalised and power-less within the dominant culture, it is particularly important in terms of procedural fairness to address ethics of cultural safety and non-oppressive practice alongside organisational and professional codes of practice. While recognising that due process takes time and is costly, Bala *et al.* (2004) argued that 'it is only with the rise of due process that parents and children have had a forum to effectively challenge decisions that profoundly affect their lives' (p. 7). Among other factors, the culture of the organisation is a vital determinant of the extent to which procedural fairness is promoted and adopted.

Impacts of the organisational context

The organisational context in which child protection practice is undertaken is gener-ally complex and fraught. Adding to this complexity, is the often fragmented and uncoordinated system in which it is embedded, characterised by:

- complementary and competing auspices, missions and roles;
- complicated legislative and policy frameworks which shape service responses that are often at odds in fundamental ways;
- diverse priorities accompanying resource discrepancies;
- cultures and climates that shape internal and external relationships;
- diverse workforce compositions with different statuses and competing profes-sional discourses and perceptions; and
- competing ways of perceiving and understanding how societal structures, rela-tions and inequalities are linked to social problems, such as child maltreatment, abuse and neglect.

These factors have a particular effect on how managerial and professional power is structured and used, and the nature of the organisational culture and climate. They are further affected by social constructions of maltreatment, and how policy and practice are developed and implemented. As outlined in Chapters 5 and 6, neoliberal ideologi-cal constructions drive punitive policy approaches, yet largely ignore the social and structural determinants of inequality and their associations with child maltreatment, abuse and neglect. Within this broader policy environment, the organisational culture shapes and influences how practitioners perceive their role, carry out their work and form relationships with service users.

Generally, the child protection organisational culture is characterised by com-mand and control approaches to management and the use of 'power over' rather than 'power with' (ARACY, 2009a; Buckley *et al.*, 2011b; Dumbrill, 2006). Further, there are parallel processes in the relationships between management and staff, and also within practitioner-service user interactions (Lonne *et al.*, 2009; Wan, 2007), and relational issues in inter-organisational coordination and collaboration (ARACY, 2009b; Munro, 2011; Ross, 2009). There is a focus on policy and procedural compliance, reduced practitioner discretion and increased accountability (blame) consistent with managerialist approaches (ARACY, 2009a; Munro, 2011). Case management systems have largely replaced casework practice (Lonne *et al.*, 2009) and there an emphasis on short-term intensive involuntary interventions that set unrealistic timeframes for parents and children to effect meaningful change (Featherstone *et al.*, 2014b). Practice has been supported by the expanded use of DMTs, often associated with concerns about inconsistent case-related decision making (Wallace, 2013). This has accompanied an increasing social surveillance role (Featherstone *et al.*, 2014a; Pithouse *et al.*, 2011; Wrennall, 2010). This requires staff to spend large proportions of their work time entering and retrieving data from information and communication systems resulting in lower priorities for direct contact with service users (see for example Queensland Child Protection Commission of Inquiry, 2013b).

In Chapter 7 we described at length the work-related stressors that impact on child protection workers such as high workloads, workforce problems and hostility from service users. Adding to this overstretched organisational environment are the often negative media portrayals, particularly when tragedies have occurred. It is unsurprising that these pressures can lead to risk-aversive cultures and routinised decision making, resulting in demands for more consistent case management processes, decision making and outcomes (see Queensland Child Protection Commission of Inquiry, 2013b). Increased proceduralism has often resulted along with the expanded use of decision-making tools.

DMTs such as Structured Decision Making are increasingly widely used in child protection and human services and entail an actuarially based risk assessment of case-related factors, although 'an SDM assessment should be tested against clients' perspectives and workers' professional judgment' (National Council on Crime and Delinquency, n.d.). Such technologies are asserted to bring increased reliability, validity, equity and utility to case management by providing an evidence base to practice, although many of these claims remain untested in robust implementation evaluations and are therefore open to challenge on a number of counts (Lonne *et al.*, 2009). Problems have been identified with their misapplication by staff who have not used them in accordance with their developer's instructions or have used them to confirm *a priori* decisions (Featherstone *et al.*, 2014b; Gillingham, 2011; Gillingham and Humphreys, 2010).

While DMT technologies may indeed prove their utility in refining assessment, practitioners cannot abrogate their ethical responsibility merely by explaining that the DMT tool determined a particular level of risk or safety. Rather, these are tools and accountability for making accurate professional assessments, and the moral deliberation and ethical decision making surrounding them, rests squarely with the responsible practitioner. In his doctoral research on the ethics of using DMTs, Wallace (2013) found that, despite their limitations and the tensions inherent in their use, 'proven DMTs are generally more consistent, reliable and valid than practitioner judgement' (p. 231). Indeed, he proposed that 'practitioners have a prima facie moral obligation to use [them] ... to enable them to make better judgements' (p. 231).

He also highlighted the agency's role in assisting practitioners to identify and interpret the values and controls embodied in DMTs suggesting these are not benign technologies, based on value free research. Practitioners should view their use through a critical lens and acknowledge their inadequacies, including their tendency to reinforce inequality and discrimination toward overrepresented groups. Importantly, Wallace (2013) observed that:

> the benefits of DMTs cannot be realised unless practitioners exercise good moral judgement and professional character. Practitioners must use DMTs, and use them properly, if they are to reduce errors and provide better assessments. They must also review assessments to ensure these are technically appropriate and thorough, as well as morally fair and contribute to the wellbeing of clients. Having used the DMT and reviewed the assessment, practitioners need to exercise professional characteristics such as persistence, courage and flexibility to follow up on the assessment and their review of it. This can mean negotiating difficult outcomes with clients or with supervisors if the practitioner concludes the DMT assessment should be overridden ... I am not, however, denying the role of systemic failure in avoidable errors ... Practitioners are more likely to disclose and engage in productive discussion if they are relatively free from debilitating and threatening professional censure ... I am arguing, nevertheless, that moral failures of judgement and character contribute to avoidable errors and adverse outcomes.
>
> (Wallace, 2013, pp. 15–16)

It is critically important that agencies provide regular, accessible and effective supervision, where practitioners receive support, and develop the reflective and reflexive practice skills that underpin ethically sound practice (see Chapter 8). While workers have a moral obligation to comply with lawful organisational directions and policy, this should always be done within a critical approach that eschews blindly following agency dictums and management directives at the expense of client well-being. Indeed, professional codes of ethics provide valuable guidance on the importance of balancing competing imperatives. It is a prerequisite of good professional practice that a critical reflexive lens is always in use. To illustrate these matters we now turn to examine a specific case.

Case example: mandatory reporting

Reeva is a paediatric nurse in her mid-20s working in a health department multidisciplinary early intervention initiative providing targeted parenting support for newborn infants. The service provides information and guidance to promote infant health and well-being and reduce hospital admissions through early problem detection.

Keira is a 17-year-old woman in the long-term care of the Department of Child Protection until she turns 18, and is participating in their transitioning-from-care programme. Her relationship with departmental workers is often strained as she mistrusts them and carries longstanding grievances. Keira looks forward to being her own boss with the department out of her life. She has a history of illicit drug use and has been on the receiving end of domestic violence from former partners. She has many problems and is prone to episodes of depression. She has attempted to take her own life several times.

Six months ago Keira gave birth to her daughter Jessie, who has medical complications from feeding problems and reflux, is often irritable, and requires regular follow up. Keira is generally a good mother but sometimes finds parenthood a burden; she loves Jessie dearly and gives her the love she feels she has never previously had. Since Jessie's birth Keira has bonded well with Reeva and the early intervention team staff, and appreciates their understanding, caring and helpful contact.

Reeva visits for the regular weekly home visit and finds Keira bloodied and bruised having been assaulted by her new boyfriend. Keira explains, she and her boyfriend, whom she recently met, got drunk last night and had a big row. He was angry and cursing at Jessie's continual crying. Keira was nursing and feeding Jessie and the boyfriend became enraged and physically abusive, pushing her around and finally pushing her head into the wall. Keira explains that it was lucky that Jessie did not get hit or injured.

Under the law and interdepartmental protocols, Reeva is required to report any situation where a child 'is at risk of significant harm as a result of the actions of an adult carer' to the child protection department.

What sorts of problems confront Keira and Jessie?

Keira has many strengths and a lot going for her. Yet, many young people in care experience conflicting emotional responses to ongoing departmental involvement, particularly when they have their own children. As outlined in Chapter 8, their life narratives shape and reflect how they behave and feel, and having experienced considerable trauma during her life, Keira may well be 'self-medicating' – using alcohol – to manage her depressive episodes. Becoming a parent poses many challenges. Keira has an ambivalent relationship with the child protection department but is strongly engaged with Reeva, whom she trusts. She is a good parent to Jessie who has feeding problems and has accessed the medical help Jessie needs.

Reeva faces an ethical–legal tension (Dickson, 2009). Up until now, she has enjoyed a good relationship with Reeva but that might well change due to mandatory reporting requirements. Reeva is well aware of Keira's mistrust of the child protection authorities and is critically aware of the importance of the support she provides for Jessie. Now she must decide whether 'not reporting' is in Jessie's best interests. She is caught between the legal requirement of mandatory reporting – and the duty to protect that this entails – and her ethical inclination to provide the support and care needed. Unless she handles this well it may result in a severing of her hitherto caring and close relationship with Keira, which could have serious negative consequences for Jessie and Keira and for Keira's ability to trust anyone in the future. On the other hand the domestic abuse Keira is experiencing places both her and Jessie at risk of harm.

What are the risks arising in this scenario?

1   The key risk is that Jessie – and Keira – may be harmed if the status quo is not changed.

2   If Reeva fails to comply with the law and policy, and if Jessie is harmed she may be liable for disciplinary and legal action. Further, the child protection department staff will be unaware of the situation and therefore unable to assess and intervene where necessary. Reeva would have to deal with her own personal guilt and remorse associated with her decision, and if serious harm results there is the potential for media backlash.

3   If Reeva were to comply with the mandatory reporting requirements, this would likely jeopardise her relationship with Keira, dent her developing trust, and increase Keira's stress and reduce her capacity to care for Jessie. At worst, Keira might sever her connection with her, potentially necessitating involuntary departmental intervention.

What legal and organisational considerations are applicable here?

While the law in this case might appear to be black and white, there is always discretion in how it is applied in specific circumstances. In some jurisdictions there may be little or no discretion about reporting domestic abuse where a child is in the household, even though there may be no suggestion that the child is unsafe. Reeva must carefully consider the laws and policies and determine her responsibilities in this situation – she is not a child protection specialist but has expertise in children, parenting and maltreatment – so consulting about the issues and options with others, including departmental staff, is appropriate. Determining thresholds for risk, harm and protective actions is not a straightforward process and involves evaluating available information to gain clarity about what the issues are and how they might be responded to. Whether or not Reeva reports this matter she is obliged to have a well-considered rationale for her decisions.

How might sharing information help this situation?

Mindful of the apparent ethical and legal considerations, Reeva decides to openly discuss her concerns and legal obligations with Keira, outlining the risks and possible consequences to her and Jessie. By dialoguing with Keira she optimises the potential for maintaining their strong supportive relationship and good ongoing parental care for Jessie. Adopting an approach where she shares power with the service user (see Chapter 11), Reeva suggests to Keira that the child protection department staff will also be concerned and that involving them could lead to Keira accessing required supports to safeguard her and Jessie from the violence. She does so mindful that if Keira refuses to take appropriate protective action then Reeva will probably have to report the matter. Because Reeva values open communication and transparent decision making, she tells Keira this. Keira confides that she is terrified of losing Jessie and that despite her reservations she will inform the department and seek their help. She asks Reeva to accompany her because she is fearful of how things will go.

Conclusion

In this chapter, we have outlined the organisational and legal complexity in child protection practice and identified a range of factors that influence practitioners' legal and ethical decision making. We have highlighted the need to appreciate this complexity within integrated agency and practitioner practice frameworks. Court processes, MR and DMTs were used as examples of regulatory requirements in use in many jurisdictions. These, along with other legislative and regulatory mechanisms, feature in child protection environments nowadays and have an important role in defining practice imperatives that assist in protecting children. They may also constitute good decision making when seen in light of broader contextual issues to which practitioners constantly apply a critical ethical lens. While laws often appear to be black and white, their application always requires judicious consideration of specific case situations and circumstances. In the next chapter, we identify key ethical issues found in child protection and family welfare practice, and examine some core principles for ethical decision making.

Reflective questions

1 How might you integrate the ethical, legal and organisational factors within your own practice?
2 What is the primary ethical question Reeva faces?
3 What is the ideal outcome you would like to see for Jessie, Keira and Reeva and why?
4 What ethical issues are evident in the case example?
5 Who is the client?
6 Who are the main stakeholders in this situation?
7 How might Reeva involve Keira in dealing with this matter?
8 What options are available for Reeva and her team?
9 How would you have handled this matter?
10 What primary ethical principles would have guided your actions?

Chapter 10 Ethical principles in child protection

Throughout this book, we argue for ethics in child protection and family welfare practice to be put centre stage. In earlier chapters, we discussed three *primary ethical principles*; namely, justice, respect and duty of care (see Chapter 4). Here, in keeping with these primary ones, we consider seven derivative *key principles* relating specifically to the stance put forward in this book on working ethically in child protection (see Figure 10.1). They are:

- the child's best interests;
- maintaining a relational perspective;
- safeguarding children;
- best available evidence;
- judicious information sharing;
- protecting the service user's interests; and
- equity, fairness and consistency.

We demonstrate the use of these principles in a case situation and invite you, through some reflective questions, to reflect on your thoughts about the practitioner's handling of the situation in terms of your knowledge and experience. Given this is not

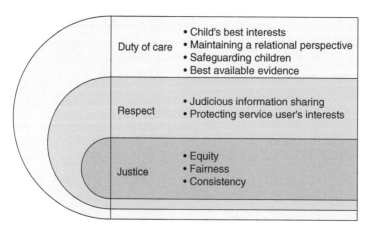

FIGURE **10.1** Ethical principles for work in child protection

an Indigenous case study, the child placement principle which states that, in as far as is possible, children should be placed within their own community and culture, is not discussed in relation to this situation. However, this is discussed in detail in relation to the case presented in Chapter 12. This chapter provides guidance as to how to integrate a range of ethical principles in a practice situation involving a number of practical and ethical issues.

Key ethical issues in child protection

Given the complexity of child protection and family welfare matters, and the multiple, multifaceted issues confronting the different stakeholders and agencies involved (see Chapter 6), working ethically in in this arena is no easy matter. There are diverse views on how child protection matters should be handled and the possibility each person or agency involved has a particular perspective or role and sees and manages the situation differently from the next person or agency is rife. Thus this is a terrain of conflicting interests and felt obligations, making it all the more necessary to have some minimal concrete guidelines to help practitioners negotiate their way through this maze.

Nevertheless, most would agree that the major issues relate to safeguarding and protecting children from harm. How this is best done is where disagreements step in, and deciding what to do is not a cut and dried matter. This pertains to how the assessment is done and the intervention that follows. As a society, we tend to place responsibility for child protection with statutory organisations without necessarily examining broader community responsibility and early intervention and community support measures. As a consequence, we hold regulatory agencies accountable to be the gatekeepers of children's safety and welfare. It is therefore left to child protection authorities to deal with serious investigations and the ethical issues involved in:

1   establishing whether abuse or neglect is present or has occurred;
2   deciding on placement options; and
3   reporting protocols.
4   these issues are discussed in turn below.

Establishing whether abuse or neglect is present

The uncertainties and tensions surrounding decisions on whether or not a situation constitutes a risk of abuse or neglect or, as in the case study presented below, whether or not abuse and neglect has indeed occurred brings further considerations as to whether substantiation of harm is warranted, notification is required, investigation is necessary, and what level of intervention is warranted. For example, if low risk of harm is indicated, then family reunification might be in the child's best interests. As Levi (2008) notes:

Ethical issues abound in child protection work, not least in relation to uncertainties surrounding the determination of whether or not an abuse is occurring or has occurred: What exactly counts as abuse? How should we understand reasonable suspicion (which serves as the trigger for mandated reporting)? How sure must we be that abuse has occurred before initiating a child abuse investigation? How much harm is acceptable before the threshold into abuse has been crossed? Is the abuse intentional? At what stage should the abuse be reported? Knowing that biases are inevitable in our assessments of risk and probability, how can we treat families fairly in our efforts to protect children from abuse? Finally, what should we as mandated reporters do when we do not think that reporting abuse is in a given child's best interests?

(Levi, 2008, p. 132)

Two other general areas within ethical issues that raise concern in decision-making processes relate to placement options and reporting.

Deciding on placement options

Placement options following substantiation relate first to *permanency planning* and the 'permanency' of placement relates to whether or not *family reunification* is deemed possible (see Chapter 6). Where not, adoption might be a possible option, otherwise, for the most part, children are placed in out-of-home care or returned to their parents under supervision. When children are removed from their family and placed into out-of-home care, there are options about what sort of placement is most suitable; *kinship care, foster care and residential care* are the usual choices. Second, where there has been a history of serious abuse or neglect and no change in the circumstances or ability of a particular family, the very serious decision to remove the baby at birth might be the only option.

Two further considerations arise in relation to placement options. First there are important considerations relating to cultural safety, cultural variations in definitions of abuse and maltreatment, and culturally appropriate approaches to forensic child protection investigations and service delivery (see Chapters 6 and 7). Second, where placements break down or concerns arise regarding standards of care or cooperation with case planning, changes in foster and kinship care placements might be deemed necessary.

Reporting protocols

The whole area of reporting in cases of abuse and neglect is fraught with tensions and contradictions (see Chapters 6 and 9). Deciding what to do when maltreatment is suspected, yet where the parents and children concerned are denying abuse or neglect is occurring or has taken place, has to be handled with extreme caution lest investigating officers open themselves up to accusations of collusion or entrapment in order to bring the matter to court. To establish facts in keeping with legal standards of evidence, due process must be followed and the *best available evidence* must be collected. However, this is easier said than done, particularly in cases of neglect, where ethical issues arise from 'knowing' that the child continues to be at risk but the worker is unable to gather enough 'evidence' to take action within the court system. This common problem leads to frustration for community agencies because they do not always truly understand just how tightly the child protection worker's hands can be tied within the maze of court and legal requirements (see Chapter 9).

Related to this, is the obligation or *duty to warn* parents that their behaviour is unacceptable and to *inform them* of the procedures workers are obliged to follow in such circumstances; this ensures that parents are adequately informed of consequences that might ensue. As much as possible, practitioners attempt to involve children, parents and significant others in decision making and sharing information, as appropriate (see Chapter 14). Parents also need to know practitioners are obliged to record their encounters with them and their children. As will be demonstrated in the case example below, reporting concerns about a child or family situation can have a negative impact on ongoing working relationships and parents need to know when reports have been, or are going to be made. McLaren (2007) noted forewarning is one way to deal with confidentiality issues in child protections:

> As a matter of formalizing this information-giving process, a number of social workers and their organizations use standardized client consent forms and/or a variety of verbal procedures to state their child abuse reporting obligations when commencing the worker/client relationship.
>
> (McLaren, 2007, p. 23)

The practitioner might sometimes decide not to disclose that the family has been reported (beyond the initial discussion of her mandatory reporting obligations alluded to by McLaren above) because she needs to maintain the relationship with the family in order to maximise safeguarding the best interests of the child, until adequate intervention from child protection services can occur. Here the parents' right to know and the worker's duty to report stand to jeopardise the child's safety, thus reporting requirements are in conflict with the child's best interests and the worker has to juggle competing ethical principles. To resolve this, she needs to decide whether safeguarding the child's interests takes priority over disclosing the report to the parents and jeopardising the relationship (see case example in Chapter 9). This example also highlights the statutory/community divide and the barriers and risks MR can in itself create; it can prove counterproductive in some situations. MR is highly contentious in child protection practice, as was discussed in Chapter 6.

Finally, often child protection investigation and follow-up intervention depends on a network of services. To ensure the best service available for children and families, it is essential that effective intra- and interagency cooperation and collaboration are maintained.

At first glance decision making around these issues must appear practical, but what makes them ethical is that they relate to the rules and principles surrounding child protection, and our duties and obligations to protect children and keep them safe in the short and long term. The onus is on the worker involved to accurately assess the degree of ongoing risk of harm to children and decide whether or not removing a child is warranted. Here, using DMTs and *holistic assessments* might prove helpful (as discussed in Chapters 4 and 9) in keeping to guidelines surrounding confidentiality, informed consent and appropriate disclosure to bring matters to court in terms of legal standards of evidence. The worker attempts to involve the child and parents in decision making, as well as other parties who are aware of the situation under investigation – building a *web of care*. Fostering and maintaining relational connections to cultural, familial, friendship and community networks wherever possible is key to building and maintaining respectful relations with those involved and taking different interests into account. Often this means workers have to reconcile competing and conflicting interests and perspectives as the example above shows.

In Chapter 6, we discussed the diverse interests of stakeholders involved in child protection matters, including parents and children immediately involved; workers and their supervisors and managers; other professionals in child protection teams; and external agencies, including legislative or jurisdictional agents, such as children's court judges, lawyers, advocates and legal guardians. In Chapter 4 we presented the DECIDE model and the broad range of concerns any decision-making model needs to take into account, including differing perspectives about child protection interventions and their outcomes for children, parents and other stakeholders including broader cultural and community groups.

This requires that practitioners need an in-depth understanding of the ethical terrain of child protection. However, core values of *confidentiality*, *openness and transparency* of decision making, *informed consent*, *procedural fairness*, *impartiality*, *harm minimisation*, *justice*, *respect*, *self-determination*, and *upholding rights and responsibilities* in the interests of the *public good* are understood, they remain crucial to working ethically in child protection. To guide practitioners in a meaningful way, some minimal principles are needed, and it is to this we now turn.

Key ethical principles in child protection

It is impossible to discuss ethical principles in child protection without reference to justice, respect and care. *Justice* pertains to fair and equitable treatment and consistency of care. *Respect* concerns treating people as you would the people closest to you, with the utmost regard (Gray and Stofberg, 2000). *Care*, like respect, is owed to everyone equally. Let us see how these primary principles and core values discussed above might be distilled into some key ethical principles surrounding child protection investigations and interventions. There might be others but we believe the following are minimally necessary for ethical child protection practice.

1   *Best interests of the child*: This principle embodies a duty of care to employ techniques and strategies of age or developmentally appropriate assessment and intervention that maximise benefits for, and reduce harms to, not only the child, but also the family. It is in the best interests of the child that they, their parents and other family members be treated with respect, that is, in such a way that their rights are respected and opportunities to exercise self-determination and autonomy are maximised (Holland and Scourfield, 2004). Engagement and involvement is preferred over coercion wherever possible. In short, the best interests of the child does not imply a 'child-centric' focus, that is, protecting children's individual rights and well-being does not mean downplaying family relationships or relational connections (Keddell, 2014). Children should be viewed in the context of their social relationships and all people in the family network are owed respect (see Chapters 5 and 11). However, in some jurisdictions this principle has been given *paramountcy*. The paramountcy principle states that parents, child protection authorities and the courts have a duty to safeguard the welfare of children and in legal proceedings it is the best interests of the child that are the primary consideration when determining what action should be taken (Crowe and Toohey, 2009) (see Chapter 9). Thus an ethical principle is also a legal prescription in certain jurisdictions and this, paradoxically, can lead to unethical practice when workers disregard parental interests in considering child protection

matters. Working ethically means parents must be respected even in situations where the paramountcy principle applies making the child's interests overriding. More importantly, it requires an appreciation of the enormity of the situation and long-term consequences for families.

2   *Maintaining a relational perspective*: Keddell (2014) notes, an ethics of care implies taking account of 'the context dependent nature of the case and the relational or caring obligations that derive from it' (p. 920) (see Chapters 4 and 11):

> An ethical decision in child protection, therefore, could be considered not only one that reflects the weighing up of universal duties to protect children and respect the self-determination rights of parents or the costs and benefits of possible courses of action (traditional justice approaches), but one that is contingent upon the nature of obligations derived from a caring and supportive relationship with the family.
>
> (Keddell, 2014, p. 920)

3   *Safeguarding children*: Related to the child's best interests, safeguarding and protecting children from harmful abuse and neglect is an overriding principle of child protection work. This includes reporting cases of suspected abuse and neglect when parents or other adults are deemed likely to cause harm to children (see Chapters 6 and 9). This principle recognises the heightened vulnerability of children not only in the family but also when they are taken into care, if such action is deemed necessary.

4   *Best available evidence*: This principle embodies standards expected of accountable workers who, out of respect for service users' rights, seek to draw on the best available evidence, rational analysis and systematic decision making to support them and justify the decisions they make in their best interests. Professional *transparency*, *responsibility* and *accountability* are important at all times, and require that service-user interests and values have primacy over organisational and worker values and interests, or workers' intuitions or emotional responses, except in situations where service users violate the rights of, or cause harm to, others. Though:

> Emotional responses are understandable given the nature of child protection, and such responses and intuitions may be morally important. Moreover, the ability to have feelings towards others and to respond to them is an essential part of any interpersonal relationships – and professional relationships are no exception. But such responses highlight rather than preclude the need for rational analysis.
>
> (Larcher, 2007, p. 208)

In such situations, as well as systematic decision making, critical self-reflection is essential. Gray and McDonald (2006) argued the deliberate use of ethical reasoning is well suited to promote the type of ethical intent claimed by evidence-based practice in considering client values and interests, but without its inherent limitations. They claimed that being concerned with morality and ethical reasoning, to some extent, demands the same conceptual skills and cognitive capacities as critical appraisal within evidence-based practice. Ethical reasoning, however, has a greater capacity to 'fit' and, therefore, inform workers' interactions with the variety of social realities and practice situations child protection presents. They further note that determining accountability is extremely complex because of the unpredictability of the people with whom workers deal, which makes the requirement of well-founded explanations and reasons all the more challenging.

5   *Judicious information sharing*: Though service-user confidentiality is protected and informed consent is needed to disclose personal information to third parties, where serious abuse and neglect is evident in statutory child protection investigations, service users forgo their right to privacy and, in certain jurisdictions, the need for informed consent (see also Munro, 2007):

> While professionals have a general duty of confidentiality that precludes disclosure of personal information without consent, this duty is not absolute. It may be neither necessary to obtain consent to share information nor to disclose that it has occurred when there are reasonable grounds to believe that the child will be at risk of serious harm as a result. Decisions to disclose information or maintain confidentiality are matters of professional and value judgements that must be reasonable and accountable and as such open to challenge, whatever their outcome.
>
> (Larcher, 2007, p. 210)

Information sharing includes the consistent provision of rights-based information in the interests of procedural fairness, as discussed in Chapters 9 and 14 (see also point 7 below).

6   *Protecting service users' rights*: Davies (2009, p. 327) notes most codes of ethics speak to the duty to protect service users' rights even when the discharge of that duty is difficult. This is carried through, among other ways, by seeking to: (i) safeguard and promote service users' rights and interests wherever possible; (ii) remain concerned about their welfare, even in risky situations where self-protection is needed, and when workers can do little to help; (iii) support families even when parents engage in harmful behaviour; (iv) assist involuntary service users to achieve as much self-determination and autonomy as the situation allows; (v) inform service users of their rights, even when they are restricted, including their right to refuse services; (vi) advise service users of informed consent requirements to share information about them with others, and situations where they forego their rights to confidentiality and privacy; (vii) encourage service users to participate in decision making about their lives and future, including children wherever possible; and (viii) acknowledge the impact of their, and their organisation's, statutory power, especially when involuntary service users have no option but to comply with requirements.

7   *Equity, fairness and consistency*: Though consideration of 'the different relational qualities in a case … are ethically defensible' (Keddell, 2014, p. 920), they need to be balanced by principles of equity and fairness, such that some consistency of service is ensured for all families. Keddell (2014) believes consistency is important ethically, arguing as follows:

> As a statutory agency, the level of protection extended to children and the level of respect accorded to the parental rights … should not intersect at a line so malleable as to make the response of a statutory social work unreliable and arbitrary. If the macro factors (orientation) are held equal and the case facts are similar, deontological ethics (that is, that the same duties are accorded to all clients based on their existence as humans with intrinsic value) would

suggest that outcomes should be consistent … Thus, either a child does or does not reach a threshold for out-of-home care or access to a therapeutic service. The home is or is not safe enough to warrant return. Decisions such as these should have some level of transferability … as an expression of the commitment to maintaining both the duty of care to protect children equally and to respect the autonomy and guardianship rights of parents. Otherwise, the law is arbitrary.

(Keddell, 2014, pp. 919–920)

Keddell (2014) distinguishes between a *child welfare orientation* and a *child protection orientation* (see Chapter 6). The former offers a broad-based prevention policy framework, based on a long-term understanding of epidemiology, rather than focusing on a single risky event; the best interests of the child are closely linked to the interests of the family as a whole; assessments include strengths, as well as difficulties; purpose is preventive; and the focus within this approach, as in Aristotelian virtue ethics (see Chapter 3), is to 'create those material and social conditions within which all children [and families] are given sufficient opportunities to reach their full potential' (Fargion, 2014, p. 2, in Keddell, 2014, p. 3).

The latter – child protection orientation – frames problems in individualistic and moralistic ways; defines children's best interests narrowly in terms of children's protection; reifies 'abuse' as something objectively apprehendable; uses standardised assessment tools; treats difficulties as signs of risks; directs legalistic and investigatory intervention types; promotes adversarial state–parent relationships; and results in the use of mostly involuntary out-of-home placement (Keddell, 2014, p. 3). There is a place for both orientations, with a child welfare orientation at the preventive end of a care continuum and child protection at the interventive end (Gray, 2014). Though the child welfare orientation tends to be more family-focused and is the realm of early intervention and prevention, and family support, child protection is implicitly 'child-focused' and concerns the development and implementation of policy that aims to promote the rights and well-being of individual children (Featherstone *et al.*, 2014b). But, as already mentioned, this does not imply a 'child-centric' practice (Keddell, 2014).

Case example: deciding whether or not to remove a child at risk of harm

Bronislawa, a 21-year-old woman with a moderate intellectual disability, was in the care of the child protection authorities from the age of five. She grew up in residential care because her mother was unable to cope with her due to a chronic mental illness. Louise has been Bronislawa's caseworker for approximately five years, first encountering her when her daughter, Anastazia, came into care at the age of six months due to her 'failure to thrive'. Louise supervised the restoration of Anastazia to Bronislawa's care and has assisted Bronislawa to learn how to parent Anastazia better. She has continued to provide the ongoing support that Bronislawa requires to help overcome her periodic lapses in care. Anastazia is now five years old and, although she remains under a care order, has been living with her mother for several years.

Recently, however, Anastazia was admitted to hospital with second and third degree burns to 30 per cent of her body after she slipped into a bath of scalding hot water she had been running for herself. She requires ongoing medical attention to treat the burns and reduce scarring. As reported in the intake worker's notes, the incident had resulted in 'a report of suspected neglect' as her mother's failure to provide 'proper supervision' had resulted in 'significant injury'. On investigation, Bronislawa had admitted to Louise she should not have left Anastazia to run her own bath. As the child protection worker with case responsibility for Bronislawa and Anastazia, Louise conducted the investigation of the report and concluded it was substantiated. She then had to determine whether or not Anastazia should return home to her mother's care once she is discharged from hospital. Louise is concerned about Anastazia's safety and her mother's ability to maintain the ongoing treatment of her burns. Louise meets with Bronislawa to discuss the investigation findings and, given this, where Anastazia might be best placed. Things do not go well. Though she has always trusted Louise and has a good relationship with her, Bronislawa is now in danger of losing her daughter once again. She flies into a rage, cursing and accusing Louise of lying and trying to take her daughter away from her. She threatens to stab Louise for being 'a backstabber' and, as her agitation and distress mounts she also threatens to kill herself if Anastazia does not come home from hospital. Louise tries to calm her down, to no avail, and, concerned about her own safety, ends the meeting, promising to meet again the next day.

What ethical and practice issues are evident?

In terms of legislation, child protection services are mandated to focus on the best interests of the child over all other considerations and, according to this mandate, the child is always front and centre. Though this might compromise equity and child protection workers do not enter into situations such as that presented in this case example lightly, they are cognisant of the 'ethic of responsibility' they bear to children. For workers not bound by this statutory obligation, the ethical principles of 'best interests' and 'duty of care' apply to all people – children, parents, families and significant others – equally.

As discussed in Chapter 11, assessing dangerousness and decisions about child removal make relational work extremely challenging. Put another way, 'harm minimisation', an ethical precondition of consequential ethics, carries an implicit responsibility to assess 'risk of harm'. Danger and suspicion threaten trust, and Louise is aware of this. She is also mindful of long-term considerations and Anastazia's developmental needs as she matures. Placing a child in out-of-home care can have unforeseen positive and negative impacts. How might a relational approach to practice help or hinder Louise in this case?

Much emphasis is placed on allowing space for multiple realities and perspectives and the importance of engaging with people's diverse life experiences. Today, with the influence of recovery-oriented approaches in disability and mental health, workers are more aware that people like Bronislawa live with disability every day of their lives. Louise understands that Bronislawa's experiences are constructed through this prism. She has always had a compassionate, caring and sensitive attitude, and believes she has developed an attuned understanding of Bronislawa. She has always treated her with respect, listening attentively to grasp how Bronislawa sees and experiences the world.

She knows that Bronislawa would never have intentionally harmed her daughter. She also knows that Bronislawa comprehends that she has done something wrong and it could happen to anyone. She remembers the child that drowned in the pool next door when the adults did not adequately supervise. Mistakes are easily made. Louise also knows how attached Bronislawa is to her daughter, and Anastazia is to her. She knows the conflict and anguish Bronislawa is experiencing, and is mindful that she trusts her implicitly. She feels trapped on the horns of a moral dilemma of immense proportions. In her jurisdiction, she is bound by the paramountcy principle. Nevertheless, she is aware that openness is the foundation of trust and her actions need to ensure her ongoing work with Bronislawa empowers her and her capacity to parent. She was pleased she had not reacted inappropriately to Bronislawa's anger and, on reflecting, is determined to find a way to include her in the decision-making process so she too is able to understand what might be the best way to proceed to ensure a positive outcome for herself and her daughter.

What ethical principles should guide Louise about what best to do here?

Louise feels as though all her training in ethical reasoning is not wholly useful, and the best decision in this case is not necessarily an ethical one. She remembers her university lecturer talking about 'ethical decision-making frames injecting a sense of certainty and handleability to the problems clients present in complex, uncertain and ambiguous situations'. Having to 'choose between alternative positions and basing this choice on sound argument' and 'having a thorough awareness of all aspects of the situation and anticipating the consequences of possible decisions and actions' suddenly doesn't feel that helpful. Louise cares deeply for Bronislawa and Anastazia and her heart aches from having to make decisions now that may hurt and anger them. Her emotions are swirling around inside as she grapples with the protective decision making inherent in her job.

Nevertheless, she knows her paramount duty is to Anastazia as this is a legal prescription in her jurisdiction. She has always felt a duty of care to Bronislawa with whom she has been working closely with for years. She recalls Bronislawa always had a good relationship with her aunt, who was very supportive of her, but Louise values working from a relationship-centred approach and is worried about issues of confidentiality if she were to contact her again now. While the legislative framework within which Louise operates would permit confidentiality to be broken to make contact with the aunt, Louise is aware that Bronislawa will likely feel she has let her down. She decides to discuss this with Bronislawa when she visits her the next day.

How might Louise best handle this situation?

In reflecting on the events of the day, Louise recalls the ETHIC model (see Chapter 4) she learned in year four of her undergraduate degree:

- examine relevant personal, societal, agency, client, and professional values;
- think about the relevant ethical standards in the code of ethics which apply to the situation, as well as about pertinent legislation and decisions;
- hypothesise about the possible consequences of the various courses of action;
- identify who will benefit and who will be harmed; and
- consult with supervisors and colleagues about the most ethical choice.

She realises her agency, societal and professional values point to her primary duty to protect the child in this situation, and it is her personal relationship with the client that is preventing her from doing what the principle of paramountcy requires. Further, the code of ethics is clear on matters of allegiance to agency and organisational policy. The legislation, too, is clear and whether or not Anastazia returned home on discharge, Bronislawa would require close supervision. Her 'gut reaction' was to recommend removal as her primary duty was to protect the child from Bronislawa's neglect and she had never before experienced Bronislawa's anger directed toward her as she had that day. She would never forgive herself if further harm were to come to Anastazia and for the first time began to believe her relationship with Bronislawa was standing in the way of the 'best decision'. She decided to discuss the case with her supervisor in the morning before going to see Bronislawa again.

Mary, Louise's supervisor, was very concerned about the events of the previous day and was reluctant for her to visit Bronislawa again unaccompanied. While Louise was with Mary, the hospital had called to say Bronislawa had visited Anastazia and made a scene with the nurse on duty, wanting to take her daughter home. Louise asked Mary what she thought about the idea of contacting Bronislawa's aunt and she wondered whether she was still around as no one had come forward to assist Bronislawa in the two weeks Anastazia had been in hospital.

Had Louise been trained in a relational approach, rather than the narrower relationship-based approach (see Chapter 11), she would realise that the dilemma she now faces arises from her limited knowledge about Bronislawa's relational network. Most of her contact has been centred on Bronislawa's history of residential care to independent living, and the lens of child protection. Apart from the aunt she remembers, Louise has very little idea what support systems beyond the service system Bronislawa draws on in her day-to-day life – what is the family's web of care? In recent years, she has been focused on Bronislawa's care of her daughter. Her ability to make the best decision now is being hampered by not wanting to appear inconsistent to Bronislawa, with whom she has always enjoyed a trusting and open relationship, and with whom she would still want to work with in a transparent manner by engaging her in future decision making. Right now, however, removing the child, which she knows she must recommend, requires having strong supports in place for Bronislawa and she does not know where to begin with this, while protecting Bronislawa's likely preference regarding confidentiality. She is happy to share information with her supervisor but feels she cannot approach people to explore their connections with Bronislawa without her consent. Failing that, perhaps out-of-home care becomes the most likely option.

How has Louise been guided by the seven principles outlined above?

1   *Best interests of the child*: Louise is acutely aware that Anastazia's best interests are intimately connected to Bronislawa's. She has long perceived the close

attachment between them, which is why the possibility of removal in light of the paramountcy principle is all the more difficult for Louise. Her heart is telling her one thing and her head another. She feels torn.

2   *Maintaining a relational perspective*: Louise wishes she had paid more attention to Bronislawa's relational network, especially given she comes from an immigrant family and knows she has some cultural connections. She vows to explore this further with Bronislawa.

3   *Safeguarding children*: Louise knows her duty of care vis-à-vis safeguarding children and that until now Anastazia has always been relatively safe in Bronislawa's care though there was always a risk that something like this might happen. She is trying to respond to the immediate crisis while considering the long-term prospects for this family.

4   *Best available evidence*: Louise knows that very few investigations are found to require drastic intervention as is the case with child removal, but this is one of them. Further, she also recalls the research on the use of ethical codes and how unhelpful these can be in situations such as this. She has researched burns treatments and knows that Anastazia is facing a long and slow healing process that requires a great deal of care. She is not sure whether Bronislawa grasps the seriousness of the situation though she knows she perceives a threat. Evidence suggests Anastazia requires short-term care while her wounds heal and Louise feels if she knew of someone who could care for Anastazia, at the same time involving Bronislawa and teaching her to change the dressings and so on, it would be easier to convince her that this is in her own and her child's best interests.

5   *Judicious information sharing*: However, as discussed, Louise feels hamstrung by her relationship-based confidentiality concerns and a resistance to explore options without Bronislawa's consent. She decides this is what she will explore with her when she sees her again and explains that short-term care might be needed while Bronislawa learns to provide the necessary treatment care. She will explain that Anastazia would suffer undue pain if her dressings were not changed skilfully and alert her to the real dangers of infection and so on. She has printed the Internet pages to share the information with Bronislawa when she sees her again – fully aware that Bronislawa might not understand all the information available and she might have to simplify and explain the important points. Fortunately, time is on her side while Anastazia is in hospital and she can see Bronislawa over the coming weeks to be sure she fully understands her decision about the situation.

6   *Protecting service user's interests*: Clearly, Louise does everything she can to protect not only the child's best interests but also Bronislawa's. In fact, it is her trusting working relationship with Bronislawa that makes Louise even more determined to make Bronislawa understand her decision. Knowing her as she does, she knows she did not mean what she said before, and she is sure her safety is not at risk with Bronislawa who has never intentionally harmed herself or others.

7   *Equity, fairness and consistency*: Louise knows that making a decision that will hurt Bronislawa will be experienced as inconsistent with her prior dealings with her. And in fairness to her, she will have to work hard to make her see that drastic situations require drastic measures. She wonders whether she shouldn't also talk to Anastazia to see how she feels about the situation and decides to discuss this with her supervisor immediately and to tell her she has decided to see Bronislawa on her own that day.

Conclusion

In this chapter, we have considered some core ethical issues in child protection and some interacting, key ethical principles that are pivotal – and minimally necessary – to the family-focused relational approach suggested in this book. Though principles and standards that ground practice in statutory child protection contexts are made with good intentions, without sound understanding of the ethical dimensions underlying them, they run the risk of being used as 'technologies', thus appearing legalistic and devoid of a care ethic. When focusing on rules and obligations, it is all too easy to forget the human dimensions of child protection work, and the need for care and compassion while protecting and safeguarding children. The following chapter examines the application of the DECIDE model and how its processes enable integration of the relevant considerations into ethical decision making.

Reflective questions

1   Which ethical principles do you believe are the key ones for child protection?
2   What do you think of Louise's handling of this case?
3   Were there ethical principles that she has overlooked?
4   If so, what were they and how might they have changed the way Louise perceived and dealt with the situation?
5   If you were Louise's supervisor and were called upon in court to say why you supported the decision Louise had made, what arguments would you provide in justification?
6   If you did not agree with her decision, what would you have done in the situation?

Part 4
Practising ethically

Chapter 11   **A relational approach to child protection**

All societies rest on the value that the family is the best place to raise a child. Therefore, attempting to keep families together is an ethical imperative, and failure to do so means there is something at fault with the system that does not provide the necessary supports and opportunities for families to raise children. Most often the main contributing factor to families struggling to raise children lies in social inequalities, which is one reason why people from poor and marginalised social classes tend to be overrepresented in the child protection and family welfare system. The twin overriding ethical imperatives of respect for persons and social justice are intimately intertwined. A society that respects people ensures they have a decent quality of life and are provided with the maximum opportunities to develop their capabilities so they can contribute to society in a positive way. Such a society prioritises social justice and the removal of barriers and restrictions to human development, or, conversely, the proactive provision of opportunities for education, work and social provision, where necessary.

Relational and relationship

A relational approach

Following on from the above, sometimes things go horribly wrong. Life dishes out hardship and people struggle to cope despite their best intentions. A *relational approach* conceptualises these struggles as coping difficulties. It does not seek to individualise problems and blame parents for not being able to look after their children. It looks for social solutions – ways to build people's coping capacities by harnessing their strengths and cushioning the family unit through providing social supports. The relational approach embraces the twin interlocking priorities of *respect for persons* and *social justice*, emphasising the importance of social relations. It sees the individual and family as embedded in a network of social relationships and uses these connections to help people restore their coping capabilities. One might see this as a *web of care*, given, for the most part, people cope within the social networks in which they are embedded, but, for some, there is a weakening of social ties and disruption of social connections – a hole in the safety net – that needs correction or fixing to restore their coping capacity. And these are the families we encounter within the child protection system.

Many parents are involved involuntarily with child protection services because they are subject to a report about their child or children having been harmed or being at risk of harm. Some parents come to these services when they are experiencing problems in coping with their children in diverse ways. Some seek help. Some come by accident. Some come because children have other issues in coping, such as learning difficulties or physical impairments. Some come with other more pressing issues, be they financial or mental health related, for example, seemingly unconnected to specific concerns about a child's behaviour. Then again, some come with worries about their child's behaviour – aggression, withdrawal, uncooperativeness and so on – seemingly unrelated to child protection concerns. In the majority of these situations, the initial contact with child protection and family welfare services is likely to involve a coping difficulty.

Relationship-centred practice is an area to which social work – as one profession within this broad, multi-professional area of practice – has paid a great deal of attention, that is, the nature of the relationship between the service user – whether it be an individual, a family or community – and its central role in the unfolding narratives of the lives of the families with whom we work. This is as important in child protection as it is within other areas of human services or social care practice, for all team members, be they police officers, psychologists, community health nurses, lawyers, welfare specialists, and so on. Where there are protective issues involved, the formation of a trusting working relationship might be severely challenged but is no less important. No matter how families begin the service encounter, its success will be based on the formation of a sound working relationship with the individual, family, significant others, and beyond in their social support network.

Relational practice adds a proviso: the success of relationship-centred practice depends crucially on how the service, and the practitioners involved, work with the individual's and family's relational connections; how they enhance their coping capacity through drawing on the ties within their social networks that bind individuals to families, communities and societies. These social connections are the glue that holds social life together and supports the individuals and families within them. Striving to fix, build or enhance these relational connections is an ethical matter if families and communities are to raise healthy children and contributing citizens together. Child protection and family welfare agencies, therefore, bear a huge social responsibility for keeping children safe while they mend the ties and restore the family's equilibrium. *How well do they do this relationally?* This is the question this chapter asks. Perhaps the best place to start is to briefly examine what people who have used child protection services have to say about the things they value in a helping or caring relationship.

Importance of a sound working relationship

How do workers apply a relational approach, based on empathy and non-judgmentalism, when they have the statutory responsibility to investigate situations involving severe abuse and neglect in situations where service users have not sought their help? There has been some valuable research examining what 'a sound working relationship' involves, and what service users have to say about what they are looking for from child protection and family welfare agencies and their workers. Many have described these services as part of a 'system of oppression'. For example, in his interviews with service users, Dumbrill (2003, 2010) heard repeated stories of their heavy handed approach. Through this anti-oppressive lens, he interpreted this as an issue of power, that is, the reason child protection services were experienced as oppressive was because some workers within them were unwilling to give up their discretionary and statutory power that prevented them from focusing on what families want for themselves. Rather than workers trying to control and direct service users' lives, an anti-oppressive service-user approach argues that workers must work to give decision-making power back to service users. Central to the anti-oppressive relationship and, we might add, strengths-based approaches, is an equalisation of power, through power sharing between worker and user.

More than this – given an anti-oppressive approach is informed by a structural perspective – it seeks to promote understanding that inequality is the root cause of social problems, since the system itself is geared to protect the privileged in society through harsh measures toward the less well off. The fact that minorities and people of colour are overrepresented in the child protection and family welfare system is given as proof of this class-based dynamic at work. Some have argued that change will only come when service users find their voice and demand self-determination. This kind of polarising, circular argument is unhelpful. Given minorities and people of colour are relatively powerless in this battleground, even if they were to find their collective voice, it is unlikely that they would be able to change the system. Ways must be found for change from within – by raising the awareness of managers and workers within the system as to what their service users say, want and need from them. Just as parents come to child protection services in diverse ways, so too can change come from multiple directions. And persistence is the key given the endless attempts from agencies working in this area to reform practice. A way has to be found through this impasse the anti-oppressive approach identifies.

Service users' perspective

There is no doubt that the quality of the helping alliance remains a key transforming variable in working with children and families. Dumbrill (2003, 2010) notes the overwhelming negativity of the experiences of First Nations people in Canada with the child welfare system, though this disdain is neither confined to Canada nor to Indigenous peoples *per se*. The majority of parents in Dumbrill's (2003) small study (*n* = 10) were, in any event, white. What we can learn from them, however, is how they experienced the 'absolute power' authorities wielded *over* them as they attempted to respond in defensible ways to protect their families. Exercising power in this way is unlikely to make for a sound working relationship, where the workers share power *with* the family. Instead, when coerced, families are more likely to become hostile and aggressive, or manipulative – doing whatever it takes to get the statutory authorities out of their lives by, for example, agreeing to everything but not changing anything – or hiding essential information (see Dumbrill, 2010).

The giving and receiving of information is an important way in which power is exercised and service users often complain about not being given the right information at the right time, especially about their rights (see Chapter 14). Workers are often not upfront and honest with them and sometimes misuse confidential information (QUT and SRC, 2013). Power is also wielded through the way resources are controlled. Those workers who formed a relationship of 'power with' that facilitated the parents working in a *collaborative relationship-based partnership* were more likely to get their cooperation. This 'helping alliance', however, is difficult to achieve, even in countries, like Ireland, where service-user representation and family participation has been incorporated into policy and practice. Buckley *et al.*'s (2011b) larger Irish study (*n* = 67) found these measures had not allayed service users' fears, shame, mortification, humiliation and anger, even when they willingly participated. Furthermore, what service users and workers wanted from the encounter was at odds: service users wanted short-term, practical help and 'freedom from the gaze of the child protection service' (p. 105). They often had very specific requests for supervised access, help in managing their child's behaviour or a violent partner. *They wanted help with coping.*

Frequently, however, support was not forthcoming and workers seemed indifferent to service users' plight. Their complaints were often ignored. The qualities they looked for in their workers were normality – being easy to talk to, reassuring and helpful. What they got instead was 'bossiness', judgmentalism and a business-like approach. Through all this, what emerged most strongly from the Buckley *et al.* (2011b) study was 'the quality of the helping alliance ... remains the key transforming variable' (p. 109). Beresford (2014), too, reiterates the value service users place on their relationship with the worker, which, he says, flows from seeing service users from a 'social perspective', seeing their lives as a whole and their strengths and abilities, rather than just what they can't do. Service users also value practical, emotional support – a shoulder to cry on, if need be – someone who listens, and doesn't judge them.

Gallagher and Smith (2010) in Scotland similarly note the importance of trusting relationships, clear, open and honest communication, and a supportive stance for service-user engagement in reducing 'conflict and discord' (Simmons and Birchall, 2005, p. 261). D'Cruz and Gilligan's (2014) small Australian study (*n* = 9) on child protection investigations found a 'domino effect', that is, 'significant practical and relationship repercussions in families' lives' (p. 239), attesting the importance of a relational approach.

In addition to the most oft cited characteristics of good relationships – mutual respect, acceptance, trust, warmth, liking, understanding, collaboration, empathy, and so on – de Boer and Coady's (2007) small in-depth qualitative study (*n* = 6) involving service users found two additional factors to be important to the development of child welfare relationships: (i) the soft, mindful and judicious use of power, and (ii) a humanistic attitude and style that stretches traditional professional ways of being (see Table 11.1).

In a more recent quantitative Canadian study, Gladstone *et al.* (2014) examined parent and child welfare worker engagement through personal interviews with 131 worker-parent dyads from 11 child welfare agencies in Ontario. The factors they found that affected parent-worker engagement are shown in Table 11.2.

Mediating factors in the worker's use of particular casework skills related to the severity of the case, worker experience, work environment, worker stress and worker burnout. Interestingly, relationship-building skills were found to be a necessary, though not a sufficient condition, for engagement. Hence, Gladstone *et al.* (2014) concluded that workers needed the skills to contribute to a collaborative relationship within an anti-oppressive approach, which they defined as involving the 'judicious use of power' with service users, echoing Dumbrill (2003), and de Boer and Coady's (2007) findings.

TABLE **11.1** 'Good' relationship responses in child welfare

Soft, mindful and judicious use of power	Humanistic attitude and style that stretches traditional professional ways of being
Being aware of one's power and the normalcy of client fear, defensiveness and anger	Using a person-to-person, down-to-earth manner (vs. donning the professional mask)
Responding to client negativity with understanding and support instead of counter-hostility and coercion	Engaging in small talk to establish comfort and rapport
Conveying a respectful and non-judgmental attitude	Getting to know the client as a whole person – in social and life-history context
Providing clear and honest explanations about reasons for involvement	Seeing and relating to the client as an ordinary person with understandable problems
Addressing fears of child apprehension and allaying unrealistic fears	Recognising and valuing the client's strengths and successes in coping
Not prejudging the veracity of intake, referral or file information	Being realistic about goals and patient about progress
Listening to and empathising with the client's story	Having a genuinely hopeful/optimistic outlook on possibilities for change
Pointing out strengths and conveying respect	Using judicious self-disclosure towards developing personal connection
Constantly clarifying information to ensure mutual understanding	Being real in terms of feeling the client's pain and displaying emotions
Exploring and discussing concerns before jumping to conclusions	Going the extra mile in fulfilling mandated responsibilities, stretching professional mandates and boundaries
Responding in a supportive manner to new disclosures, relapses and new problems	
Following through on one's responsibilities and promises	

Source: de Boer and Coady (2007).

TABLE **11.2** Key casework skills for parent–child engagement

Factors affecting parent engagement	Factors affecting worker engagement
The extent to which workers ignored problems parents saw as important	Workers including parents in planning
	Workers being caring and supportive
The extent to which workers asked parents to do things that the parent did not feel would be helpful	Workers praising parents for their efforts, ideas or achievements.
The worker's skill in locating appropriate services	
Workers making or returning telephone calls	

Source: Gladstone et al. (2014).

How does what service users have to say inform a relational approach?

The discussion has thus taken us into the terrain of what service users are looking for in their workers. Clearly, relational skills are essential. Yet, as Ferguson (2014) found, some workers do not have the skill set necessary to comfortably engage with children and families. Though most North American studies have focused on 'communicative-interaction' skills, Ruch (2005) in the UK accords immense importance to the worker's self-reflective skills. However, rather than focus on what workers do, let's briefly examine the idea of a relational approach and how this informs the work to be done, and the worker's role, rather than get mired in what workers are not doing.

A relational approach assumes a facilitative role for workers. It sees helping as a social process concerned with solution finding, or at least creating the relational conditions for change at various levels. How we create the relational conditions for one-on-one engagement is informed by the US model of clinical practice and its core conditions of effective relationships, but that is where the association ends. The clinical model best fits the work of therapists within the child protection and family welfare team, who draw on relational psychotherapy and see the clinical role as involving pathology identification or diagnosis. This psychological model sees a direct causal relationship between pathology and behaviour such that solutions cannot be found without first identifying underlying causes. As Saari (2005) explains, the roots of contemporary developments in relational practice lie 'in cognitive and constructionist theory as well as in psychoanalytic ideas' (p. 3).

Contemporary relational theory also has synergies with the core values and practice principles of the holistic 'person-in-environment' perspective and the long held dictum of 'starting where the client is'. These approaches capitalise on 'relational theory's intersubjective stance', which lends a 'new coherence' to 'the process aspects of evidence-based … practice' (Segal, 2013, p. 376). For the most part, the child protection and family welfare practitioner's job is not clinical. It is not about diagnosing psychological or emotional problems but, rather, creating the relational conditions for their solution at various levels. Truax and Carkhuff's (1967) pioneering research on the core relationship conditions for effective helping – warmth, empathy and genuineness – became central to psychotherapy in the 1970s and was widely adopted in clinical social work (see Fischer, 1978).

The relational approach which we see as best suited to child protection and family welfare work rests on a *social* rather than a clinical model. As Folgheraiter (2004, 2007) described it, a relational perspective is the social divested of the clinical: 'from the relational perspective, we are faced by a *social* problem when a broader capacity for action – that is, action undertaken by a 'group' of people – is insufficient' (p. 27, emphasis in the original). The 'group' in this instance might be parents who are not coping with, or do not have the abilities to cope with, their familial or parenting responsibilities. Here a relational perspective has some synergies with a narrative approach, where problem is 'externalised', that is, it is seen as deriving from external pressures. Understanding the problem 'from the outside', as it were, enables the conceptualisation of the problem within a structural framework such that service users – and workers – can see themselves as a product of circumstances shaped by external social conditions and pressures. This became an important route via which issues of equity were brought into the interpretation of the problem such that it was the social conditions and not the service user that needed changing. This, too, is the nub of a relational perspective, as we shall see.

Starting with the problem

The true nature of the problem lies in how it is felt by the person who has it. The worker's role is to foster the relational conditions in which the service user's insight into, or awareness of the problem, is the first step in making change possible. How the 'problem' is evaluated is the starting point of a relational perspective. It wants us to be aware that the mere act of problem definition requires a moral evaluation or judgment, and the very idea of a 'problem obviously implies a negative judgment' (Folgheraiter, 2004, p. 30). A moral evaluation is made when the judgment inform-ing the perception – problem – concerns the goodness or badness of the phenomenon – person, behaviour, and so on – thus perceived and judged. This construction of something as a 'problem' takes place 'silently' in the mind. Though one observes the external data in the decisions and actions the worker takes, the 'inner mechanisms' that render a situation a problem cannot be observed, but is trusted to be objective based on the evidence the worker provides. The worker, in other words, takes 'what appears to be' the case as an objective, rather than a subjective socially constructed reality. This is reinforced in child protection by the requirements of normative assess-ments based on policy, legislation and regulations on harm, safety and protection (Folgheraiter and Raineri, 2012).

However, we define and assess problems in accordance with our moral sentiments and make moral judgments that compel us to take action; thus perception–judgment–action and decision are related processes motivated by moral sentiments:

> They are the deep-lying 'archetypical' motivators of the practitioners' action. The social policies of the welfare state that frame these routine actions have arisen from a moral impulse in society. They spring from a sense that certain situations are unsatisfactory or intolerable. This moral rejection by the collective conscious-ness is symbolically embedded in every individual dealt with by every institutional practitioner, or more in general in every administrative act performed by the wel-fare state.
>
> (Folgheraiter, 2004, p. 32)

Besides this moral code, there is a technical code in operation when practitioners make judgments or diagnoses. Implicit in the process of assessment or diagnosis is a search for a problem or dysfunction that is *defined* as a problem through 'a specific act of reasoning, an intentional cognitive process' (Folgheraiter, 2004, p. 32) to iden-tify a predefined dysfunction or pathology, as in the clinical model described above. And, as Horwath (2007) notes, in this reasoning process, practitioner's factor in their own perception of what neglect comprises, their 'gut reaction', as well as evidence, the views of colleagues and team managers, and perception of available services, not to mention 'their own personal feelings such as fear, guilt, over-empathy and anxiety' (p. 1285) (see Chapter 9).

However, the point Folgheraiter (2004) is at pains to make is that the status of something as a 'problem' is not inherent or intrinsic to the phenomenon, but is attrib-uted to it by an act of *judgment*, taking relevant factors into account. Given the subjective element involved in decision and judgment, there is no knowing how many problems workers fail to see, and how many problems they see that are not prob-lems from other standpoints, or within different sociocultural conditions. Mostly, however, practitioners deal with predefined problems, such as child abuse, which is 'not an objective condition but a social construction, the meaning of which arises from ever-changing values' (Reder and Lucey, 1995, p. 14, in Folgheraiter, 2004, p. 35). Hence, an:

> important field where the *relative* nature of social problems – even those dramatic ones that seem self-evident – is apparent is child abuse. Cases of this kind are constantly on the increase, but one may ask whether child abuse is objectively more common, or whether it is statistically increasing because those who carry out assessments are more skilled at detecting the problem.
>
> (Folgheraiter, 2004, p. 35)

Whether or not problems are socially constructed makes no difference to the practitioner, who has to deal with them 'as if' they were real. The key is what they do once a problem is perceived. Some problems are best left alone. Good intentions – acting solely on compassionate impulses – often lie at the root of many practitioner errors. There is a chance that doing the right thing from the practitioner's perspective is not necessarily right for the service user. This is the nub of a relational approach because it is not primarily about the practitioner but, rather, their understanding of the problem from the service user's perspective. The spotlight is on the service user, not the practitioner factoring in their perception of abuse, and what their peers have to say and so on. Folgheraiter (2004) tries to emphasise this by posing an important question: 'problem for whom?' In relational terms, the service user's problem must become the practitioner's problem, and *vice versa*: 'this intuition goes well beyond the classical notion of *empathy*' (p. 39) to meaningful engagement, to an alliance between practitioner and service user.

The entreaty seen as the beginning of the helping relationship – 'start where the client is' (Goldstein, 1983) – is central to empathic understanding, and lies at the heart of the relational ethic of care (see Chapter 4). Unless the service user feels understood or cared for, or helped, he or she is not cared for, helped or understood. Goldstein (1999) wrote eloquently about this:

> there are few human relationships in which meaningful understanding is not a product of a true, give-and-take, dialogical exchange: *Can I indeed understand you if you don't understand who I am, how I think, and what I believe or, to borrow the popular idiom, know 'where I'm coming from'?*
>
> (Goldstein, 1999, p. 386; emphasis added)

Practitioners need to know where service users are coming from. As Kierkegaard (in Folgheraiter, 2004) observed: 'helping somebody implies your understanding more than he does, but first of all you must understand what he understands. If you cannot do that your understanding will be of no avail' (p. 40). *The true nature of the problem lies in how it is felt by the person who has it*, and this is best understood when we are mindful of the limits of our own understanding:

> We need to go beyond reason alone to use our own greater curiosity and imagination, a sense of 'What is it like for you?' and seek sense of and find meaning in persons' lives. This is where the artistry of practice dwells that shifts the focus

from what I need to understand to how. The difference between the what and how of understanding mirrors the difference between theory and practice. The theorist strives to universalize and reduce, to fit the human condition within an explanatory framework: that is science. The practitioner, in contrast, strives to particularize and individualize, to find meaning in – if not become part of – the peculiar, diverse, and the fugitive aspects of the human condition: that takes art.

(Goldstein, 1999, p. 386)

The helping relationship is also relational in the sense of seeing problem solving as a shared process. As Folgheraiter (2004) says, 'creating a shared problem means creating better conditions for its solution' (p. 40). The worker must take time to foster the motivation for change: 'to enable the problem to emerge in the mind of the person afflicted by it' (p. 41). This is where client-centred practice begins, with fostering the relational conditions in which the service user's insight into, or awareness of, the problem is the first step in making change possible.

To return to the *relational basis* of the professional helping relationship, 'a problem exists when the practitioner sees it, when the user sees it, and when each of them knows what the other knows or sees what the other sees' (Folgheraiter, 2004, p. 42). This 'reciprocal awareness' requires a shared sense of the problem and it takes work to create it: it renders 'unilateral definition by the expert ... meaningless' (p. 42). The relational perspective sees the expert and user as mutually interconnected – and *extends this connection to all the people in the user's network that feel the problem.*

Shifting the focus to the social

A key tenet of this chapter is to appreciate the social is always relational. Folgheraiter (2004) wants to shift the focus from the clinical/psychotherapeutic – systemic – relational approach to a 'relational view purged of clinical content' (p. 57), that is, the focus on pathology or dysfunction as inhering in the structure of human relations surrounding the individual. Attachment theory fits this clinical model where pathology is said to stem from broken attachments (see Chapter 6). In the clinical model, relations are seen as the causes of *individual* problems. Relational workers, however, are concerned with *social* problems and 'actions necessary for' their solution: 'to say that a problem is *social* or to say that it is *relational* is exactly the same thing ... It is the inadequacy of the social' (p. 61), of persons standing in relation to one another, trying to manage and cope with a difficulty. The practitioner engages parents, children, extended family, and so on in the network, to work together to resolve the difficulty through joint problem solving.

However, the dominant child protection model still uses an individualistic logic with the task assigned to a single organisation or practitioner, rather than a relational network of service users and (team of) professionals. In other words, child abuse and neglect is not just an individual behavioural failing, but a social-relational one, where the family is unable to cope due to a disconnection in the social links and relationships within its network. Networks fail because they do not possess the resources or capabilities relative to their life tasks or due to inadequate interconnectedness. Connectedness is crucial to the efficient functioning of a network at all levels, whether that be the family, organisation, or a group of organisations in a community offering wraparound or integrated support services (see Chapters 5 and 6). Thus, rather than isolating the parent as neglectful, or only focusing on the best interests of the child, the focus should be on the family as a network with all its significant others, and enabling them to engage in joint problem solving and action.

A practitioner is not using a relational approach because she is acting on relations. The focus is not the neglected child or looking for interactional pathologies, but the dysfunctional system of persons standing and acting in relation to one another. The focus is on the interactions among numerous interconnected individuals in a 'web of care'. The child is embedded in this system of relations and:

> networking means operating synergically [synergistically] 'with' systems, not try-ing to repair them one to one. It starts with their strengths; it does not diagnose and attack their weaknesses. It creates involvement, movements and autonomy of action in the social field; it does not isolate one system (the family) from others (other families, other interested parties, etc.) in order to skew[er] it with thera-peutic manoeuvres and counter manoeuvres in a therapy room. It creates care, maturation or development (and thereby also reduces or heals the 'pathology'), proceeding laterally to possible pathologies. It creates the premise for wellness, it does not bring it about directly.
>
> (Folgheraiter, 2004, p. 101)

The influence of the non-directive Rogerian client-centred approach of the 1960s freed helping professions, such as social work, from a psychological culture and made the 'client' a subject with a role and a voice, and saw the solution as inherent in the situation – the client had the potential to change but it was hidden by the problem. Self-determination comes close to the meaning of 'relational' here. The client speaks, the practitioner listens, and even while seemingly doing nothing than just listening, the worker is actively allowing the client to discover his or her inherent potential. This is the strengths base the worker draws out. But Rogers's approach shared with the psy-chological approaches he eschewed a unidirectional flow from client to worker rather than the other way around. The relational approach (Folgheraiter, 2004) we envisage is neither practitioner- nor client-centred. It is one where solutions are worked out in the course of time *through the synergies created by the dialogue and interactions between all the parties.*

The *relational attitude* means being aware that every problem has its own intrinsic logic and knowing that none of those involved in the problem possess the key to its solution. In child protection, problems frequently persist because family members within the family system repeatedly engage in unproductive interactions. Once they understand the dynamics of actions and reactions in setting up unhelpful communica-tion, and see the problem as systemic and relational, they can begin to see how each person plays a part in maintaining the unhealthy dynamic. The problem thus becomes shared and, as such, requires joint action. It takes a practitioner with inner psycho-logical strength to recognise strengths and find solutions in desperate situations. As Goldstein (1999) put it:

> if the nature of the client's condition is refracted by my lenses such that I capture strengths and resilience, then my expectations will see change as movement in more affirmative directions that echo, not my own vision and goals, but rather my client's values, choices, hopes, and powers. Understanding in these inductive

terms will necessarily be elusive and hard to pin down, since I will need to be ever mindful of the ambiguities and uncertainties (and often the contradictions) of the client's mutable worldviews.

(Goldstein, 1999, p. 388)

The relational attitude means accepting there are no ready-made solutions and having the self-confidence to cultivate creativity in finding solutions. Drawing on Joseph Epstein, Goldstein (1999) noted, such 'artistry and understanding lie in "the triumph of character over psychology. Psychology wants to know what a man's problems are; character has to do with how he surmounts them ... life is a work of art not a case study"' (p. 388). The practitioner's authenticity is crucial, and the process of solution finding that thus ensues has been variously described as a journey, an unfolding narrative, an empowering process, and so on; that is, one in which nevertheless the means are found to seek unknown ends, or solutions. Who knows where the relationship might lead? How the problem might be solved may just be the right question to ask when we enter the realm of relational work. But is it? Can work with children and families in contemporary times – characterised by the need for certainty, for evidence-based practice – afford to push the barrel of relationships thus conceived? Is there still room for artistry?

New directions

Folgheraiter (2004) takes the relational perspective in a new direction drawing on different ways in which the 'social' has been theorised through notions like *social capital*, *social inclusion*, *social networks*, and so on. He picks up on all relations as embedded within networks – the family, peer groups, and other forms of social groupings to which people are connected or belong:

> Relational ... work engages with existing networks to enhance their resilience and capacity to resolve difficulties. It does this by addressing the identified problem, and by engaging, mobilising and developing both supportive and problem-solving networks. These networks can include family members, friends, teachers and any other significant actors who have a contribution to make. The participative approach offers a way of translating policies that aspire to social inclusion into practice.
>
> (Folgheraiter, 2007, p. 265)

When the practitioner enters the family, or any other social grouping, they are entering already existing networks of relationships, with functional and dysfunctional elements, shared and conflicting values and interests, capabilities and deficiencies, strengths and weaknesses, and so on. They have to see strength in naturally occurring or natural, helping networks formed by spontaneous relationships (see Chapters 5 and 8). These existed before the practitioner stepped in due to the perceived problem. Given the problem, like the network, already exists, the network would already have begun a process of adjustment or maladjustment, as the case may be. The network also comprises weak and strong bonds or ties, or degrees of connectedness and disconnectedness. Where strong ties exist, the family might band together to conceal the problem making it more difficult to gain their trust. This is what makes the determination of severe child abuse and neglect so difficult, especially where an external report is made, as the family might try to hide the problem from the worker.

A 'natural network' then might be seen as 'a force in motion' (Folgheraiter, 2004, p. 174). The practitioner enters the network with a purpose of using her knowledge to influence it in some way, and provides 'relational guidance' and, from an empowerment perspective, seeks to enhance the network's capabilities to cope with the problem or fulfil people's needs and interests. This relational role is facilitative. The practitioner facilitates this process of empowerment or capacity building to strengthen the network and the individuals connected to it by enhancing linkages and internal interactions for joint problem solving, cognisant of issues of confidentiality and informed consent.

Techniques used for joint problem solving include defining the problem, brainstorming, generating and analysing possible solutions, choosing a solution, anticipating new problems, implementing the solution, perceiving further problems, monitoring and evaluating progress, in an ongoing cycle of change and improvement (Folgheraiter, 2004, pp. 216–217). Often networks have little sense of the community development process and these connections have to be fostered (see Chapter 5). Problems have to be seen as shared and solutions need to be seen as best generated through joint or collective problem solving. Awareness raising is needed for community action to become possible. This is the realm of community work, which is carried out through groups or networks that share a role in providing a safe and supportive environment for families raising children (Gupta et al., 2014; Holland et al., 2011; Jack, 2004; Jack and Gill, 2010; McLeigh, 2013; Melton, 2010b, 2014).

The practitioner also works with networks where there are high levels of obligation, such as long-term caring networks. The goals here are not communitarian but personal, and have to do with the dignity and survival of those concerned. In other words, the practitioner develops a caring network around the individual, as in palliative care work. Often in these situations the worker managing the case is part of a professionalised helping network and 'must work together with a mix of agencies and also assess their importance' (Folgheraiter, 2004, p. 223).

Inter-professional collaboration through networking and teamwork is a complex top-down process usually initiated by a 'statutory duty of the public welfare system where objectives must necessarily be achieved in the face of limited formal resources' (Folgheraiter, 2004, p. 224). Here there is little voluntary action and the worker is duty-bound to conform to the prescribed roles within statutory intervention with formalised relationships prescribed by regulatory guidelines.

The relational is participatory

Engaging networks is crucial to better outcomes for children – they are better protected when practitioners and parents are able to develop collaborative working relationships in which the worker listens and hears the service user's voice. The onus in a relational approach is not on the practitioner to find solutions, but on the interaction between the parties involved to explore issues in dialogue so that solutions emerge from the interaction. Morris and Burford (2007) talk about the child's network being engaged inclusively, that is, including all significant others within the family network, not only in assessments but most crucially in the joint search for solutions. The relational approach is solution focused only when all involved participate in finding solutions. However, they found professionals were 'struggling to promote participative practice ... [thus] traditional exclusive forms of practice [tended] to be sustained' (p. 209). Why is this the case?

Morris and Burford (2007) found workers often underestimated service users' ability to collaborate as partners in joint problem solving and 'engagement of networks and communities was still relatively underdeveloped' (p. 214). This would seem to suggest that 'giving over power to users', as Dumbrill (2003, 2010) suggests is easier said than done. Given 'professionals view full active engagement with those who may use services as a high risk activity for which they feel ill-equipped and unprotected' (Morris and Burford, 2007, p. 215), what would seem to be needed for this to eventuate is better support for workers.

The culture of the system moulds the practice and it is within the nature of systems to be self-sustaining. Even when new approaches, such as early intervention and prevention are added, they tend to interlock with pre-existing formal services. Hence, early intervention and prevention is coupled with a child protection culture that tends to target families from disadvantaged groups in the usual ways. With only a small proportion of children who are maltreated coming to the attention of formal child protection services it begs the question: where are all the others receiving support? Clearly, the support they receive comes from their social networks. This leaves marginalised families, who lack access to the strong supportive networks of the better off in society, with no cushion against the might of the child protection edifice and its heavy-handed responses.

Case example: removal at birth – risk and relationship

Nina worked for some years as a drug and alcohol counsellor and recently graduated in social work. She is now working as a social worker in a public maternity hospital and has just received the surprising formal advice from a seasoned team leader, Keith, from the statutory child protection authority, that they have obtained an interim court order to 'apprehend' the not-yet-born baby of Jane, who is currently giving birth in the delivery room – two weeks early.

Nina had been in weekly contact with the primary caseworker in the statutory department but had not communicated with this team leader. She had been working with Jane, aged 23 years, since she commenced attending the antenatal clinic five months ago. Jane was in care in multiple foster homes herself as a child, and as a result had experienced a lot of difficulty trusting people. She had reconnected with her mother and was, until recently, estranged from her again as her mother had vehemently disapproved of her new partner, Jordan. This week, Nina had met with Jane and her mother to discuss plans following the birth of the baby and all three had been optimistic about the future, which heralded a bolstered relationship between mother and daughter.

Jane had given birth to her only other child when she was 16 years old; this child had been adopted at birth – a fact that had haunted Jane and her mother. Just prior to coming into the maternity hospital, Jane had charged her ex-partner, Jordan (the father of her baby) with breaching the restraining order he had received three months previously, and had breached the previous week. Jordan was in police custody awaiting a court appearance.

Jane had a history of illicit drug use and had regularly been attending drug counselling since discovering she was pregnant. She attended counselling once a week and also attended a support group at a local church. She was 'clean' and would not return to the flat she had previously shared with Jordan as he was only on remand and had often threatened to kill her if she tried to leave him.

Nina's assessment, and that of the multidisciplinary hospital team, was that Jane was deeply bonded to the unborn baby, was desperate to avoid this child 'going into welfare', and had engaged energetically with support services, although emotionally she was very fragile at this time and could well 'do a run with the baby' if provoked. She provided her assessment and was upset by Keith's confronting response:

> It's my job to focus on the risk to this baby, and we have my professional opinion supported by a court agreement now that the baby will be at risk; it's your job to find the mother some accommodation and ensure her safety – and if you do so then we might see if she can get the baby back – but only then!

With a focus on relational matters, as well as risks, what are the facts relevant to this situation?

As noted at the outset, there are two essential aspects to a relational perspective: (i) relationship-centred practice; and (ii) relational practice. It is apparent that Nina is aware of the first and has developed a strong working relationship with both Jane and her mother and is very mindful of the other external relationships, such as those of the church group in which Jane is involved. In the short time she has been at the hospital, Nina has also used her relational skills and has established a strong working relationship with the nursing and medical team, where she is highly respected. However, she now faces a new relational context – that of co-workers in the statutory authority, where the ultimate duty to protect the baby and the power and authority reside. The following are just some of the most relevant facts to which you could add more:

1 Jane has had one child removed and is aware of the risk of her baby being removed; she has worked with Nina to avoid this risk and has been developing trust in her.
2 Jane is frightened for her own safety and has been engaged with a safety plan.
3 Jane and the unborn baby are both highly vulnerable and the priority of the child protection officer is, and must be, on the safety of the baby.
4 Although Jane is drug free at present, she was a relatively long-term user of illicit drugs and was using immediately before entering treatment after discovering she was pregnant.
5 Nina knows that mothers who have been drug users and whose children are removed by a statutory authority are highly likely to spiral into drug use again; and, with new permanency planning legislation worldwide, therefore, babies removed at birth are more likely to end up in alternative care permanently.
6 Nina also knows, from her experience and from research, that the primary bond between the mother and baby is realised fully at birth. If the baby were removed at birth, there would be a risk to both the baby and Jane remaining separated.

This is particularly so as the public policy move has been towards permanency planning and adoption unless children are reunited within a year.

7   Nina is a relatively new worker and, although a most competent practitioner, and in the face of surprising information, has a limited sense of her own authority in this situation versus that of Keith who has the power and authority situated in his statutory position and experience, as well as a court order.

8   Nina knows Jane well and has a good relationship with her. She likes her and trusts her. Neither she nor any of the medical and nursing team had anticipated this action on the part of the statutory department as she had been working with Jane to organise ongoing care of the baby and accommodation options that included Jane and the baby living with the maternal grandmother.

9   Nina has assessed Jane as having determination to provide care for her baby, to have some strong relational networks, including her mother, the counsellor and the members of her church support group, and is protective of the baby to whom she has displayed strong feelings of attachment throughout the pregnancy.

Of particular relevance are the relational matters between Nina and Keith. Nina has developed strong relationships with Jane and her mother and the multidisciplinary hospital team. However, relationship-centred practice is not just about our relationships with service users and team colleagues, it must include relationships with other services. In this instance, the statutory authority. The real power sits with Keith, who has the primary obligation to protect the safety of the child whom he has assessed as being at too high a risk to leave in the care of Jane. Nina had indeed focused on the hospital-based relationships and had not realised her assessment, supported by her team, could be so dramatically derailed. She knows she has very limited power to stop this 'apprehension', is angry and has no idea how to deal with Keith or to advise Jane and the team and manage of the consequences, including the relationship fallout. Nina will have to tell Jane her baby has been apprehended and will experience this as a violation of the trust she placed in Nina even though it has not been Nina's decision and she does not agree with it.

Which ethical issue would you address first?

Nina's professional opinion and that of her team is that all the gains Jane has made, her relationships and her chances of mothering her baby are being jeopardised by the decision of the child protection worker and his legal advisers, who do not appear to have been aware of the planning that has gone into ensuring the safety of the unborn baby to date. Keith's priority is child safety and it appears he has not been apprised of Nina's role. Further, he has never met Jane. The court order is in place and Nina cannot change or subvert this. In her estimation, there is no immediate risk to the baby. Jane will have to be advised immediately of the order. The question in her mind is how to maintain Jane's trust, engage with Keith and with her team, and ensure all views are heard before a final decision is made about 'placement'. There is still the likelihood the baby could be placed with Jane's mother, as Nina had planned.

What options does Nina have in relation to the situation?

Nina could react explosively and express her anger at Keith. She could resort to feelings of intimidation and berate herself for ignoring the strength of statutory authority and her own naivety. She could accept the court decision and go immediately to tell the team and Jane. Or she could take stock and seek the advice of her supervisor. Nina is an experienced practitioner and she starts with some self-reflection. She is well aware of the facts of this situation and is secure in her own capacity to make judgments. She is feeling a range of emotions, including rage and despair, but remains convinced that the arrangements in place for Nina and her baby are robust and any risks to the baby will be well-mediated in the relationship networks that are being organised. She determines to seek her supervisor's support for a crisis meeting of the hospital team, to which Keith will be invited, along with the caseworker with whom she has had ongoing communication to date. The outcome she hopes for is to convince Keith that, despite the court order, there are sufficient plans in place to enable Jane to safely maintain care of her baby. She remains unsure when to contact the maternal grandmother and this provides her with another ethical question: should she share this information with Jane's mother before she talks to Jane?

Conclusion

There is a wealth of literature on the importance of interpersonal relationships and the value of building strong relational networks. Person-centred work is as important as social support and community work to build strong communities. Strong social networks and connections are important to people's resilience when they are faced with problems in coping. At the same time, it is important to build strong interpersonal relationships, especially in child protection, given the system's adversarial nature. Though there are power imbalances built into the system with powerful agents, and disempowered disadvantaged parents at the base of investigations, there are also parents who are dangerous and who must be subjected to forensic investigation.

While the child protection system is focused to deal with these kinds of cases, applying a heavy handed investigative approach to all families in the system is neither needed nor just. For a relational approach to be truly possible, the system must change from within, building practices that are respectful and just. This means, no matter how service users come to the attention of child protection and family welfare services, the development of a sound working relationship with the family is essential to the success of the work. Further, it means thinking relationally, that is, seeing people as embedded in social relations and social relationships, and viewing these networks as resources. And, as the case example vividly shows, it also means understanding and being able to manage relationships in the service network in which the worker is embedded, if the worker is to safeguard the best interests of children.

Reflective questions

1 What issues does the emphasis on relational practice described in this chapter present for you?
2 How might you balance relational considerations with statutory obligations to safeguard children?
3 What might have enabled this case example situation to have been addressed differently from the start?

Chapter 12　Applying an integrated framework: the DECIDE model

The challenges all practitioners face in child protection decision making is by now abundantly clear. Applying an *integrated framework* to such decisions does not provide an immediate answer. No framework, however integrated, does this. None provide reasoned and responsible answers if all we do is logically and rationally follow a book of rules or a code. All ethical decision making is a deeply practical exercise and it is circular, and linear, and contextual, all at the same time and requires *discernment and reflexivity* at every turn. In child protection and family welfare, it involves a seriously practical discipline that seeks to resolve problems of profound importance to children, families and communities. Consequently, it requires an appreciation of the *value laden and moral dimension* of the work and the important place our values, trust and personal beliefs have in mediating our responses. It obliges us to harness this understanding in an ever-changing environment in which no situation is ever the same as another, in order to make well-reasoned decisions that offer the best possible outcome. And it requires that we are ever mindful of the political, legislative and organisational context within which families live and we work.

To add to this complexity, assimilating all of these matters must be mediated by an understanding of self and an ever-developing reflexivity and wisdom. The understanding is not just about one's own values and beliefs but also includes learning from previous decision making, and other evidence from research and practice. Writing about the difficult role of public health nurses in this sphere, Marcellus (2005) skilfully highlighted the significance of the capacity for developing relationships in this work. She observed that those working with 'at-risk families' simultaneously support and police the family and must develop trusting relationships with families experiencing powerlessness and oppression. They must also do this while paying attention to the protective needs of the child, as well as the vulnerability of adults. As is apparent in all the chapters to this point, and explored more fully in Chapter 11, relationship skills are crucial – and so is the ability to think not just about a particular relationship but to *think relationally*. Yet, Ferguson (2014) noted from his ethnographic study of social workers doing direct child protection practice in England that some struggled to work creatively within the *emotionality of this environment*, portraying the challenge of integrating the head and the heart *in situ* with children and parents. As discussed when we introduced the DECIDE model in Chapter 4, three core concepts undergird this decision-making framework: (i) competing ethical principles; (ii) unequal power relationships; and (iii) complex stakeholder responsibilities. In this chapter, we begin with underlining the core contextual issues to be taken into account when applying this integrated decision-making model: (i) awareness of the pervasiveness of power relations; (ii) acknowledging legislative and public mandates; (iii) mediating evidence and social context; and (iv) discerning organisational obligations, thinking relationally and managing professional relationships.

Core contextual issues

In applying the DECIDE model, the practitioner needs to be mindful of at least four core contextual matters relating to integrated decision making:

1 awareness of the pervasiveness of power relations;
2 acknowledging legislative and public mandates;
3 mediating evidence and social context; and
4 discerning organisational obligations, thinking relationally and managing professional relationships.

Though these matters have been addressed in some detail and in different ways in other chapters, all need to be understood now within the context of applying the DECIDE integrated decision-making framework.

Awareness of the pervasive presence of power relations

Emphasised in all chapters, and a central theme of this book, is the need to appreciate the way power is present in all forums for decision making, and to discern how to manage it in all its diverse forms and vagaries. We have noted the identification and *management of power* imbalances are crucial components of good ethical practice (see Chapter 4). This, we have said, is not as simple as acknowledging the *relative powerlessness and vulnerability* of the populations represented by the primary service users (see Chapter 7) vis-à-vis the professional and statutory power held by those in authority. Certainly such awareness is vital. So, too, are the need to differentiate the power between various service users and stakeholders within the family/community; to acknowledge children generally (but not always) have little power; people who abuse others may be very frightening and powerful; and many people are rendered easily immobilised and helpless by their circumstances, particularly by the debilitating effects of poverty and intergenerational trauma.

Add to this the power complexities within organisations, which are sanctioned by state legislation to intervene in the most sacrosanct of personal spaces – family life. These organisations and associated legislative frameworks bestow huge power on workers. Ironically, they are often described as *command-control* agencies (Harris, 2008), where workers feel dominated by authoritarian regimes, and ruled by procedures and rules that reduce their capacity for professional judgment and *ethical discernment* (Trevithick, 2014). In these environments, independent thinking is prevented, compliance is a priority, and cultures can feel intimidating and bullying.

Acknowledging legislative and public mandates

Child abuse is a legal construct outlawed by societies to enable the protection of children. A vast international patchwork of covenants, legislation, procedures, guidelines,

policies and recommendations from inquires, as well as case law, exists to author-
ise the work of people responsible for ensuring the safety of children from families
thought to have abused them, or deemed likely to harm them. This complexity is
local, as well as national and international. Practitioners across a range of disciplines
are expected to know and understand the abundance of obligations therein, at the
same time as they are negotiating the daily demands of highly demanding work, and
managing the important sensitivities of children, families and communities. These
laws are a societal response and have emerged from what might be called a public
consensus that families must not be immune from scrutiny and 'something has to be
done to stop children being abused in families and to save them'.

Directives associated with these legal obligations generally include reporting
requirements, definitions of types of abuse, duties of investigation, response procedures, and evidential requirements and, for example, with laws associated with MR,
they establish significant sanctions if not followed. However ambiguous they may
sometimes appear, the plethora of rules and regulations provide severe constraints on,
as well as possibilities for, the role of workers.

It is vital that all practitioners appreciate the 'facts' of the situation, about which
they must make a decision, in terms of the legal, policy and procedural requirements
and the options they have for discernment (see Chapter 9). For example, in many
jurisdictions, legislative principles attempt to balance the right of the child to his/her
family with the duty to ensure stability in other care arrangements. Similarly, some
legislation includes a *principle of least intervention,* which requires consideration to
be given to minimising disruption to the lives of children. What this highlights is the
ethical duty to be knowledgeable about legal duties, not in order to 'blindly follow'
dictums and procedures, but to be accountable for including them as elements of the
decision-making process. Indeed, at the centre of any ethical decision-making process
is the requirement to discern and to challenge, as well as to seek advice. Professionals
have *a duty to challenge* laws, regulations, procedures and other dictates that they see
as harmful to the people they serve. Within the context of the jurisdiction in which
you work, some reflective questions might include:

- How strong is the public mandate to protect children at any cost?
- How does your contemporary legislation present this mandate?
- What are the legislative requirements you would need to consider in determining
  any initial action in a situation such as this one?
- What procedural requirements might influence your choice of initial assessment
  and action?

Mediating evidence and social context

As elaborated throughout the book, the social context of child protection is that of
concerned societies that have mandated governments to police families in order to protect children from abuse therein. To a greater or lesser extent, in different jurisdictions,
this mandate is balanced with a requirement to assist families to resolve the problems
that might lead to maltreatment (Parkinson, 2000). The history of this endeavour to
protect children has been troubled, and a number of authors have identified distinct
periods characterised by particular orientations to children, families and to the very
understanding of the meaning attributed to abuse and neglect (see Chapters 5 and 6).

For example, Scott (2013) identifies the original historical 'wave' as that of rescuing destitute children; the second 'wave' as the discovery of physical and sexual abuse; and the third wave (current) as one in which we are recalibrating our thinking about intervention in the light of painful historical legacies, and evidence of unintentional harms to children, families and communities by over intervention. At the same time, as she notes, there are significant harms associated with under intervention. Most importantly, she indicates the evidence is clear that the system we have is no longer sustainable as demand has outstripped supply, and we need a new public health model to replace the forensic and investigative one that embodies the second 'wave'.

Research data and new understandings about the context in which child protection practices have been experienced have been provided throughout. The *painful historical legacies* have been noted and include evidence from a multitude of adults who were in care as children; families who have been subject to debilitating scrutiny and disruption; children who have experienced multiple traumas associated with investigation and removal; and, communities, in particular, Indigenous peoples, people of colour and people from marginalised groups, whose cultural identities have been compromised and often shattered. Matters of inequality and impoverishment of targeted families and children, as well as the disastrous consequences of racism and colonisation have been underscored as evidence of system failure. All are relevant in this case study.

The big question is how do practitioners incorporate all the evidence available and use it in their decision making to keep children safe to the best of their ability? And, of course, how do they do this when the pressures of work are enormous and when the risk of public opprobrium if one 'fails' is an ever-present fear?

Within the context of the jurisdiction in which you work some reflective questions you might ask at this stage are:

- Which large macro issues in public policy surround this decision right now, for example discrimination, inequality, recent inquiries and media attention?
- What are the cultural issues relevant to your decision making?
- What are the requirements, if any, for cultural engagement?
- What are the protocols for speaking to cultural elders?
- What are the relevant gender issues in this scenario?
- What evidence is there about outcomes for Indigenous children placed in out-of-home care that might be relevant to this situation?

Discerning organisational obligations and managing professional relationships

As identified in Chapters 6 and 9, there are obligations for child protection and family welfare practitioners associated with their organisational membership and allied legal duties such as those enunciated in child protection laws. There are other obligations associated with legislation such as antidiscrimination, workforce safety, child care standards, employer regulations, and public sector codes of conduct, and there are additional regulatory requirements connected with particular organisational mandates. Regardless of individual mandates, almost all organisations are structured to achieve the outcomes their charters demand and the literature is rife with evidence of NPM discourses to ensure work is coordinated, managed, measured, marketed and aligned to clear objectives and outcomes. These *managerialist imperatives* have proven particularly difficult for professional decision making because, to some extent, the controls and procedures have been developed in light of what are seen to have been professional failures in judgment and decision making (Munro, 2011) and so, in some regards, they replace professional judgment at the very time that we are imploring workers to increase their professional discretion, discernment and reflexivity.

Given practitioners work within very different organisational structures across a wide range of specific mandates and philosophies, it is no surprise that there are substantial difficulties in managing interagency and intersectoral collaboration, particularly as the pressures have emerged to work collaboratively and in integrated ways to achieve outcomes (see Chapter 6). Horwath and Morrison (2007) identify five different 'levels of collaborative endeavour' in safeguarding children each of which requires different skills on the part of workers: communication between different disciplines; cooperation on individual casework; formal coordination of joint working partnerships; coalitions of structures that require the sacrificing of autonomy; and integration in which entities are created to form new hybrid organisations.

All of these arrangements require attention is paid to the building of worker relationships and trust – and yet, as Horwath and Morrison found in their research, these relational elements are the very ones that are neglected as organisations attempt to collaborate. It is somewhat ironic that agencies focused on working with children and families in which trust and relationship are so central, appear to ignore intra- and interagency trust and relationships. Understanding the need to work relationally in child protection requires practitioners to appreciate relationships and social networks at every point and level of their work, including working across agencies to develop trust (see Chapter 12).

Additional to the interagency relationships needing to be managed by workers who are assessing complex situations involving fragile families and vulnerable children are the internal relationships that need to be managed. Supervisors, colleagues and managers coexist in work worlds to which they bring very different experiences, values and understandings, let alone disciplinary backgrounds, knowledge and discourses (see case example in Chapter 12). In each exchange there is the potential for issues to be clouded by *power differentials* that get in the way of the reflexivity required of the decision maker. The now ubiquitous case conference and case review arrangements so common in child protection work provide hothouses for interpersonal difference and dissent. The powerlessness of families in these situations has been well described in Chapters 7 and 8. What also needs to be acknowledged is the presence of *power dynamics* between different workers that can profoundly alter the processes and outcomes for children and families. The way intra- and interprofessional relationships are managed by workers will undoubtedly affect the outcomes of their entire decision making. It is vital that power differentials and lines of authority are understood, acknowledged and challenged when necessary if clarity about the facts, risks and priorities are to be enunciated and shared openly.

In our view, while regulatory standards, risk assessment tools, DMTs and procedural regulations have their utility, they have largely crowded out the more distinctive skills required of professional judgment in ethical decision making. It is a requirement of an integrated ethical framework that these professional skills need to be re-honoured and re-established as a matter of some urgency for children and families, and for the workers who are responsible for the decisions. The following case study highlights the key matters discussed in the application of the DECIDE model.

Case example: permanency planning and cultural safety

David is a six-year-old boy who, along with his then two-year-old sister, Jemma, was removed on a court order by the statutory authority from his family home in a remote Aboriginal community two years ago following three substantiated reports of neglect, the last one involving the risk of sexual abuse. This community is severely disadvantaged and scores high on every level of health and social inequality. It is isolated, impoverished, has very low employment levels and income, poor and overcrowded housing, low school attendance, and high morbidity and mortality rates many of which are associated with colonisation and the intergenerational impacts of trauma.

At the time of their removal, the two children were living with their mother, Glenda (28 years), her new partner, a 'white fella' called Bill (35 years), and other extended family members, including the children's maternal grandmother, Violet (56 years). The children had been reported by the school as living in 'squalid conditions' in a house with no running water and left unsupervised in the house used by numbers of extended family including a maternal uncle (Doc). This uncle had previously been named, but not charged, with sexual abuse of a minor as there was insufficient corroborating evidence to proceed to trial. Violet was assessed as unprotective as a grandmother as she regularly went drinking with Glenda, Bill and others.

Glenda has three other children from an earlier relationship – all in kinship care in the community. Jemma is the daughter of Glenda and Bill and has been placed in kinship care with her maternal aunt and family in a nearby community. David was placed in foster care with the Bligh family, a well-respected, well-known and 'good' Christian non-Aboriginal family in a more distant regional town.

David's father, Bruce (44 years), is an emerging 'tribal elder' in the community. He had been the sole income earner in his extended family and had continued to contribute financially to David's care (albeit intermittently) – working for the local government, a key employer in remote communities. He is in prison following a two-year sentence for violent assault on a policeman during a drunken spree in a nearby town three years ago. He is due for release in three months. Bruce had no previous convictions and is very attached to David, whom he regards as holding the future safe in terms of his Aboriginal ancestry. He was only informed after the event, while in prison, of the child neglect complaints, the statutory action to remove the children, and their subsequent out-of-home care placement. Bruce has persistently expressed his determination to accept treatment for his alcohol abuse and to assume care of David.

With the support of the Aboriginal Legal Service (an advocacy and legal representation organisation that is an ardent fighter for social justice), Bruce is appealing against the care order which involves David being in the care of the state until he reaches 18 years of age. He is particularly angry (as are his lawyers) that David has been placed with a 'white' family and notes this is against the 'Aboriginal Child Placement Principle' – a policy of all Australian statutory child welfare authorities, aimed at ensuring cultural continuity and safety for Indigenous children in care. He sees this care arrangement as a violation of the rights of his son and his people, and another example of 'stealing' Aboriginal children. Bruce's mother was a member of the 'Stolen Generation', having been removed from her mother and placed in an institution when a small child. She ensured her three children were well educated before she died aged 48 years. Bruce has no other children and his two sisters live far away in the city with their families. His father was a tribal elder who died of 'a heart condition' when Bruce was in his teens.

You are a child protection worker in the child protection department with responsibility for David's case. There is a staff complement of eight, four of whom are new to the job. The office covers a wide, sparsely populated, largely poor, geographical region and is situated in the large mining town where David lives with his foster parents and two other foster children. You have met David and Mr and Mrs Bligh twice in two months and are impressed that David appears happy, is attending school and is well-nourished. He does not appear distressed that he has not seen any of his family since being removed from their care. At the same time as you are wondering how to manage the large number of cases on your list that are awaiting investigation (some of them urgent), you are informed by Joan, your very experienced (and pushy) team leader, that there is a legal challenge being launched by Aboriginal Legal Services to repeal the care order and return David to the care of his father once he is released from prison. Joan is your direct line manager and supervisor. She tells you that you must do everything possible to ensure David stays in the placement because 'his mum did not object in the first place, and the Blighs are our best foster parents'.

This case study is factual (although anonymised) and aptly captures the multifarious nature of complex decision making in Indigenous child welfare. To reiterate the DECIDE model provides a framework for thinking through the key ethical issues surrounding a case. It is not prescriptive in any sense and the questions generated by one's immediate reactions and further reflection open up possibilities for deeper ongoing reflection as the matter proceeds. Questions help to highlight the fact that, while the stages of decision making need always to be used, it is in the iteration of new questions at each stage that we get successively closer to a comprehensive understanding of the situation at hand. Thus questioning lies at the heart of the DECIDE model. Questions in this case might include:

- What are your immediate emotional reactions and intuition?
- What are the facts of the situation?
- Who are the key stakeholders?
- What is the major ethical question for you at the outset?
- What other ethical concerns do you have about this situation?
- Where does most of the power appear to lie?
- What is your understanding of the extent and limitations of your role in relation to reviewing David's placement with his foster family?
- To whom do you owe ethical duties and responsibilities and what are these?
- What factors will influence your decision about whether or not to prioritise David's situation versus other pressing matters?

- What is your understanding of the authority of your team leader (supervisor) to determine your assessment of the situation?
- What power and authority do you have to make an assessment and make a decision about optional actions?

DECIDE integrated decision-making model

So, how does the practitioner aspiring to be thoughtful, reflective, virtuous, wise and relational manage situational complexities? The integrated DECIDE model emphasises the pivotal place of self-reflection and reflexivity as necessary professional learning tools as practitioners navigate the iterative journey of ethical decision making. To recap, the process followed in embedding the DECIDE model in ethical decision making in organisations involves:

- understanding the issues at stake in a case – the exact problem and its nature;
- determining those who have a stake in the case situation;
- disentangling and accommodating primary ethical principles and derivative key ethical principles in decision making;
- weighing up the myriad considerations involved, and prioritising ethical principles for specific cases;
- incorporating legal, policy and procedural requirements within decision making;
- managing interorganisational disputes and role conflicts;
- resolving ethical issues; and
- learning from outcomes.

One of the most important skills for practitioners to develop, is a reflexivity that enables them to connect with their own knowledge, values, morality and rules, and apply these to the problems they confront at work in a systematic way. Thompson *et al.* (2006) encapsulated this by explaining competence in making ethical decisions as involving the ability to make judicious decisions, for which practitioners can provide a well-reasoned justification that can be publicly articulated and 'stand up in court' (p. 66). The DECIDE model starts with the understanding that practitioners need to *clarify personal and professional values* and *show insight* into their *own values* and the *values of others*. They also need to understand fundamental ethical principles and derivative key ones, and apply these to the very practical situations they face. Additionally, they need to be able to use skills to enable the views and perspectives of various stakeholders to be represented and, finally, to make decisions and articulate their reasons in ways that capture the complex vagaries of the context of people's lives. Woven through each of these competencies is the appreciation of how power is exercised and/or wielded, and how it is then managed for the benefit of the people we serve.

The way the model is methodically portrayed in a somewhat rational and linear fashion is done only to capture its essential elements. It is indeed a circular and iterative process in which each stage informs others. It is not as tedious and pedantic, or indeed as overwhelming, as it might seem at first glance. Many of the elements are easily identifiable and spring to mind immediately for the reflective practitioner. In teaching this model to students and practitioners over the years, we have been told that for many, even novice practitioners, some of the processes are already 'second nature'. The important message is that each element, however obvious or obscure, must be part of the decision making in a way that can be shared and public. In the following section, we recapitulate the model and link it to the situation facing David's worker.

DECIDE framework

Define the problem

Before expressly defining the ethical problem to be solved (and there may be a number), the facts of the situation need to be ascertained. What are the facts that have a particular bearing on the situation and what ethical issue/s demand a decision? Some of the 'facts' may include such matters as organisational factors, cultural perspectives, personal anxiety or political pressures. In identifying the facts, the people involved and those who have a stake in the decision are more easily identifiable. Name the important stakeholders. In doing so it might be useful to pay attention to some of the following:

1   Who has an interest in the process and outcomes of solving this problem?
2   From what theoretical, ideological or professional perspective might these stakeholders operate?
3   How do different stakeholders define the problem?
4   What kinds of action/intervention would they propose or be promoting?
5   What outcomes do you think different stakeholders expect?
6   Taking these different perspectives into account, how do you think the problem should be defined?

Defining the problem is almost always the most difficult part of this process and often a number of problems can be named before the priority one is established. It is useful to compare notes with colleagues at this stage to be alert to the different ways problems may be perceived. However, ultimately, as a decision maker, the worker must have a particular ethical question in mind. It is useful here to be clear about:

1   who exactly has the primary decision-making role for resolving the particular situation;
2   what the primary duties of the decision maker are in the situation; and
3   what ethical problem(s) emerge as the most urgent to be addressed.

In relation to the case example above, among the many facts confronting David's caseworker are some salient ones:

* The geographical community in which he is working is one dominated by evidence of gross intergenerational poverty, inequality, and racism, much of which are related to the outcomes of earlier (and some would argue, ongoing) colonisation.
* David is an Aboriginal child in the care of the state and for, at present, unknown reasons he has been placed in long-term care in a non-Aboriginal family, and this is contrary to the placement principles applied to all Aboriginal children in out-of-home care.
* David has apparently been in stable statutory care for two years where he appears happy.

- David's mother agreed to this placement.
- David's foster family are important people in the local town.
- David's biological father was not consulted about his care arrangements (as required under the Child Placement Principle), and is mounting a legal challenge to his guardianship removal and wants him returned to his care.
- The worker is 'new' to the area and has a large caseload of overdue investigations.
- The worker's team leader has been there a long time and has considerable authority which she wields with some ease, and does not believe there is a case to be resolved as she wants David to remain in his foster placement.
- The Aboriginal Legal Service is unlikely to mount a case without some chance of success.
- The worker feels (uneasy, worried and concerned) ... about the situation.

There are many others facts that can be discerned and all influence the way the problem is defined. In terms of stakeholders, there are a large number: the child, David; his mother, Glenda; his father, Bruce; the Blighs; the team leader Joan (representing the department); and the Aboriginal Legal Service lawyers. It is hard to determine who the most salient ones are but, arguably, having to reduce these to the four most significant ones, the worker named:

- David, the child in question;
- the Blighs, David's foster parents;
- Bruce, the child's father; and
- the Aboriginal community represented by the Aboriginal Legal Service.

Unarguably, David's mother and the supervisor are important stakeholders and some might also identify the other children on the worker's caseload as important stakeholders. Deciding who the key stakeholders are is a decision the worker has to make. We have accepted the decision made by the worker in this case at the time.

In terms of naming the problem, what are the optional ethical problems and which is the one you decide is the most pressing? In this particular situation, the new worker decided the most important ethical problem he faced was 'how to ensure David's situation was adequately dealt with without risking his own employment as a new worker'. A more 'seasoned' worker may have identified a different ethical problem, such as 'how to ensure the rights of David and his father were balanced for the benefit of David's immediate and long-term care'. Alternatively, and in the light of an emphasis on relational practice, the worker might focus on an ethical question, such as 'how to ensure I am sufficiently relational in this context so that I can facilitate what is in the best interests of Bruce, and his family and community, and engaging my team leader in the process'.

Ethical review

Here the task is to identify which particular ethical principles are relevant to this problem/decision and reflect on which of the principles have priority for which stakeholder. In all child protection matters, the dominant stakeholder is the child or children, and to them a dominant duty of care is owed and, of course, the 'best interest' principle has paramountcy (see Chapter 10). However, the parents are inevitably stakeholders and, particularly if young, ill, vulnerable or otherwise disabled, will require a duty of care on the part of those in authority. The matter of context and, in particular, power relationships, is critical here. Identifying the structural factors that are influencing the problem assists in understanding the relevant social justice matters and human rights, and in balancing duties of justice owed to all to maximise equity and fairness. All people are owed respect, which involves attending to relational integrity with all stakeholders. And nuancing these three primary principles in the light of derivative key ones always proves helpful. In this context, cultural safety and continuity are crucial derivative ones. The process of identifying dual, and sometimes complex, responsibilities and balancing competing principles and duties is always difficult. However, practitioners who have used an ethical framework for their decision making will already be used to such discernment.

In David's situation we have tentatively identified four key stakeholders (alongside his mother and the supervisor). What are their dominant rights and what are the worker's dominant duties and responsibilities to each of them? It is useful at this stage to list these and scan the various rights and duties while acknowledging the duties are often in tension with each other in relation to each stakeholder. Rights and duties are generally the mirror of each other (see Table 12.1).

In this situation, the worker was particularly concerned with what he articulated to be the systemic injustice to Indigenous families and communities that were already disadvantaged alongside the intergenerational results of colonisation, forced removal, abuse and poverty. As a young man he was also perturbed by the way Bruce's legal and moral rights as a father had been totally overlooked in the processes that led to the removal and placement of David. He had had a similar experience in an earlier relationship of his own. And, in being reflexive as he had been trained to do, and reflecting on his own earlier responses to his visits to David, he noted how he did not inquire with him about his situation, and accepted a superficial observation about

TABLE 12.1 Primary rights of stakeholders and duties of the worker

Stakeholder	Rights of the stakeholder	Duties of the worker
David	Care: • Safeguarding • Best interests Justice: • Cultural safety	Duty of care to most vulnerable Ensuring cultural safety
The Blighs, David's foster parents	Respect: • Information sharing • Relational perspective	Respect and protection of their interests
Bruce	Respect: • Informational sharing Justice: • Equity • Cultural safety	Respect for persons and maintenance of relational perspective while ensuring attention to equity and cultural justice
The Aboriginal community represented by the Aboriginal Legal Service	Justice: • Fairness	Respectful information sharing Justice: ensuring equity and fairness

him appearing happy. He now wondered about why David had not had any contact with any of his immediate or extended family for two years, and the cultural as well as the psychological impact of this.

Consider options

With the ethical question at the forefront, the stakeholders named and the principles and duties owed to various stakeholders identified, it is possible to recognise fairly quickly the options available and the practicality of the choices therein. Brainstorming the choices and how they accommodate the principles and duties will lead to options that are easily excluded, or otherwise listed as real options. The chosen options must recognise legal and procedural constraints while not using these as the sole determinant of action. The question is what are the most reasonable, ethical and practical choices available. It is important to brainstorm all the possible ways to deal with the problem and to spend time focusing on the most sensible and practical options, as well as those that feel intuitively to be the best. In relation to the question facing the worker in David's case, these are some options he could list:

- Accept the recommendation of his team leader and get on with important investigative work and await the receipt of the formal legal challenge.
- Tell his team leader she is wrong and familiarise himself with the facts of the situation in readiness for the legal challenge.
- Don't say anything to his supervisor and familiarise himself with the facts of the situation in readiness for the legal challenge.
- Decide the real issue lies with the rights of David's mother, Glenda, whose needs may have been over-looked, and organise a full case review.
- Engage the team leader in a dialogue about the situation and persist with emphasising the cultural imperatives and the long-term, intergenerational consequences in this situation.
- Acknowledge his rage with what he sees already as an unjust situation for Bruce and David, and investigate options for contact between David and Bruce.
- Contact the Aboriginal Legal Service to express an interest in supporting their intervention.
- Decide child protection work is just too hard and commence a search for less demanding employment.

These are not whimsical options but, among others, are ones that flitter across one's consciousness as one faces ethical challenges. They are all options – and were to this caseworker – however fanciful! In the context of complex decision making in the midst of bureaucratically demanding arenas, and without compromising child safety, practitioners have to prioritise what is in their own best interests sometimes!

Investigate outcomes

In listing options – perhaps around three – consider the likely consequences and outcomes for each. Some considerations might include: will anyone be harmed and if so, how can that harm be mitigated and what are the highly charged concerns framing this decision and how are they influencing my choice. Identify the likely ethical consequences, outcomes, costs and benefits of each choice. Check each of the options against the principles, rights and responsibilities named, and review that outcome to see which of the options is the most ethically acceptable, or, at worst, least harmful. In doing this, the worker also had in mind what he called his own moral compass and sense of moral safety, and he could name that as a consequential factor in his decision making. In the caseworker's situation, he might prioritise three options (as noted in Table 12.2) and now needs to identify how they fit or otherwise with ethical duties, the likely outcomes and the implications of these.

Decide on action

It is important at this stage to decide and to develop a clear plan – one that has a certain objective in mind and that plainly articulates the reason for the decision, and the balancing of principles and priorities required in the process. At this point it is important to remember there are never absolutely 'right' answers, only answers and plans that are well-reasoned and somehow recognise and accommodate the emotional tensions in the decision making and lead to the best decision possible in the case.

TABLE **12.2** An optional outcome analysis

Options	Fit with ethical duties to each stakeholder	Likely outcomes
Accept the recommendation of his team leader and get on with important investigative work and await the receipt of the formal legal challenge	OK as David remains safe although not sure about cultural safety	David is physically safe
Tell his team leader she is wrong and familiarise himself with the facts of the situation in readiness for the legal challenge	Hardly respectful or relational with supervisor	Likely to escalate the problem
Don't say anything to his team leader and familiarise himself with the facts of the situation in readiness for the legal challenge	Not respectful to supervisor or to David and foster parents	Likely to alienate all but the Aboriginal Legal Service and Bruce Impaired relationships
Go back to basics and engage the team leader and colleagues – including foster parents – in a carefully constructed dialogue about the important aspects of this situation and the imperatives therein	Respectful to all Courageous Focused on important principles of justice and respect while keeping David safe	With skilled relational capacity, could work to free stakeholders to think about both short- and long-term interests of David and his cultural security as well as personal safety

Evaluate results

In the frantic world of frontline practice, this endpoint of the decision making is often left out, or is addressed at a much later stage when the best, or worst, of outcomes are sometimes incidentally raised. Ideally, at as early a stage as possible, it is important to learn about what worked well or otherwise, and to learn from successes and mistakes. Evidence of outcomes is often slow in coming and in the area of protecting children is particularly fraught because of the potential dissonance between short- (immediate safety) and long-term (life chances, family integrity and cultural security) outcomes about which so much recent literature is being addressed. It is at this stage that reflection and reflexivity are paramount and yet, with the demands of work, are often left out within the work arena (workers report this is what they do at home or in a bar!). We urge practitioners to use supervision and team discussions to reflect on process and outcomes and evaluate these in a regular way and to entrench this practice.

Conclusion

Integrated ethical practice in the way described above may appear daunting and, yet, surely it is no more daunting than the appreciation of the substantial responsibilities sitting on the shoulders of people who are making serious decisions about the immediate and long-term impacts on the lives of children, families and communities. All practitioners know they are expected to practice ethically as well as within the confines of the law, and generally do so, although many find it hard to name the elements of such practice in any comprehensive way. What we name and integrate in this chapter are all the elements that can, and should, be taken account of as one grapples with inherent complexity. In the case example above, the pervasiveness of power relations, the significance of legislative and public mandates, the importance of appreciating social context and organisational obligations, and, of thinking relationally are very evident. In being able to name these elements and act reflexively, transparency and public accountability for our professional decision making is ensured.

> ### Reflective questions
>
> 1   How does the idea of an integrated model of ethical decision making sit with your own training in ethics so far?
> 2   What are the key elements of this approach that appeal to you?
> 3   What are the elements you find most difficult to accept?
> 4   What did you learn from the worker's conceptualising of this situation?

Chapter 13 **Working ethically across cultures: a focus on fathers**

We have shown that working ethically across cultures is challenging and, in many countries, conducted against a historical backdrop of imperialism and colonisation that continues to resonate in contemporary practice and in the circumstances of Indigenous peoples, who tend to be overrepresented in child protection interventions. Gender issues are threaded through policies and practices, obliging consideration of the causes and consequences of abuse and neglect, as well as who takes responsibility for the protection and welfare of children. This chapter focuses in particular on a practice culture within child protection and family welfare systems, where the bulk of practitioners and service users are female and where men or fathers often tend to be overlooked. It explores the issues involved in working with men/fathers. This area offers important ethical challenges and is experienced as such by women workers who see men's violence and abuse as central to the difficulties women and children often face. Oppressive behaviour by those who are themselves oppressed is filled with ethical challenges and the chapter offers some thoughts on elements of respectful and relational practice in such a context.

Fathers, men and child protection

In the last decades, a small but growing research-based literature emerged exploring some of the issues in relation to fathers and the child protection system. In particular, there was a focus on why low levels of engagement by practitioners are a feature of the work. Differing and often competing imperatives have underpinned this focus on the need for engagement. For example, some feminists pointed out the unfairness of women bearing the brunt of the protection task, especially if the risks were posed by men who were abusive to them as well as to children. A pragmatic imperative prompted a concern to *engage fathers* in order both to assess the risks to, and the resources for, children's welfare and protection (Ashley *et al.*, 2006; Daniel and Taylor, 2001; Featherstone, 2009; Roskill *et al.*, 2008). The importance for fathers themselves of being supported to fulfil their role positively was also emphasised, particularly by *fatherhood organisations*, given the overwhelming evidence of such men's economic and social marginalisation, and historical practices of child removal which resulted in many Aboriginal and Indigenous men not knowing their own fathers.

However, before examining these matters, we must first discuss *terminology and its complexities*. The term 'father' is not straightforward, particularly when thinking about practice issues. Is it just birth fathers, or father figures, or indeed any man with whom the child has some form of connection usually through the mother? This is not at all straightforward in societies where there is considerable diversity in family practices and household composition, and researchers have pointed to the difficulties that can be posed for practitioners where there are multiple fathers and/or father figures (Featherstone, 2009). Indeed, researchers in Canada who took an inclusive approach in the sense of talking to men of any status living in households where there were children present were challenged by birth fathers for adopting such a stance (Brown et al., 2009).

In turn, stepfathers challenge the way that term can be used. For example, child deaths can support unhelpful discussions suggesting bifurcation between 'safe' birth fathers and 'dangerous' others invoking the trope of the stepfather (Revans, 2009). However, as Batchelor (2003) has pointed out, methodological problems are rife in the work examining child abuse and stepparents. Not only is there inconsistency in the definitions of abuse used, there are difficulties around the term stepparent: 'if abuse is attributed to a stepparent, was he or she a longstanding member of the child's household or one of several transient adults in that child's life?' (p. 203). As she noted, men who have problems in forming close attachments and who have a history of violent relationships might have had a series of relationships with vulnerable women, some (or many) of whom might have been sole parents. These men might come into contact with and abuse a series of children, any or all of whom could be classed as their stepchildren, regardless of whether they had taken on what might be considered to be a parenting role. Similarly, men seeking to sexually abuse children might seek out and build relationships with single parents as a means of having access to children; their sexual abuse might figure in research as abuse by a stepfather. Research into child murders by men has suggested the importance of understanding how men and women made vulnerable by repeated experiences of economic, emotional and psychological deprivation abuse and trauma could develop very damaging relationships with each other (Featherstone et al., 2014b). In this chapter, the term father is used mainly because the issues dealt with mainly concern birth fathers.

Engaging fathers

Research in the UK has noted that birth fathers who were unmarried and non-resident were at particular risk of not being engaged with by practitioners (Ashley et al., 2006; Roskill et al., 2008). This was partly linked to the following: the *household focus* adopted by busy practitioners who dealt with whomever was in front of them; assumptions about women's responsibility for child welfare; and a lack of understanding of the legal responsibilities and rights of birth fathers. An audit of case files found 80 per cent of birth fathers were not part of the household where their child was living and that only 12 per cent of children were living with both birth or adoptive parents, with 54 per cent living with a single parent (mother) (Roskill et al., 2008). However, basic information on fathers, including their contact details and their legal status, was missing from a significant number of files. For example, 20 per cent of children's files audited did not have the birth father named on the file, with the figure being 31 per cent for looked after children.

While there is a lack of rigorous research on this, it is clear that such trends towards lone motherhood and 'absent' fatherhood have been found across caseloads in many countries. As Featherstone (2009) noted, this must be located in an understanding of the demographic features of marginalised and impoverished families more generally. In terms of whether birth fathers were likely to be non-resident, the risks were not spread equally throughout the population and it was not that surprising, therefore, to find high rates in the populations involved with child protection services. In research on 'modern fatherhood', Poole *et al.* (2013) sought to develop an evidence base in this area because of the difficulties in developing accurate evidence. For example, historically and currently, men have not always known that they have children with whom they are not involved, or conversely, may be 'fathering' children who are not their birth children.

Poole *et al.* (2013) data were collected from men including those who did not live with their children, and therefore relied upon self-reports which, as indicated, tended to underestimate numbers of children or reflect denial on the part of men. However, in the absence of other evidence, the findings are of interest. The focus was on non-resident fathers of children of dependent age (under 16 years). Their estimate was that five per cent of all men aged 16–64 had non-resident children aged younger than 16 years, equating to 980,000 men in the UK.

Poole *et al.* (2013) showed that a father was more likely to have non-resident children if they: were white British compared with an Asian ethnic group; were in a black ethnic group compared with a white British ethnic group; had a lower level of educational attainment; were not in paid work; belonged to the lowest socioeconomic group; rented a property rather than were owner occupiers; and had married or cohabited three or more times.

Losing contact with children, moreover, was linked to poverty and attendant deprivation, with the availability or otherwise of suitable housing an important factor. Poole *et al.* (2013) found that those who were in contact, compared with those who had rare or no contact, were more likely to: provide financially for their non-resident children; live less than half an hour away; have multiple bedrooms; be a home owner; be in paid employment and belong to a higher socioeconomic group; and have educational qualifications (at least GCSE).

Reynolds (2009) specifically examined the issue of Afro-Caribbean and West Indian non-resident fathers and questioned assumptions that non-residence assumed non-involvement or lack of support. She noted that such fathers had been traditionally constructed as absent from parenting and unwilling to take responsibility for their children. However, she argued it was necessary to see parenting practices contextually, and as informed by cultural and historical factors and intersecting identities of race, ethnicity, social class, gender, age and generation. She argued that fathering policies that specifically focused on non-resident fathering tended to emphasise the social inequalities resulting from fathers living apart from their children, and neglected the wider issue of structural inequalities resulting from Afro-Caribbean and West Indian fathers' racial-ethnic identity and racial divisions in society.

The research in Poole *et al.* (2013) provides some important background information when seeking to decode the issues for fathers whose children were involved with child protection services. It is important to reflect again here on the evidence of the links between deprivation and involvement with child protection systems. However, we lack a rigorous evidence base that explores not only the demographic features of families but also the characteristics of the relevant men. There are some suggestive studies. For example, a secondary analysis of data collected for another purpose showed that they were usually economically marginalised and often had histories of childhood trauma, and significant physical and mental health issues (Featherstone, 2004). Featherstone used analyses of masculinities to explore with, and understand, the issues fathers in the family services faced. She argued for the use of the term 'vulnerable' to signify their often very precarious connection to labour markets, and histories of abuse and physical and mental health difficulties. However, she noted there is much more rigorous research needed to understand what is happening in the relationships between the men and women whose children came to the attention of child protection and family welfare services. For example, are those who suffer multiple deprivations and traumas arising from sexual violence, for example, singularly ill-equipped and supported to overcome toxic histories of distrust and establish more lasting bonds?

In terms of Indigenous fathers, there is considerable evidence not only to support the picture above, but there are further concerns as well. For example, the Aboriginal Fathers Project in Canada was a research study of the roles of Aboriginal fathers (Manahan and Ball, 2007) which investigated the ways community programmes could support fathers' involvement with their children and increase their participation in family-centred programmes. Those fathers interviewed highlighted the lasting generational impact on them of colonisation and assimilation practices. Their traditional role as protector of the family and the community was suppressed brutally without supports being put in place to access other valued roles. They considered the trauma of residential schooling had had lasting generational effects on their parenting skills, power to communicate and ability to show affection to their children. Many who had never set foot inside a residential home themselves also felt the impact on their own fathers had meant they had not experienced positive father figures growing up. The HREOC (1997) inquiry found similar impacts on Australian Indigenous peoples.

Misunderstanding and misrecognition

Featherstone and White (2006) explored young fathers' experiences of health and social care services. Eighteen young fathers were interviewed within a focus group. All but one were from minority ethnic groups and were aged between 15 and 29 years. Their children were mostly under five, with a number having a child under a year old. While the majority were still in relationships with the mothers of their children, their living situations were fluid in that they were not cohabiting or were intermittently doing so. A key finding concerned their perception of the state as being on women's side and the contrast the men drew between being a man in the UK and in the USA where they saw men as having more rights and status. While the men made no overt reference to racism, they spoke of having no 'rights' and saw the state as only interested in them when seeking child support or as perpetrators of domestic abuse. Social workers were considered to be unpredictable and inconsistent with them, and, as women, to side with women and be suspicious, if not hostile, towards them. Overall, there was a strong disconnect between how they felt they were perceived as fathers and how they perceived themselves. In relation to the latter, given the ages of their children, much of their talk was necessarily aspirational but the vast majority expressed a strong commitment to having an ongoing emotionally connected relationship with their children. A key issue in terms of social work practice was that the fathers' investment in a language of 'rights' meant that encounters with social workers were likely to be problematic as rights talk on the part of parents, especially fathers, is considered selfish and irresponsible in a context where parents are expected to invest in a language of 'responsibility' (Featherstone, 2009).

Ferguson and Hogan (2004) in their research on practices with fathers in Ireland explored excluded young men's tendency towards protest masculinity:

> Men's practices of drinking, violence and criminality … constitute a public acting out of a 'hard man' image. Their status and definition of themselves as men is given meaning through protest, an acting out of being against everything that is seen as socially valid.
>
> (Ferguson and Hogan, 2004, p. 136)

The boys put a lot of effort into performing a powerful persona in contexts where they had very little power in reality. However, in their research, Ferguson and Hogan noted the complexities here, some of the young men were at ease with non-traditional gender roles and nurturing their children. There was a lot of concern with façade which they suggested social workers needed to get beyond but struggled to do so.

Men's investment in models of masculinity that stress their need to be in control may leave them particularly vulnerable to feeling shame and being shamed by encounters with professionals in contexts that are deeply imbued with classed and racialised assumptions about appropriate dress and behaviour. A lack of understanding about culturally appropriate modes of greeting and engaging can mean engagements start from a position of perceived disrespect from the onset. Ashley *et al.* (2006) and Ferguson and Hogan (2004) found that fathers felt judged by social workers in terms of their appearance (e.g. having tattoos and being big in build). They felt assumptions were made about their potential to be violent based upon their appearance.

Fathers also reflected on their inability to engage in processes that they felt excluded them and made them feel inferior. They spoke of how they got angry in meetings and did not feel able to communicate in ways that were considered suitable by professionals. They spoke of professionals employing unfair standards in terms of assessing their conduct. For example, if they were late for a contact visit, it was evidence of lack of commitment, but if the social workers were late, it was because of traffic problems. There was evidence that the work commitments (not just of fathers but of adult family members generally) were not respected and facilitated for when arranging meetings. This is currently a very serious concern as welfare changes in the UK mean the sanctioning of welfare claimants, including single parents who have no child care, for not attending job interviews.

Practical help with securing suitable housing, for example, is increasingly not seen as part of the social work task, and there is evidence of practice that sees fathers' inability to secure suitable accommodation, even in extremely expensive cities like London, as evidence of 'their lack of commitment' to their children (Gupta *et al.*, 2014). This exemplifies the way need has become framed in a neoliberal society as individualised and evidence of risk (Featherstone *et al.*, 2014b). It also signposts the continuing retreat in the UK from a social work history rooted in an understanding of structural disadvantage and its inequities, and any conception of the social work task in child protection as being concerned to support families as distinct from detecting and dealing with child maltreatment.

There is a rather dated literature on the occupational discourses that circulated within social work offices in Wales that supported women as oppressed by men but also as ultimately responsible for children's welfare and protection. There are also discourses that support constructions of the absent/present men as dangerous and/or no use. There is evidence, however, that occupational identity overrode gender identity in that women and men social workers felt much more in common with each other than they did with same gender service users (Scourfield, 2003).

There is a much more recent research-based literature on the effects of widening inequality upon relationships within societies. Levels of trust are lower in more unequal societies as people cease to inhabit the same material and moral spaces (Wilkinson and Pickett, 2009). According to Clark with Heath (2014), policy reactions to the economic crisis have intensified such divisiveness. It is likely, according to Featherstone *et al.* (2014b), that such divisions have impacted upon social workers' sense of connection and solidarity with service users whatever their gender although empirical research is urgently required here.

Fathers, ethnicity and Indigenous communities

As indicated throughout this book, across many countries the issues in relation to ethnicity and Indigenous communities cast in sharp relief tensions around how services operate. In the UK over the years many authors have examined the experiences of black and other minority ethnic children and their families within the child protection system.

In terms of the representation of black children in the child protection and 'looked after' systems the evidence is unclear. Owen and Statham (2009) found that while overrepresented among children in need and in the 'looked after' population, black children were not overrepresented on child protection plans. However, recent research by Bywaters *et al.* (2014) found that a child's chances of being on a child protection plan (CPP) or a looked after child (LAC) was strongly statistically related to measures of area level deprivation. A child in the most deprived decile of neighbourhoods nationally had an 11 times greater chance of being on a CPP and a 12 times greater chance of being a LAC than a child living in the most affluent decile. This research only looked at area level deprivation and there is an urgent need to drill down to understand the issues at the level of individual families. The relationship between deprivation and ethnicity requires further sustained attention in light of the finding by Bywaters *et al.* (2014) that, after controlling for deprivation, black children were less likely than white children to be a LAC, contrary to prior evidence.

This supports a well-rehearsed hypothesis that black children and their families may be more *or* less likely to be subjected to child abuse investigations by English child protection authorities and allied practitioners – also referred to as a 'hands on/hands off' dilemma. On the one hand a *pathologising* approach to black families may lead to unnecessarily coercive intervention, as well as a *cultural relativist* approach, which leads to non-intervention when services are required. Either way, a particular set of dynamics operate to stigmatise black families' identities, devalue their experiences and foster professional discourses which are skewed towards a deficit focus, rather than a strengths-oriented approach, to interventions with black families (Bernard and Gupta, 2008).

In Canadian research, Brown *et al.* (2009) explored how fathers were manufactured as 'ghosts' in child welfare services; they pointed to particular issues linked to class disadvantage and those arising from Indigenous status. They suggested 'an analysis of gender, class, race and culture of child welfare discourses shows how these fathers are seen as deviant, dangerous, irresponsible and irrelevant' (p. 25). Thus they were frequently either invisible to practitioners or rendered invisible through practices that forced them to move out of the family home rather than engage in purposeful work to change.

Case example: men's participation

The following case example from the UK is of relevance in this context. Hasina lived with her husband Jai. They are black British with three children. Jai drank, had gambling problems and had been violent towards Hasina. She attended every meeting with the social workers and always made the children available so they could see and speak to them. Jai was angry and unwilling to meet with the social workers and had not taken up the offers of help with his drinking and gambling. There is no doubt this was not an easy situation for anyone concerned. In our research, which involved interviews with all the adults involved, it became apparent that, because the social workers had focused attention on the mother and not worked with them both together, an impasse had been reached (Featherstone and Fraser, 2012a). It is perhaps unsurprising that he resented an intervention that focused on 'empowering' the mother. While men resist social workers literally by not engaging or disappearing, social workers also 'disappear' men, thus placing the women who love them and/or are afraid of them, in very difficult situations. Women like Hasina can end up being categorised as 'passively compliant', an example of language use that renders the complexities of her situation invisible and also obscures the power/powerlessness nexus she is in (Featherstone and Fraser, 2012a).

Domestic abuse and child protection

Awareness of the physical and sexual violence experienced by women within and outside the home, coupled with a growth in understanding about the consequences of many women's economic dependence, has been a key achievement of the women's movement. In the UK in the 1970s, attempts to get social work to address violence for the sake of women's welfare were to prove unsuccessful. It was the linking of the abuse women received with the implications for children's welfare that was to prove of enduring significance culminating in legislative change and the linkage with emotional abuse.

While there have been some gains, we would argue that the insertion of domestic abuse into a child protection paradigm has been problematic for women, children and men. The majority of agency responses have tended to focus on the role of the mother in securing the protection and welfare of the children, and encouraging women to leave or to get the men to leave. This is a position that Mason (2005) called 'unsafe certainty'. While an illusion of certainty is pursued, the reality is that these men do not just disappear, they may hide, they may go onto other families and, moreover, their physical absence does not connote emotional absence in the lives of women and children. They leave traces of yearning as well as pain, traces that may be very difficult for mothers to manage as they deal with their own and their children's sense of loss and disappointment. The growing understanding that domestic abuse has harmful implications for children has often placed mothers in very invidious positions (see Chapter 6). Consider the following case example.

Case example: women's participation

Julia had experienced a childhood of sexual abuse and had been in care. She had three children and had been subject to domestic violence from a partner from whom that she had since separated. When she found herself sinking into depression, she approached children's services for help and they made her children subject to a child protection plan, an action she described as 'bullying'. This is a far from unusual response in recent years to situations where women experience domestic abuse. Because of increased awareness of the harm done to children when domestic abuse is occurring in families, it has been decisively reframed as a child protection issue with the consequence that many women end up being positioned as responsible for abusing their children because they are being beaten up.

Separation from an abusive partner is usually considered to be evidence that women are taking appropriate responsibility, although this ignores the inconvenient reality that separation can up the stakes dramatically and lead to an intensification of abusive behaviour. But in Julia's case her decision to separate was not considered enough evidence to show she was taking responsibility for her children's welfare as she had become depressed. This selfish behaviour on her part needed monitoring because of the well-established links between maternal depression (interestingly paternal depression is not usually assessed as a risk factor for fathers) and neglect. Perhaps unsurprisingly Julia expressed to the researcher that she felt she had been 'bullied all her life', by her abusers and the services supposed to protect and support her. She felt strongly that the decision to make her children subject to a plan was stigmatising and punitive in a context where she had freely sought some help for herself personally and as a parent (Featherstone et al., 2014b).

There have been gains for children because of the recognition of domestic abuse, in the form of developments such as therapeutic support, but they are often outweighed by the punitive focus taken towards their mother which can mean they lose both parents. Over the decades, researchers have noted that children sometimes blamed their mothers for 'putting fathers in prison' and there was a degree of idealisation of absent fathers (Featherstone, 2009). Such findings underscore the importance of developing relational and systemic understandings and approaches, and working on children's relational needs and identities. There are examples of practices with women and children such as the project run by the NSPCC in York, UK (Radford, 2013). This helps mothers and their children separately, and together, to explore their complex and conflicting feelings and journey towards healing together. But these projects are in a minority. There are also projects that use family group conferences (FGCs) but again these are not common. Daybreak is a charity that uses a FGC approach with domestic violence using a whole family approach.

There is a history of developing programmes that work with men who are violent to women in intimate relationships, although service developments tend to be patchy, and there can be reluctance in times of austerity to develop such resources because of beliefs that scarce services should be focused upon women and children. Moreover, such services are often reserved for those mandated by the courts and involve men who are highly abusive. While, as we note below, there are examples of services that are focused on early help seeking, these remain underdeveloped and difficult to access.

Programmes have usually been named *perpetrator* programmes and have their roots in the therapeutic, anti-sexist men's movement, and the women's refuge movement in the USA (see Featherstone *et al.*, 2007). Historically, it is the latter that emerged to set standards for treatment and safety as a result of concerns that those with a more therapeutic focus were in danger of excusing men's behaviour. Moreover, they were considered to be too isolated from mainstream services and, therefore, unable to ensure the safety of women and children (Rivett, 2010). The Duluth programme emerged over time as the main programme, reflecting a feminist perspective on the causes of violence as rooted in men's control and power over women in a patriarchal society, and masculine socialisation practices (Pence and Paymar, 1993). It was, and is, designed to be embedded within a coordinated community response and is not supposed to be a stand-alone programme. It has its origins in community reaction to the murder of a woman in a specific locale. This history is of relevance in understanding the apparent high level of anxiety about moving away from a set format. Safety planning for women and children is central. It comprises a set format where power, control and equality issues are systematically addressed and where cognitive behavioural therapies are used.

Over the years, Duluth programmes have been subject to a number of criticisms. Their set format is considered to be too prescriptive and insufficiently sensitive to the diverse needs of differing men attending programmes (Rivett, 2010). The question asked was whether they were suitable for men from different cultural backgrounds with different histories of oppression and racism. An allied critique contested the underlying theoretical approach as it assumed singular explanations for why men were violent (Gadd, 2004). A linked critique contested the reliance on cognitive behavioural approaches and argued for psychosocial approaches that engaged with unresolved childhood pain and trauma. A range of writers suggested the importance of recognising that not all violent men were the same (Gondolf, 2002) and that not all violence was the same (Johnson, 1995). Moreover, it is argued that the role played by factors such as mental health difficulties and substance misuse needs more consideration than is found in Duluth (Rivett, 2010).

The originating impulse of the Duluth model was to explain the violence in singular ways and to see any other explanation as part of men's attempts to excuse or minimise their behaviour. Thus poverty and racism were screened out explicitly as valid factors in understanding abusive life trajectories. This reflected a tendency towards dichotomising approaches as if one level of description or explanation necessarily excluded another. However, 'to say that violence, domination, subordination and victimization are psychological does not mean they are not also material, moral or legal' (Goldner *et al.*, 1990, p. 345). The importance of addressing the injuries arising from class, race and colonisation in men's lives is reinforced in this perspective.

In the last decade, as a result of a number of developments, men's identities as fathers *and* perpetrators of domestic violence have been highlighted and there has been a growth in interventions that engage with men who are violent as fathers. Featherstone and Fraser (2012b) conducted an audit of interventions in this area. A key reason for the growth was:

> Children's services are struggling to get a grip on the issue of domestic violence in families and one of the key problems is that it's such a widespread problem. They're really struggling to find an appropriate response because you know they recognize that they can't take every family where children are exposed to domestic violence to a child protection case conference. So you know sending fathers on perpetrator programmes is a very sort of attractive solution for children's services.
>
> (UK academic)

There has also been a growth in interest in engaging with fathers and domestic violence because of changes in public law, with contact between both parents seen as desirable even in circumstances where domestic violence was present. An influential development from Canada has been the 'Caring Dads' programme, which has a both/and philosophy (Scott and Crooks, 2004). It relates to men as fathers and as abusers; it contains gender reflections and assumes men can change, and explores men's maltreatment of children generally. While the originators of the programme see it as having a 'fatherhood' focus *and* a 'perpetrator' focus, this is strongly contested by those who would emphasise the need to stress the identity of perpetrator as primary and the necessity of adopting the Duluth format (Respect, 2010).

A degree of defensiveness and policing of programmes is evident with strong moral injunctions that experimenting may imperil women and children's safety. But innovation is also evident. For example, Strength to Change is a public health approach in the UK. It works with self-referrals and uses a variety of formats and theoretical approaches (Coulter, 2013).

Across many countries, such as Australia, Canada and the USA, where the traumas and injustices of colonisation have been uncovered, a range of projects that work with men around developing healthy fathering identities and practices are to be found. These address domestic abuse in ways that move away from a focus on blame and criminal justice responses (see Ashley, 2010 for details of programmes from Canada, New Zealand and Australia). These incorporate features such as healing, therapy and spiritual dimensions. In Australia, Aboriginal approaches emphasise the spiritual needs of families generally, as well as communities, and advocate the use of spiritual knowledge and developing 'circles of trust' in order to bring about change. This poses significant challenges to the highly rational blaming approach often found in some of the programmes seeking to engage fathers based on Western approaches.

Overall, an important conclusion from the literature on engaging fathers who are violent is their clear desire to be fathers whose children love and respect them, and who are not afraid of them and/or afraid for their mothers. Indeed, it is this that projects such as Caring Dads key into and build on to promote change.

Developing respectful and relational practice

> The tragedy is that none of us automatically responds to hardship, humiliation or the abusive exercise of power through noble resistance, we are just as likely

to turn our sense of grievance upon ourselves or innocent others. This is suffering turned upon itself and it is this double suffering which is often the subject of professional practice in welfare work.

(Frost and Hoggett, 2008, p. 455)

Frost and Hoggett (2008) have developed an important analysis of responses to social suffering using the concept of 'double suffering'. The notion of *social suffering* as developed by Bourdieu (1999) emphasises not just the unequal distribution of material goods in society but also people's lived experiences of oppression, and the feelings of humiliation, anger, resentment and despair that can accompany oppression: 'using material poverty as the sole measure of all suffering keeps us from seeing and understanding a whole side of the suffering characteristic of the social order (Frost and Hoggett, 2008, p. 4).

Frost and Hoggett (2008) argued that some experiences threatened to go beyond our capacity to digest them because we lacked the resources to symbolise and give meaning to them. They were more likely to be experiences that have been forced upon us rather than ones we had freely chosen; those we faced as powerless objects rather than as active agents. The most extreme examples were where people were forced from their land and their histories and languages suppressed. Frost and Hoggett (2008) suggested that, when experience could not be thought about, then we would have an unreflexive relation to it. If suffering could not be thought about, it would be somatised and embodied, acted out or projected.

In terms of somatised or embodied practices, Frost and Hoggett (2008) believed social suffering was inscribed on the body: The low self-esteem, low status, lack of social capital and lack of power to direct one's own life were written on the body and manifested in health inequalities and also self-destructive behaviours. Suffering was enacted, for example, through behaviour that was damaging or harmful to self and/or the environment. Suffering could also be projected onto others including, most obviously, those more vulnerable:

> Subjects of social suffering may not draw easily upon our compassion if they do not present themselves as innocent victims, but as aggressive, resentful or suspicious people whose hurt and loss is directed at others rather than at themselves.
>
> (Frost and Hoggett, 2008, p. 453)

Frost and Hoggett (2008) named the ethical challenges in *double suffering*, especially when we encountered those who were profoundly marginalised, who were harming others, and it was the difficulties here that could lead to the taking of seductive short cuts, such as 'I'm only here for the child!' (Featherstone et al., 2014b).

This is, of course, highly problematic, not least for Indigenous people who have consistently argued that Western approaches to 'the child' have little or no synergy with Indigenous values of family, community and the connection with land (Lonne et al., 2009). This does not mean that the violence and abuse that may be happening should not be dealt with, but short-term and individualist approaches need to be carefully reflected upon. Can appropriate help be provided? If not, why not? What might be the consequences? Above all, it is incumbent upon workers to reflect upon the fact that they are but 'brief visitors' in families' lives. Nonetheless, the consequences of what they do, or do not do, will endure.

Case example: children's understandings of their lives

Early in 2014, Claire, a social worker, received a phone call asking whether she was willing to meet two children, Tom and Joe. Five years previously she had initiated care proceedings that led to their being placed away from their father, with a long-term plan that they be placed for adoption. They were then four and three respectively. The children had requested the meeting because they wanted to know exactly why they were taken into care. They were seeking to re-establish contact with both their birth parents, but especially their father, as they had lived with him and had some memories of him.

Claire explained to the children when they met that it simply was not safe to leave them with their father as he was not supervising them properly, and there were no appropriate bedtime or meal time routines. A number of accidents had occurred in the home due to poor supervision, and they were both often very late for nursery school because of the lack of sleep routines. There was little doubt about his love for them, but he was 20 years old, and the assessment was that he was too immature to look after them. Moreover, he was estranged from his own birth family as he had been in care himself because of his parents' abuse. The children's mother too was only 20 years old and had been in care. She had left soon after Joe was born and lived in another town with a boyfriend who was very violent towards her, and there was a fear that he might, in turn, harm the children if they were placed with her. Claire told the children that the local authority felt the children needed a 'forever' family who had the resources to commit to securing their long-term welfare.

The children were very curious about what their parents had been like, and were particularly keen to know what help social workers had actually offered the parents to help them care for their children. They asked Claire many searching questions in this regard. In the following few days, Claire found her thoughts returning again and again to the children. She felt so relieved that they seemed happy and, although a plan for adoption had not been realised, partly due to Tom's increasingly difficult behaviour, they were together in a long-term foster placement. She was pleased that their connections with each other had not been severed and wondered what would happen in the current climate where the focus on adoption is even stronger than it was then.

Would the children be split up in order to maximise the chances of at least Joe, the younger and 'easier' one, getting adopted? She also reflected upon her own life since she had left the office where she had then worked. She had become a mother to a little girl now aged three, the age Joe was when she removed him, and this made her reflect with a great deal of pain on the ethical and emotional implications of her work. She found herself telling her husband about it that night after he had finished reading their daughter a good night story, and was taken aback by the look of utter pain that crossed his face. Claire wondered as she lay awake that night about the ethical aspects of her practice. Did she put enough effort into supporting the father and mother to break the cycle of care and loss they were in? Had she operated with enough care for the relational and lifelong identities of the boys?

Alternative approaches

We have argued that a relational understanding of children's needs and identities can only be fostered and promoted successfully when their parents' struggles in society, riven by inequalities, are recognised and supported. Calls for *father-inclusive practice* are crucial but must be located in this context. There are examples of practice approaches that offer possibilities for voice to be exercised by all family members, such as FGCs, avoiding the cul-de-sacs of a focus on the child as purely an individual. As discussed in Chapter 7, with their origins in Māori culture, FGCs are a response to widespread concerns from within the Māori community about the disproportionately high numbers of their children being removed from their families, and a sense that 'traditional' decision-making and problem-solving approaches were not being used to engage more positively with children's difficulties. While its potential in relation to developing and supporting inclusive models of family – rather than normative and restrictive notions based upon a particular model – has been highlighted (Featherstone, 2004), it is with its potential for engaging fathers and men more generally with which we are concerned here. Holland *et al.* (2005) in their study of FGCs in Wales found that 'one encouraging development – from the point of view both of those who want to take pressure of women and of those who want to improve men's access to services – is the high incidence of men's attendance at conferences' (p. 69). Clearly, getting more men there may not always be desirable, but exploration of process issues in this research suggested, for example, that fears of men dominating were not borne out, for a variety of reasons, including the 'style' of the conference. While this aspect of their evaluation was minor, there is increased interest in continuing to develop FGCs as a possibility for increasing men's participation in decision making about their children and in encouraging men, women and children to develop more 'democratic' models of relating (see Ferguson (2004) for an extended discussion on the role of welfare workers in fostering such practices and the theoretical premises underpinning 'democratisation').

Family Rights Group (FRG), a charity that operates in England and Wales offering support to parent and family and friend carers so that children may be enabled to be cared for safely within their networks, provides a professional advocacy service. The service targets parents whose children are particularly at risk of suffering significant harm, and being removed from their family. Direct face-to-face advocacy is provided from the point of initial investigation to the first child protection review conference. Indirect advocacy is the practice of professional advocates negotiating by letter, email or telephone on the service user's behalf, or with the service user on an ongoing basis in the name of FRG. The advocacy projects developed by the FRG draw upon the evidence of a qualitative research study on specialist advice and advocacy for parents in child protection cases (1997–2001) and are informed by the associated protocol funded by the Department of Health (Lindley and Richards, 2002). The authors drew on relevant policy and research literature to inform this work. Key themes from the protocol developed by Lindley and Richards (2002) are offered here.

It is crucial that advocates are independent of all agencies involved in child protection work, but independence needs to be worked at rather than assumed, and vigilance is required to ensure it is not jeopardised. It is not the advocate's responsibility to make enquiries where there is a suspicion of harm to children, but it is essential that they do not conceal information about any continuing or likely harm to a child. While there are no MR legal responsibilities to report information about such harm, advocates with a professional qualification (e.g. solicitors or social workers) are under a professional duty to do so, and others are under a moral duty to do so. Advocacy services need to provide training and supervision to support advocates making judgments about harm thresholds. Advocates are there for parents and are therefore partisan, but should be supported to remain dispassionate. An advocate's intervention is on behalf of parents and not by the advocate in their own right. Even if invited to, the advocate must decline to give their personal opinion about risk or the likelihood of particular case outcomes, but an advocate should not withhold information from the parent.

There is a sense in which advocates operate within an ethic of care; they offer rights-based advice in a context of stressing the importance of working within relationships, whatever the individuals may have done, or are suspected of having done. This is complex work in a context where there are multiple stakeholders. Evaluations have highlighted the possibilities it offers to service users to exercise voice and experience being heard, and recognised, in very daunting and frightening circumstances (Featherstone et al., 2011; Featherstone and Fraser, 2012a).

Returning briefly to the case example of Hasina and Jai highlighted above, the involvement of an advocate was considered by Hasina to have improved communication in the family, not least because the advocate had included Jai from the onset and seen him as part of the solution, and not just a problem to be removed. Of interest here is that this respectful and inclusive intervention not only engaged Jai, but was experienced much more positively by Hasina than a model of practice overtly focused on 'empowering' her by getting him to leave. Women may not only want practitioners to work with men for their own sakes, but also be for the sakes of their children. In research with women on whether they felt interventions should be directed at men, the majority said yes, and some spoke of their sadness that their children did not have the fathers they deserved, and asked for help to make such services happen (Roskill et al., 2008).

Clearly, working across race, gender and class divides are areas of cross-cultural practice that require reflective self-awareness to identify cultural, class, race and gender blind spots. In closing, we have placed another case example below for readers to further explore the issues raised in this chapter.

Case example: maintaining connection

John is a 21-year-old man of Jamaican parentage, born and living in London. He has little contact with is family of origin and was in care from the age of ten. He has a two-year-old son who he does not live with. He had a relationship with the mother which broke down after the child's birth because she became very depressed and went to live with her mother. Her mother does not like John and considers that he is not a good influence on her daughter because he is not employed and hangs around with other young men who have been in trouble with the law and do drugs. So it has been difficult to get contact with his son and he has not seen him for a year. He has heard that child protection workers are involved because his former girlfriend has got a new boyfriend and has moved out to live with him. She has left their son with her mother who is now seeking to be approved as a kinship carer for the little boy. John is very worried about his son growing up without his involvement or indeed any knowledge of him and arranges an appointment with a social worker to discuss what his rights and options are.

John is a young black man who has been in care:

* What might the issues be for a practitioner to consider in terms of race and gender when meeting and seeking to engage him?
* How might a practitioner convey respect and openness to John?
* What assumptions might inform professional assessment about John as a father or as an ongoing carer for his son?

Conclusion

In this chapter, the focus has been on the issues raised by working with fathers across cultures. It has also addressed some of the difficult issues raised by domestic abuse and highlighted some of the messages emerging from research, particularly that with families themselves about their fears and desires in relation to respectful and relational practice. Case examples have been used to highlight the complex issues and relational aspects of practice. The following chapter explores the ethical use of information within child protection practice.

Reflective questions

1　How might you work in culturally safe ways with service users and others who are different to you?
2　How might gender differences affect your own practice framework?
3　Are there ways that your own organisation could further develop its approaches to working across class, gender and cultural differences?
4　What approaches might you take to learning more about working cross culturally?

Chapter 14 Using information ethically

While the focus of this chapter is how practitioners use information, including how they gather, record and share it, we commence by examining how service users might view the *sharing of personal information*. This does not necessarily come easily. Why might this be? First, it is *potentially embarrassing* for service users sensitive about 'washing their dirty laundry in public'. Second, there is a lot at stake, thus openness is a risky business given the potential consequences. Third, their *relative powerlessness* (as discussed in previous chapters) balances the scales against them, thus the requirement of *openness* might seem unfair and unwise in these circumstances. In a submission to the Queensland Crime and Misconduct Commission inquiry into Queensland's child protection department, Lonne (2003) explained:

> Put simply, if parents can form a trusting relationship with departmental staff they are usually able to work productively to address the factors that led to abusive or neglectful behaviours and events. On the other hand, if staff poorly exercise their power and authority, parents can be put offside and find it difficult or impossible to establish a trusting working relationship. The appropriate use of power is fundamental to good child protection interventions.
>
> Furthermore, the establishment of effective working relationships is primarily the responsibility of departmental staff, because it is extremely difficult for parents to be trusting when they have so much at stake. Most are fearful of losing their children. Hence, they tend to be very reluctant to fully disclose information about the abuse and other private family matters, fearing that if they disclose they will be subject to criminal charges and lose their children. Being distrustful, they can usually quickly sense if a departmental officer is comfortable and appropriate in their use of power, or is instead prone to adopt a bullying or overly forceful approach.
>
> Having someone a lot younger than you who is professionally trained (and likely earning more than you) ordering you around and holding all the aces can be very unsettling for parents and may prove fatal for developing trust. These factors can significantly affect the nature of the helping relationships.
>
> (Lonne, 2003, p. 3)

Sharing information: a risky business?

When service users, particularly parents, are responsible for child maltreatment, working with child protection workers places them in a quandary: if they are wholly

178

truthful, there is a real possibility they and their children will face severe impacts; if they withhold information or act deceptively and are found out, they risk serious consequences. Hence, many service users use strategies of obfuscation or 'tell them nothing' as the way forward (Dumbrill, 2006); this further complicates an already complex situation. Even those who have not caused harm to children face uncertainties and anxieties when confronted with an official interview about how they care for their children.

Child protection workers have a key role in giving service users *bad news*, or at least, 'unwelcome news', particularly the assessment that abuse or neglect has occurred, or is highly likely to occur, or information relating to injury to their child in out-of-home care (see Chapter 10). Despite legislative and procedural guidance defining maltreatment, reconciling the evidence with situational and cultural variables can be challenging (Lonne, 2015). While some incidents are unambiguous, many are not. Personal and cultural thresholds raise thorny issues in establishing what is in the *best interests of the child*. This sort of situation makes it very difficult to build the kind of trusting relationship needed to achieve clarity about the risks to children. The responsibility to build an authentic and trusting relationship in which open dialogue can occur rests with the practitioner (see Chapter 11).

Truth telling or deception

Truth telling is essential and must sit alongside respect for people's legal rights and privacy. Lying and deceiving, however, can give people a sense of power over others, though is fatal to the building and maintaining of trusting relationships. A conundrum exists for child protection workers undertaking investigation and assessment interviews with service users. Reliable assessments require the collection of all the relevant information from those involved – the child, their parents and relatives, and significant others, such as teachers, neighbours and health professionals. People may be unwilling to divulge their full story if they do not have faith in the fairness of the process, feel their information will not be treated confidentially and will be used against them. More often than not, child protection workers are unable to promise complete confidentiality; they are duty bound to pass information on to others in child protection matters. For example, approximately one in four child protection parents participating in Victoria's Child and Family Services Outcomes Survey believed their private information had been used inappropriately by child protection workers and confidential information was released and used against them in legal proceedings (QUT and SRC, 2013). Many felt aggrieved by this. Dale's (2004) English study of parents' perceptions of child protection interventions identified their appreciation of being treated fairly and openly by police, in contrast to their relationships with other professionals, such as social workers, who were perceived to fabricate, distort and exaggerate concerns.

Procedural fairness and due process requires that the details of allegations against people suspected of harming children be provided to them, and that they be afforded the opportunity to respond to these allegations (see Chapter 9). However, this raises several perplexing questions: what if someone who has provided information does not wish others to know what they have said? What if the information received is vital to the protection of the child but sharing it will likely cause harm to someone else? For example, a parent discloses information about their partner and thereby places

179

themselves at risk of a vengeful response. And, what should be done when someone makes a report to the child protection department, which is, by law, confidential, and during the subsequent investigation the outraged parents conclude, rightly or wrongly, that they know who reported them and decide to confront them?

Confidentiality, informed consent and relational practice

Clearly, withholding and sharing information requires a consideration of the ethics of confidentiality and informed consent and, despite mandatory reporting policies, there are legal consequences for withholding information or sharing information inappropriately (see Chapters 6, 9 and 10). Most child protection legislation calls for information that identifies reporters to be kept confidential and used only for the purpose of putting the law into effect, through authorised protective interventions such as when child protection workers arrange for a child to be placed with foster parents; in such situations they need to provide sufficient information about the child, his or her family history, behaviour that may place others at risk of harm, or that is necessary for ensuring the child's well-being, including medical and health issues, and other matters related to the care-giving role. Importantly, information should only be used for the purposes for which it was collected, and provided to others to enable them to properly undertake their role and perform their duties. Deciding how much detail people need requires judicious consideration of service users' rights to privacy, the sensitivity of the information and the benefits and costs of sharing it (see Chapter 10). Kennedy *et al.* (2013) note there are competing demands for such decisions: 'one set of imperatives protects information, and the other allows or compels disclosure' (p. 100).

As well as keeping information confidential, records need to be stored securely and accessible only to those with authorised access (Kennedy *et al.*, 2013). Releasing and sharing information with others is often done on a 'need to know' basis and most agencies have organisational policies on client access to their records and confidentiality requirements. Implicit in a 'need to know' regime is that judicious discernment is required to determine what exactly people do, and do not, need to be aware of to carry out their duties. A guiding standard is ensuring the release of information will not cause significant harm to anyone; this requires consideration of all those with a stake in the matter, as well as the potential risk and seriousness of harm that could result. Prior to releasing information, seeking consent from those who have provided it typically entails exploring with them the merits of this and negotiating what exactly should be released and how. Even when the law allows practitioners to release information without informed consent, there are real benefits in seeking their consent, not least because it enables broader participation in the decision-making process and the sharing of power. Such dialogue facilitates ongoing relationship-based work and enables service users to have some control over the information shared and confidence that they will be informed prior to any release. Parton and O'Byrne (2000) suggested a constructionist and narrative approach is respectful of service users' rights as it:

> does not privilege professional, disciplinary or expert knowledge over clients' knowledge. On the contrary, a person's knowledge of his or her experience (local knowledge) is viewed as an essential element of the work. In order to understand a human situation we must go to the actors themselves and the act

of telling their stories not only becomes the focus of the work but a central way in which their situation can be improved … In this view, a … relationship is a partnership, with each party bringing something of value to the conversations. A constructive approach emphasises process, plurality of both knowledge and voice, possibility and the relational quality of knowledge … Through conversation we explore, evaluate and engage with each other and the qualities with which we imbue this dialogue affect the process. Compassion, respect, affirmation, permission and interest are all likely to increase the chances the dialogue will realise its creative potential.

(Parton and O'Byrne, 2000, pp. 184–185)

This dialogical approach forms a platform for participatory decision making in the use of information, and gaining informed consent for its release. As Parton and O'Byrne note:

… it is an approach that recognises not only the importance of dialogue but that language is crucial for constructing the experiences and identity of both the self and the interaction, and which takes seriously the diverse elements of power which are involved.

(Parton and O'Byrne, 2000, p. 187)

Working with service users and sharing the issues surrounding keeping or sharing information with them is a very powerful exemplar for the judicious and ethical use of power. Information gives people power, withholding it can increase their power and sharing it can enhance relational equality.

Rights-based information sharing

Using a *rights-based approach* to information sharing and release enables practitioner cognisance of the need to ensure they have well-founded reasons for collecting, sharing, using and storing client information. This is part of the integrated framework for child protection practice advanced in this book (see Chapter 9). A rights-based framework ensures checks and balances to the misuse of power and requires practitioners to:

- know the legal and organisational requirements relevant to child protection work, including principles and processes for treating people fairly and impartially (see Chapter 9);
- understand universal human rights protocols, including the obligations and protections to prevent discrimination and infringement of people's citizen rights (see Chapters 5);
- hold values consistent with the pursuit of social justice and equality (see Chapter 10);
- practise in ways that embody integrity and relational practice (duty of care, respect and justice) (see Chapter 10); and
- embrace personal reflection and reflexivity to assist in the practitioner's development and organisational learning (see Chapter 6).

Practising from a rights-based framework ensures a critical lens. As outlined in Chapter 5, human rights are a liberal Western invention; they are individualistic in nature, and frequently the rights of some conflict with the rights of others (Connolly and Ward, 2008). Nevertheless, there is such a thing as collective rights, such as the rights of service users:

> ... the more focused the practitioner is on the service user's human rights, the more likely it is that an environment will be created which fosters positive change. We therefore see a focus on rights-based ideas, including those that impact on the relationship between practitioners and service users, as central to achieving good outcomes.
>
> (Connolly and Ward, 2008, p. 176)

Rights-based practice sits comfortably with the principles of procedural fairness, whereby service users are informed in a timely way of decisions that affect them and the reasons why they have been made. If practitioner assessments could reasonably be perceived as detrimental to the service user's interests, the reasoning behind these assessments should be explained clearly, and an opportunity provided for clients to dispute or challenge the conclusions reached by providing new information that was not available to the assessor. They should also be advised of the legal avenues for appeal available within the organisation and the broader child protection system (Kennedy *et al.*, 2013).

Sharing and recording information

A rights-based approach has implications for how records are kept. Language and its construction is vitally important (Parton and O'Byrne, 2000). Practitioners should use plain, easily understandable language, uncomplicated by technical, professional and legal jargon. Hence, recording entails the exercise of discretion and *judicious consideration* of what to include and exclude. Different parties articulate their perceptions of facts in various ways, and agency records need to accurately capture these differences. 'Facts' can be disputed, or their interpretation within practitioner assessments can be hotly challenged, and record keeping should identify areas that are contested. Information should be described in ways that do not shut down discussion about how events and conversations might be interpreted. Rather, there needs to be a *clear separation between the facts and professional opinion*, understandings, and interpretations of the facts. Professional opinions are based on specific understandings of the disciplinary, organisational and practice context in which assessment is conducted and any biasing effects should be made explicit. The logical reasoning used to assess the case should be clearly articulated, including aspects that are unclear or unknown. Changes to dated previous assessments should also be recorded. Most importantly, sufficient information needs to be recorded at key decision points to ensure service users, particularly children, are kept properly informed (see Chapter 13). Describing why particular decisions were made may be just as important as why others were not.

Formal records need to provide a reliable and complete account of events and ensure transparency and accountability (see Chapter 10). Records should be in sufficient detail to enable the relevant and important information to be quickly ascertained, but not so detailed as to include extraneous material. All information should be written or recorded in a way that is accessible for review by service users and accountability forums reviewing cases. Records are sometimes made available to criminal or civil courts adjudicating matters involving maltreatment. Nothing should be put into formal records that practitioners are not perfectly comfortable having examined by these bodies and service users. Nonetheless, case records can sometimes contain information or opinion that is defamatory or hurtful and practitioners need to avoid this when recording events (Kennedy *et al.*, 2013).

Records have material impacts on the lives of service users and therefore need to be reliable and complete. When service users access agency records it can be quite emotionally confronting, and the language used by practitioners, for better or worse, can have a long-lasting impact. Service user's narratives about their dealings with child protection can be hardened or softened by what is written in official records (see Chapter 8). There are many reasons people access these historical records, but often it is for sense-making purposes, related to their identity and need to understand the events that have shaped their lives, or to reconnect with their past (see Chapter 13). Service users should be assisted to have the official record altered when it contains factually incorrect or untrue assertions, and this includes having the records include their rebuttals to practitioner assertions and assessment conclusions. It is critical to get record keeping right and this entails practitioners being upfront, transparent, accountable, dependable and reliable in recording their encounters with service users and others. Tobin (1994) noted virtue 'ethics is about doing the right thing and … about being the kind of person who can be relied upon to do the right thing' (p. 55).

Case example: releasing information (part 1)

Lui Chen is a children's hospital social worker who has been working closely with Maria Lopez and her four-year-old daughter Betty. Maria has another three children aged 12, 10 and 9 years. Betty has a moderate intellectual disability, and some other significant physical health issues, including lupus. Lui has become increasingly concerned about Maria's deteriorating care of Betty resulting from her need to hold down three part-time jobs since her welfare benefit was cut off by the government. Maria has shared with Lui that, at times, she has left Betty home alone while she went to work because she could not afford childcare, and she needs the work for the family to survive. Maria also disclosed to Lui a very recent event where the children were home alone in the early evening as she had to work a late shift, and Betty wandered off by herself, eventually being returned by a stranger who found her wandering a nearby street.

Lui knows that the child protection department have previously investigated Maria's care of the children. Lui meets with Morgan, who works in the department about other protection cases, and spontaneously shares her concerns about Maria and Betty, explaining that she wants the matter to remain strictly confidential as she is seeking to organise support services. She outlines recent episodes of the children being left unattended, sharing identifying details as she seeks to find out whether or not there is any current departmental contact with them. She is, however, clear with Morgan that she is not making a formal report of suspected maltreatment and expects him to treat the matter as confidential. Morgan tells Lui that he is unaware of the family but that other staff in his office may be having contact with them.

What ethical issues are evident here?

There are a number of ethical issues evident in this scenario. However, all these issues will be perceived differently depending on the organisational and legal context of particular stakeholders. There are some key ethical issues: establishing whether abuse or neglect is present or has occurred, and reporting measures (see Chapter 10). The determination of the occurrence or risk of maltreatment is primarily, but not exclusively, the remit of the child protection authorities and, as shown in Chapter 9, there is much complexity and discretion evident in decision making about this. A related ethical issue is the duty to protect and safeguard the vulnerable, particularly concerning Betty who has higher needs due to her disability.

A central ethical concern surrounds the family's access to the necessary supports they require to flourish as a family, and the standards of care provided by Maria and the hospital, which has a duty toward Betty and her mother. As we have noted, particularly in Chapter 5, the redrawing of the welfare settlement and the prioritising of paid work for all can place mothers such as Maria in very difficult, almost impossible, circumstances, caught between differing and competing imperatives; child protection services require her availability to care for her children, while welfare systems require her to be engage in paid work. Moreover, in neoliberal policy contexts safe and adequate child care provision is often considered the responsibility of the individual parent. In this scenario, Maria is between the proverbial rock and a hard place, and welfare regime requirements to work, in presumably low-paid employment, to ensure she gets needed state support for her children seemingly disregard the realities of her children's needs to have an accessible parent and carer available.

The confidentiality of the information shared is also a key ethical issue, along with the seeking of informed consent from Maria for its release. Because informed consent was not sought by Lui, there is potentially a breach of the respect owed to Maria. Finally, the maintenance of cooperative and collaborative interagency relationships may be at risk due to the informal information-sharing process used, and damaging collaborative arrangements presents ethical issues to the ongoing provision of aid and support to other families.

Who has a stake in this situation?

As outlined in Chapter 6, there is a diverse range of stakeholders in child protection work, with various interests and concerns constructing the ethical, legal and practical issues differently. Some will have a specific interest in the child's health, for example, while others, like social workers, might differ on the consequences they perceive, and whether these are more immediate or longer term. There are, of course, Maria, Betty and her three siblings who are centrally involved and who have a material interest in the process and outcomes. Lui and Morgan are also primary stakeholders, along with their supervisors, and organisational colleagues and leadership more broadly. Other stakeholders, including politicians, managers and community members, also have a stake in the outcomes, including organisational reputations concerning confidential records maintenance.

What other options did Lui have for dealing with this matter?

While Lui opted to discuss the matter informally with Morgan, other options were available to her. Lui recognised she needed guidance about how best to respond.

The DECIDE model identifies the importance of defining the problem. Assembling relevant information can help to clarify exactly what is at issue and, subsequently, which ethical principles are relevant, and the options that exist. Gathering information about what the problems are enables clarity to emerge, and Lui could have first sought information and perspective from within her own organisation, and used her supervisor as a sounding board to understand better the case and its complexities. This would have enabled her to assemble information about the organisational and legal context and its requirements upon practice, as well as defining the problem and the key ethical principles. Similarly, seeking guidance from her professional association using non-identifying information about these would have helped Lui. Gaining perspective about the matters at hand is essential for sound ethical decision making and is in keeping with the use of reflective and reflexive practice.

Another key option not taken up by Lui was to consult with Maria about her situation and her concerns, using their existing strong relationship as the platform for dialogue. A dialogical approach to the exploration of issues at hand builds the client-worker relationship (see Chapter 11). Importantly, it seeks to reposition the power within the helping relationship and enable unseen solutions to arise from the ensuing discussion. By not discussing her concerns about the care of the children with Maria, Lui kept the issues within a professional realm of decision making, thereby depriving Maria of awareness of the concerns, but also a constructive role within the process of option exploration and solution. A rights-based approach would see Lui's decision to not engage with Maria about her concerns as antithetical to the recognition of her rightful part in the decision-making process around protecting her children. Maria could likely be very receptive to information about the concerns held, and the sorts of changes required to prevent maltreatment, as well as the roles and responsibilities of the child protection department. Not involving her precludes this except in an otherwise reactive context, where Maria would likely feel left out of discussions about her family's situation.

Lui could have also reported the matter to the child protection department using existing protocols. If formal policy or legal requirements to do so was in place Lui would have a duty to do this, presuming that the facts of the situation meet the necessary definitions and thresholds. Doing this would not have necessarily precluded an ongoing productive relationship with Maria and the family, particularly if she advised them about her obligations prior to making the report. She could then continue to advocate for the family to access the needed supports and assistance (see Chapter 13). It is arguable that such an option would necessitate an open and honest discussion with Maria, and that there are no guarantees that reporting will lead to anticipated outcomes. There is real tension between this option and the one involving constructivist dialogue with Maria, and this could have been openly acknowledged and its characteristics explored.

> *If you were Morgan in this situation, how would you describe the ethical issues, and what options would you have for dealing with them?*

The ethical issues for Morgan are similar in many respects to those perceived by Lui as they entail the potential occurrence of maltreatment, reporting obligations and confidentiality requirements. Yet, because Morgan is employed by the child protection department and carries specific legal duties and organisational responsibilities, his perspective is likely to be focused upon the risk of harm to the children, particularly Betty. His duty to carry out the law, exercising appropriate discretion and assessment skills is integrally linked with his duties, legal and ethical, to protect the vulnerable from harm. We know that ethics and the law can be in conflict (see Chapter 9). But what about truth telling? Did Morgan advise Lui of whether he was able to keep the information she provided confidential? If not, why not? Did he attempt to clarify his legal responsibilities about the use of information? The issue of the confidential nature, or otherwise, of the information that Lui provided has arguably become a key issue that requires attention. Does Morgan require prior consent before he can, legally or ethically, pass this information onto others? Should Lui have got prior consent from Maria before passing on details of the family situation? The ethical use of information is now front and centre for consideration in this case, and ought to have been part of Maria and Morgan's initial discussions.

Within a child protection paradigm the focus of intervention can be unnecessarily narrow and largely ignore other important considerations, such as the inequality and harsh welfare measures that underpin this family's situation. In Chapters 5–8, we outlined the individualised nature of child protection that holds parents and caregivers entirely responsible for their children's situation. Risk of harm is the key criterion, and notwithstanding the tension that exists with other considerations, this will likely dominate consideration of the issues and options. Nonetheless, the ethical issues identified by Morgan should also include those inherent in the very complexity and uncertainty we have outlined earlier. These include the impacts of investigation on the family such as stigma and increased stress, the potential damage to the hospital and community support system for the family from increasing Maria's suspicion about being put under surveillance rather than helped, and the consequences upon interagency relations from the tensions between the various statutory and voluntary intervention options. As outlined in Chapter 10, should interventions subsequently include removal of the children from Maria's care, then there should also be an active consideration of the ethics in doing so, particularly in light of the negative impacts of placement disruption and failures in the standard of care.

The DECIDE model entails identification and analysis of the key ethical principles prior to consideration of the options. Doing so allows proper reflection concerning the tensions that exist between principles, such as safeguarding, judicious information sharing, protecting service-user rights, and equity and fairness aspects that exist in this case. Moreover, the model facilitates the incorporation of both a logical reasoning process and the emotional and relational aspects to a situation, for example, the strength of the helping relationship between Lui and Maria. Taking statutory action with respect to the identified risks will likely have a consequence for the trust that Maria places in her future relationships with formal sources of support, thereby impacting upon the well-being of the children. Morgan should not ignore these considerations when exploring the issues and options available.

Case example: releasing information (part 2)

When Morgan returns to the child protection department office, his team leader, Serena, advises him that as a departmental officer he has an overriding duty to protect children who may be at risk, and therefore no agreement to confidentiality can be given. She instructs him to make a report out of the information he has received and to organise to visit the family residence, investigate the situation, and assess the risk to the children, especially Betty. Morgan does so. The next day he receives a call from a very irate Lui who accuses him of unethical behaviour for using without her consent the information she shared. She tells him that Maria has accused her of breaking professional rules by releasing without her prior consent confidential information shared by Maria with Lui, and she vows to never see her again. Maria has also reported Lui's actions to the hospital management. Lui tells Morgan that she will report his behaviour to the department's head office for breaching professional confidentiality. She tells him to forget about any ongoing interagency cooperation. Morgan is taken aback by these events and meets with his team leader to work out what to do.

Is there an ethical issue facing Morgan now? If yes, what is it?

This scenario illustrates how protective interventions can set off a train of unforeseen events, particularly when consideration of the options has not included their possible consequences. The ethical issues are not substantially different for Morgan than what they previously were, although they are different in nature, for example, they now clearly involve relational aspects that affect the cooperative working of the central stakeholders, and may therefore impact upon the risk to, and well-being of, the children. While Morgan may see the potential risk to Betty and the other children as the primary ethical issue, this does not give licence to ignore other related issues.

To be responsible, open, and accountable as a practitioner one has to be able to explain fully and justify the actions that have been taken. In this case, the key ethical issue now facing Morgan is the use of information he received and, specifically, the perceived breach of confidentiality. As outlined earlier, the matter raises issues of truth telling and the process used by both Lui and Morgan in sharing details of the case with others, while not first seeking informed consent for its release. The disputes that have arisen go to the ethics rather than the legalities – that is, what is the right thing to do with information perceived as private and confidential? The actions taken by Lui and Morgan have impacted negatively upon their working relationships, yet these are essential foundations for effective protective work. The perceived breaches of confidence are also likely to affect the reputations of those involved and the extent to which others see them as trustworthy.

What sorts of legal and organisational matters should be
considered concerning the claims about confidentially?

As Dickson (2009) notes, tensions exist between what is legal and what is ethical (see Chapter 9). While the law in the particular jurisdiction may allow the release without prior consent of information about risk of harm to children, this does not necessarily mean that doing so is perceived by others as ethical. Clearly, in this case, Maria and Lui are unhappy with the release of the information to others without their prior consent. They believe that their information has been misused and reputational risk has resulted. Sometimes individual cases can highlight bigger systemic issues and failures.

These need to be closely examined so that lessons can be learned. Organisational reputation is important and conflicts need to be managed so that their 'good name' does not unnecessarily suffer.

Moreover, statements from Lui indicate that ongoing interagency cooperation and collaboration may cease. There is an ethical implication from such a stance, namely, that other unrelated service users and families may not receive the sorts of integrated service responses that they need because frontline practitioner relations have soured. System integrity is a fuzzy concept but nonetheless real. It entails notions of ethical practice and dependability in the delivery of services that meet both individual service users' needs but also that of the broader society; hence, when questions arise about defensive and risk-aversive practice, these not only concern individual cases, but also system-wide mandates and responsibilities. This case raises questions about practitioner and organisational trustworthiness, and therefore requires action by the hospital and the child protection department to resolve the matters in dispute through appropriate forums that are respectful and ensure people's rights are assured.

What ethical principles might apply to this scenario?

Referring to the key ethical principles identified in Chapter 10, we can see that those that apply here include: the child's best interests; safeguarding children; judicious information sharing; protecting the service user's interests; maintaining a relational perspective; and equity, fairness and consistency. Applying these in decision making, though, entails recognising that there are tensions between them, and they may be in conflict, particularly when stakeholders have different organisational missions, values, roles and perspectives. As we have argued elsewhere (see Chapters 9 and 10), it is inappropriate to just cite a single principle as the be all and end all in practice considerations. Unfortunately, this has often happened with the misuse or misapplication of the 'best interests' principle. Even where legislation identifies this principle as the paramount one, this should never mean that it is the only one ever considered.

Child protection decision making involves assessment of complex human behaviour, ethics and legal and policy requirements, as well as situational specifics that defy simplistic approaches such as the exclusive use of the 'best interests' principle. Understanding the need to safeguard these children does not give licence to ignore the duty to protect service users' interests, or ensure equitable and fair responses. The laudable ends of protecting children do not give practitioners carte blanche to justify the means used to do so. Practitioners should not, like Pontius Pilate, wash their hands of responsibility for adverse impacts on others by merely resorting to the asserted benefits for the protection of children. Rather, workers need to use their moral and logical reasoning to identify the problems and issues, determine the relevant facts and primary ethical principles, and assess the merits of the available options, all within a process that values relationship in protective outcomes.

What options might Maria, Lui and Morgan now have to deal with this matter?

The advent of conflict here might well be the prompt for dialogue around weighty ethical and protective issues. As we have explained, differences in perspective about the ethical problems, issues, principles and options can legitimately arise from the various roles and responsibilities that exist. Dialogue is needed to facilitate deeper appreciation and understanding of these by all stakeholders, shared understandings, as well as to realign the use of power within the relational contexts of various interactions and responsibilities.

Maria is likely to remain relatively, but not completely, powerless in this situation because of the impoverishment she experiences, her gender and the 'othering' that occurs for many people suspected of causing harm to children. Her issues around the breach of her family's privacy and the conduct undertaken in the release of information without her involvement or prior consent are, nonetheless, critical to the options to be explored. These are legitimate issues that demand resolution, and advocacy by others can be of great assistance. Resolving Maria's issues provides an opportunity to re-build trust and the working relationships necessary to protect the children and safeguard their well-being. Within such a dispute-resolution process associated matters can also be addressed, including the stigma associated with investigation, the power imbalance, ensuring her rights, and recognising her emotional reactions to the perceived betrayal of trust. 'Clearing the air' is likely to be essential for the protective issues to also be addressed. Extra support for Maria may also be necessary to assist her to deal with the added stress that will have probably resulted.

Lui's options include taking the issues up through her own organisation to seek resolution to them through more formal processes. Why? Because the organisations are stakeholders with their reputations at risk. The questions surrounding the legal and practice definitions and thresholds for intervention also need to be addressed, uncertainties clarified and differing perspectives recognised. Dispute resolution processes for the relationships between Maria, Lui and Morgan are also required, so that the working relationships can be restored, or if this is unattainable, for other suitable working arrangements to be employed. This may require a change of practitioner for Maria. Lui will likely need support as these sorts of conflicts can be quite stressful, not the least because they require significant attention to providing detailed records of the events and decision-making rationale.

Morgan will have similar options and requirements to help him deal with these stressful events. As noted earlier, merely relying on a legal justification for his actions will often not be sufficient if significant ethical issues remain unaddressed. It may be likely that Morgan will be advised to hand over case responsibility to someone else if the relational aspects remain problematic despite attempts to resolve them. It is important for both Lui and Morgan to have close supervision that enables them to deconstruct these events, and to develop greater reflective and reflexive capability that will facilitate their learning and professional development, not the least being their own parts in the creation of the matters at issue.

Case example: recording and sharing information

Aalia is a practitioner working at a faith-based fostering service that is contracted to the child protection department to provide support, training and guidance to a range of foster parents and kinship carers who care for children in the care of the department, and support and casework for the children in their care. There are strict legislative, policy and contractual requirements to be complied with concerning the standards of care provided in the placements, and the safeguarding of children. Aalia takes these matters very seriously and is aware of the tensions that can exist in trying to meet the needs of all concerning proper standards of care.

Aalia undertakes regular casework with an 11-year-old girl who, along with her three younger siblings, has been placed with her maternal aunt and her male partner for the past several years when it became clear that her mother's drug habit and related criminal behaviour led to them being exposed to her criminal associates and abused. It meant that they could no longer stay at home as the 11-year-old girl was sexually abused by one of her mother's many boyfriends, and her younger brother, who is physically disabled from cerebral palsy, was physically abused.

Aalia has become concerned about some matters the girl has raised with her about her aunt's partner, who has a diagnosis of Asperger's and presents as having difficulties interacting socially with others, and lacks non-verbal communication skills. The girl tells Aalia she is really worried about how he behaves around her siblings, particularly the physical games and wrestling that occurs, which she thinks is rude and 'really weird stuff' that leaves her feeling highly anxious about whether they are at risk of sexual abuse. The girl describes the games and demonstrates the sort of touching that goes on during these regular games which makes her feel uncomfortable. She begs Aalia to keep the information she has shared secret as she doesn't want to jeopardise the placement or hurt her aunt who has been very good to them. The girl fears that the placement would end and that the family would be broken up and sent to unknown foster parents. She says she would rather kill herself than see the family split up.

Aalia is unsure about what to do, particularly as finding placements for large families is very difficult and from what she knows of the aunt there is a strong likelihood that the placement would end if the matter comes to light. The regular three-monthly report to the department is due and Aalia feels uneasy about what she should include.

- What is the key ethical question facing Aalia?
- What are the most relevant facts?
- Who are those with a stake in this situation?
- What are the ethical duties stakeholders carry and to whom are their primary duties owed (in particular focus on confidentiality and respect)?
- What options might Aalia consider to address ethical and risk issues?
- How do these resonate or otherwise with the identified duties and principles?
- What information, if any, should Aalia record here (and in so doing explain and justify the ethical decision making)?
- What information, if any, should be passed on and to whom?

Conclusion

In this chapter, we have examined the process of ethically using information in child protection, and the legal and organisational contexts that come to bear upon decision making about sharing and releasing information. The relational impacts surrounding information use are critical. We have shown how there are legitimate stakeholder differences in the perspectives that can be taken concerning the presenting problems, the ethical issues and the options available. A case example has been used to unpack and explore the intricacies involved in the complex matters arising from sharing information and understandings of confidentiality. In Aalia's case example above we have outlined relevant questions for readers to discuss, and below we pose some further reflective questions around the complexities of ethically using information. In the final chapter we overview the key points made about ethical practice and using the DECIDE model, as well the implications for the ever-changing institutional and community environment for child protection practice.

Reflective questions

1 How might practitioners negotiate the legislative, organisational and ethical considerations relevant to the use and release of information?
2 How can practitioners manage ethical dilemmas arising from wider policies that mean individual parents have to manage very contradictory demands in the context of information sharing?
3 What might be some of the complexities in a truth telling approach?
4 In what sorts of situations do you believe it is ethical to break confidentiality?
5 How well does a rights-based framework fit with your personal and organisational approaches to information sharing?

Chapter 15　**Travelling hopefully**

Interventions in the lives of children, families and communities are hugely consequential and profoundly ethical in nature. Such interventions involve human connection and engagement in the personal and family lives of citizens who are themselves embedded in their own network of relationships. Practitioners face a vast array of often confusing situations and ethical questions as they balance multiple demands, emerging ideas, new perspectives, available evidence and numerous competing interests in complex relationships, while working to a risk-averse societal mandate that is increasingly focused on protecting children from an ever-expanding array of harms. Indeed, as we write, there is a storm brewing about the actions of the police and child protective services in Maryland investigating parents for neglect as they allowed their children (aged 6 and 10 years) to walk home unaccompanied from a park (Greenfield, 2015).

The definition of neglect has expanded dramatically in some Western countries in recent decades and, as this example demonstrates, continues to expand within a child protection mandate that seems to be operating under authoritarian and, indeed, paternalistic norms (Lonne, 2015). There are, of course, many situations where children are manifestly suffering but what should be done cannot be decided by simply applying numbers to a 'risk template', adding the figures and calibrating what this numeric character means in terms of safety.

In this book, we have proposed a comprehensive and integrated ethical approach to dealing with what is now often referred to as a 'wicked problem' (ARACY, 2009a). Applying this approach and framework to difficult decisions does not give practitioners immediate answers. There is no simple formula, which, if followed, gives precise answers to vital matters of huge human concern, such as guaranteeing the safety of children. We have presented ethical decision making as a process requiring critical discernment around the contextual elements to determine the ethical issues present, name the questions, and work out which ethical principles pertain most suitably to finding solutions that achieve the best outcomes possible. All practitioners have to use critical reflection. All ethical decision making is deeply practical and circular, as well as linear and rational, and, particularly in situations involving children and families, highly emotion laden. It involves the head and the heart, and demands personal awareness and professional judgment, and reflexivity at every turn.

New ideas emerging from research, scholarship and practice in the social and natural sciences contest the ways in which we think about how to respond to individual problems and collective trauma. The neuroscience discourse that is now heavily cited to support either risks or opportunities in child protection and family welfare practice – depending on who is translating it – provides significant insights and challenges to practitioners and policy makers alike. Additionally, there is growing evidence on health and welfare inequalities associated with demographic vicissitudes, the effects of colonisation, racial discrimination, and extreme poverty, and the implications of these findings for child and family well-being. In addition, there have been significant and far-reaching developments in public policy that have increasingly embraced and promoted community development and public health approaches to deal with the implications of these inequality data for children, families and communities. Added to this contextual mix are changing community attitudes, including changes in community perspectives and values on matters to do with childrearing, gender relations, racism (and racial inequalities), addictions, and health and illness. These research findings require us to engage in constant review of our theoretical base, and robust cross-disciplinary and intersectoral collaboration in decision making.

Importantly, the demands for accountability to all stakeholders in the human services have increased markedly in recent years. The voices of children, care leavers, their families and communities, as well as other communities of interest, have provided a quality and type of evidence not previously understood, and coupled with rising costs and poor outcomes of many protective systems, this evidence has added a new urgency to the need to clarify decision-making practices and review policies in child protection and family welfare. Throughout this book, we have sought to name and highlight how these changes have affected ethical debates and decision making for practitioners and policy makers concerned for the welfare of children and families, particularly those at the vanguard of child protection practice.

Noted throughout previous chapters is the growing awareness that child protection is at least at a watershed, if not in crisis. This is evident in multiple ways – in the now extensive knowledge of the unintentional harmful outcomes to whole communities, as well as individuals, of much intervention; the escalating numbers of reports of abuse and children removed from families; the failure of, and abuse in, institutional care; the unavailability of sufficient and safe foster and kinship care options; the dramatic burnout among child protection workers and failures to retain workforce numbers; and, unsustainable cost increases alongside many poor outcomes for children, families and communities.

Practitioners cannot be expected to manage alone this highly emotionally politicised work, and the processes and consequences. In order to find answers, managers, policy makers, legislators and families must become partners with them in their efforts to understand and deal effectively and ethically with the challenges we collectively face. An appreciation of this changed context at the micro, meso and macro levels is essential if we are committed to ethical practices and wish to participate in responsible deliberations that are open to public scrutiny about the values and evidence for our decisions.

In the remainder of this chapter, we briefly capture the essence of the contemporary environment for practitioners, families and communities under the heading *Distance and danger*. Our focus, however, is on the possibilities of what we have called *The alternative story* that captures our hope for a future in which service user, stakeholder and community find a place in professional decision making, and where children's well-being and safety are located as much as possible within the context of their ongoing relationships.

Distance and danger

In Chapter 1, we recounted a story from England that provides a compelling example of how a singular focus on the safety of a child can lose sight of the broader contextual and environmental issues vital to ethical decision making. In so doing, we identified the important theme we call *distance and danger*. In this context, we underscored the contemporary 'omnipresent focus' on risk that is a feature of contemporary child protection practice. We argue this is one important theme, among many, that is contributing to an increasing distancing between statutory practitioners and families and communities; this, we argue, can impede enlightened ethical decision making and potentially risks engaging in the 'othering' of service users (see Chapter 8). This case study also highlights the organisational mandates and constraints on practitioners and recognises the signals of danger that have become endemic in system design, and which so profoundly influence practitioners and alienate service users and other stakeholders.

In the contemporary environment, facts are gathered and decisions are made in locations very distant from the life worlds of children and their families and communities. Practitioners and their managers can be distanced from their own values and professional principles by rampant proceduralisation and the ever-present threat of making a decision that leaves them publicly, morally, organisationally and legally vulnerable. Relentless attention to structural change following endless inquiries seems to have been at the expense of the attention that needs to be paid to the more subtle aspects of present relationship and culture so central to the child's family and community life – and to their connection and identity.

In terms of these continuing structural changes, we note the significance to all service users and stakeholders of the escalating worldwide policy directions toward privatising child protection services, which involves placing the welfare of children in the hands of private enterprise. For practitioners, child protection practice often feels like dangerous territory to work in, even though their motivation is enlightened and the rewards for ensuring child safety are evident. For many practitioners, privatised practice suggests more danger in an already fraught environment. Who will set priorities and whose voice will be heard? How will the very real tensions between maximising profits and ensuring safety and well-being of the vulnerable be resolved? What checks and balances are needed to ensure that the institutional priorities do not override the moral obligations to protect and serve? How is the public good to be maximised within these private-capital governance arrangements? We have noted that we work in an environment in which, despite the best of intentions, lip service is often paid to the voices of service users – be they children, young people, parents, families or communities. And it is an environment in which the participation of service users and other stakeholders is often precluded (and distanced) by the relentless pressure of work and the need to make urgent decisions.

Many stakeholders talk of the distancing alienation they feel as a result of dashed hopes for a renewed social contract in child protection, which appeared to be promised following public apologies for earlier child protection practices that accompanied previous child rescue approaches. Nowhere is this distancing expressed more powerfully than in the reports by, and research work with, Indigenous peoples and those from communities of colour. In a powerful way, they capture the essence of the requests from many service users and stakeholders to return to engaging with a respectful place for community, harnessing caring families and coordinating care networks. All research and reports recognise the need to protect children from danger and many also observe the acknowledged failures of the state to care adequately for children, particularly the Stolen Generations in Australia. There is scant evidence that the state has proved to be a good parent for the children in its care. Having engaged with the wisdom of the 'private realities' of Indigenous parents, researchers Ivec, Braithwaite and Harris (2012) talk about the loss of the hope of families and communities in promised new directions, and the urgent need to acknowledge past and present dangers and deal in hope and renewal:

> The well-being of children is of concern to parents who have lost their children, to carers who have become surrogate parents, and to child protection authorities that regulate both parents and carers. For this reason, harnessing the caring networks should not be as difficult as it has become.
>
> (Ivec *et al.*, 2012, p. 99)

The alternative story: commonality and community

Our hope in this book is that we might support moves from a story too often characterised by distance and danger to one that stresses commonality and community. Hope has been central to the stories human beings construct for themselves over the ages: hope in a better after world, in the hereafter or for the one we currently inhabit, or indeed both. Richard Rorty (1999) understood hope as a metanarrative, a story that serves as a promise or reason for expecting a better future. While he was dismissive of many of the most powerful of longstanding metanarratives, he recognised the importance of what he called 'social hope'. We echo this and make common cause with those who advocate that such calls are rooted in debate and deliberation rather than exhortations supported by reference to absolute principles.

This book is rooted in a concern to restore the deliberative and dialogical in this area of work and to open up this way beyond practitioners who cannot and should not carry such a project alone. Indeed, we would suggest it is profoundly unethical to ask them to do so and agree with Warner (2014) that change is only possible through alliances with others who have a stake in the system. She notes that the most problematic of these constituencies, at present, is the established conventional media but actually this is the one about which we should be least concerned. We agree that, while it is an important mediator of opinion, a focus on the media may not be the most pressing of our concerns, and the most important constituency comprises the parents, children and families who come into contact now or in the future with child protection and family welfare services. The most powerful of the constituencies includes the politicians whose rhetoric and actions have a profound impact and who may well construct scandals to satisfy short-term political objectives.

In engaging all concerned, the following questions are central: why should families be supported to care safely? Indeed, this is the most profound question of all. How can social supports be developed and provided in ways that recognise and foster already existing strengths and protective capacities within families and communities? What kind of policies and practices are required to counter the poverty and disadvantage that makes good parenting so much harder to achieve, especially for those with histories of cumulative trauma? As we have identified through the book, there are considerable policy practice examples that can help us with addressing these questions:

> In the morning of 16 March 2011 it was raining in New York. Nevertheless by 9.30 Arnhold Hall at the New School University off Sixth Avenue in Manhattan was filled with close to 200 leaders of the city's child welfare system. The city and state commissioners, foster care agency executive directors, caseworkers and parents had gathered to talk about parent advocates in the foster care system. Parent advocates are mothers and some fathers whose children have been placed in foster care. Whereupon, these parents changed the behaviour that caused them to lose their kids, regained custody of them, underwent training, and were now working in foster care agencies helping other parents struggling with the types of problems they had overcome.
>
> The forum was the culmination of 20 years of parents organizing on the outside, moving to the inside, fighting to have their needs addressed and their opinions heard, and finally having their work valued and funded by government and voluntary agencies. The forum was an acknowledgment that parents and the parents' movement had played an important role in reforming New York City's child welfare system.
>
> (Tobis, 2013, p. ix)

As Tobis notes, the movement lifted the pessimism that affected the parents concerned but he also notes the broader populations' responsibility to join with them, increase their strength and, crucially, to destroy the wider pessimism that things would not improve. We would suggest that this pessimism concerns not only families in the system and their supposed intractability, but also the ability of welfare institutions to deliver social goods. Tobis asks his readers to imagine what it is like for families trapped in the system:

> Anyone who has experienced their own difficulties might think about the times we have been depressed, have not had enough money, have drunk too much, or have broken promises to ourselves. Think about the mistakes each of us has made while parenting. Imagine what our responses might have been without resources to fall back on – skills, money, family, friends, and connections. And think of what would be seen if our lives were constantly scrutinized.
>
> (Tobis, 2013, p. 217)

His is a plea to move beyond the process that occurs in societies where those with difficulties are seen as 'other' and their suffering not recognised or hidden behind a technocratic and abstract language of expertise and risk. Kleinman and Kleinman (1991) argued that the process of writing the details of personal experience in the language of expertise adds to the suffering as it sanitises the 'brute' facts. While economic indicators of suffering may be necessary in terms of rationalising resource distribution, they all too often lead to people being treated as problems and instrumentalised. Featherstone *et al.* (2014b) argue the language that is often used, particularly in policy documents and guidelines, and associated research reports on child protection, not only instrumentalises people (especially parents), but also actually removes them as real, live, breathing, intelligible beings, with whose meanings we need to engage in the context of their lived experience. Indeed, not making them visible (warts and all) compounds their exclusion and suffering. The role of families themselves is of vital importance in increasing visibility, emphasising strengths and capacities, and advocating for changes rooted in the everyday realities of living with poverty, discrimination and a lack of respect.

ATD Fourth World (http://4thworldmovement.org) is a human rights-based, anti-poverty organisation with more than 40 years' experience of engaging with individuals and institutions to find solutions for the eradication of extreme poverty. In the UK, it is working with academics, politicians and practitioners seeking to influence how policies and practices in the area of child protection can be developed in a more respectful way, fully cognisant of the human rights of all concerned. This ongoing work is engaging a variety of constituencies in workshops, training events, education and conferences to examine all aspects of practice, highlighting how disrespect is conveyed at the most basic of levels (for example, in practitioners constantly being late for meetings). Deficit-based approaches sap confidence and demoralise people already struggling with considerable difficulties. By contrast, recognising people's strengths in 'getting on and getting by' provides a respectful platform from which further change might be possible.

Practice focused largely on seeing the individual family, and what is happening within such families, should not be dismissed. Categorical thinking can strip the humanity from the person seen as an instance of class or race, for example. However, such practices can miss the bigger picture and, crucially, the common threads uniting families struggling with multiple adversities to care safely, often in very challenging local environments. Community development approaches offer important possibilities in this respect, as we have noted in this book. Jack and Gill (2010) suggest a number of practice examples to counter individualistic and reactive approaches to safeguarding children and young people. These proactive approaches take a broad view of the factors affecting children's health and safety and aim to develop a community which is informed and thoughtful about child protection, and emphasises that high levels of poverty, unemployment, traffic and crime provide the context in which most safeguarding concerns and childhood accidents have to be understood. They developed neighbourhood-based family support, community action with young people and positive action to build on the strengths of families and communities.

In the USA, Strong Communities for Children is a large-scale example of a neighbourhood-based child protection system (Melton et al., 2008). It has demonstrated effectiveness in mobilising large numbers of volunteers and organisations in diverse communities (Melton, 2014). But it is also showing potential usefulness not only in promoting child safety but also in meeting other important goals for community health. Indeed, it emerged from the US Advisory Board on Child Abuse and Neglect's collective view in the early 1990s that the challenges posed by the ongoing crisis in the child protection system and the generational decline in social capital were intertwined, thus necessitating community-based approaches. This is a clear difference from approaches that locate the harms children experience solely with their parents' or caregivers' acts of omission or commission, as a result of either their poor characters or their poor choices. The focus on community also acts as a necessary corrective to approaches that locate maltreatment solely within poor attachment patterns or poorly functioning brains.

An interesting example provided by Melton and Andersen (2008) relates to the role of religious institutions. These are often considered, with good reason, as sources of risk to children. However, they note that religious institutions can be leading resources in the development of community-wide safety nets for children. In the Strong Communities for Children initiative in the upstate region of South Carolina, multiple indicators show that, even in an area dominated by theologically conservative congregations, churches have been most heavily engaged in protective action to strengthen families and thereby prevent harm to children. They also point to Safe Families in Chicago, another faith-based project providing support to ensure the safety of children with positive results.

Protective interventions should supplement rather than supplant these tapestries of informal familial, neighbourhood and community care that provide the vast bulk of protection, support and tangible assistance for children and families. Yet, despite the political rhetoric that 'child abuse is everyone's business', child protection policy development has led to widely expanded functions for professional practitioners, with the role for the broad community often relegated to that of social surveillance and reporting (Melton, 2005). We argue for transformation through increased recognition of the centrality to family life of this vital web of care and significant investment to re-build community-level capabilities through community development strategies. Such approaches offer much better value regarding the reinvigoration of community capacity and connection than do the prohibitive costs of continued expansion of child protection and family welfare systems that seem increasingly aligned with punitive welfare policy formulations. Indeed, there are very real risks that without a fundamental re-alignment of contemporary child protection approaches that these systems will collapse under the 'dead hand' of highly bureaucratised and proceduralised approaches, persistent net widening and immobilised helping processes.

In conclusion, we hope we have shed some light on embedding ethics into child protection policy and practice and the thorny question of how we practise ethically in the highly regulated organisations that bear the important responsibility of protecting the safety of children and families in society. We hope this book opens spaces for dialogue on what it means to work ethically in child protection and that due recognition is given to the role and resources of families and communities in serving the best interests of children everywhere.

We recognise that this transformation is a task for all stakeholders. There is a shared responsibility in embedding ethics into our protective and welfare systems. Indeed, leaving it solely to child protection workers and associated health, human services and education practitioners is itself, in our view, unethical. Policy makers, executives and managers have critical roles in setting the organisational and programme parameters that enhance the public good through providing accessible and effective services for vulnerable children, families and communities. System leaders have both the authority and the responsibility to guide the required policy development and change processes.

Ethics should not be assigned the role of 'optional extra' for our current approaches. Rather, working ethically is a necessary foundation for the protection of the vulnerable and the rendering of assistance to those in need. Embedding ethical considerations into policy and practice frameworks should be a cornerstone for ensuring that there are proper checks and balances upon the necessary function of exercising state power in intervening in family life in order to protect children from maltreatment. We remain optimistic that this book will provide students, practitioners, managers, policy makers and stakeholders alike with renewed passion for dialogue around ethics in child protection. Hence, we champion the quest of 'agents of hope' to play their part in the ongoing reform of our child protection and family welfare systems. Dialogue of the issues presented in this book and the model for ethical decision making is a necessary part of this transformation into more humane protective and caring interventions. While there are risks, clear benefits are also evident. We are travelling hopefully in our quest for a better way for all concerned.

References

Allan, J. (2004). Mother blaming: A covert practice in therapeutic intervention. *Australian Social Work, 57*(1), 57–70.

Anscombe, G.E.M. (1958). Modern moral philosophy. *Philosophy, 33*(124), 1–19.

Aristotle (1954). *The Nichomachean ethics of Aristotle.* Tr. Sir David Ross. London: Oxford University Press.

Arney, F. and Scott, D. (eds). (2013). *Working with vulnerable families: A partnership approach* (2nd edn). New York: Cambridge University Press.

Ashley, C. (ed.). (2010). *Working with risky fathers.* London: Family Rights.

Ashley, C., Featherstone, B., Roskill, C., Ryan, M. and White, S. (2006). *Fathers matter.* London: Family Rights Group.

Asquith, M. and Cheers, B. (2001). Morals, ethics and practice: In search of social justice. *Australian Social Work, 54*(2), 15–26.

Australian Institute of Health and Welfare (AIHW). (2013). *Child Protection Australia 2011–12,* Child Welfare series no. 55. Cat. no. CWS 43. Canberra, ACT: AIHW.

Australian Institute of Health and Welfare (AIHW). (2014). *Child Protection Australia 2012–13,* Child Welfare series no. 58. Cat. no. CWS 49. Canberra, ACT: AIHW.

Australian Research Alliance for Children and Youth (ARACY). (2009a). *Inverting the pyramid: Enhancing systems for protecting children.* Canberra, ACT: ARACY.

Australian Research Alliance for Children and Youth (ARACY). (2009b). *What is collaboration?* Canberra, ACT: ARACY.

Bala, N., Zapf, M.K., Williams, R.J., Vogl, R. and Hornick, J.P. (eds). (2004). *Canadian child welfare law: Children, families and the state.* Toronto, ON: Thompson Educational Publishing Inc.

Banks, S. (2006). *Ethics and values in social work* (3rd edn). Basingstoke: Palgrave Macmillan.

Banks, S. (2008). Critical commentary: Social work ethics. *British Journal of Social Work, 38,* 1238–1249.

Barclay, P.M. (1982). *Social workers: Their roles and tasks.* London: Bedford Square Press.

Batchelor, J. (2003). Working with family change: Repartnering and stepfamily life. In M. Bell and K. Wilson (eds), *The practitioner's guide to working with families* (pp. 147–168). Basingstoke: Palgrave Macmillan.

Bauman, Z. (1993). *Postmodern ethics.* Oxford: Blackwell Publishers.

Beauchamp, T.L. and Childress, J.F. (2001). *Principles of biomedical ethics* (5th edn). Oxford: Oxford University Press.

Beckett, C., McKeigue, B. and Taylor, H. (2007). Coming to conclusions: Social workers' perceptions of the decision-making process in care proceedings. *Child and Family Social Work, 12*(1), 54–63.

Ben-Arieh, A. (2015). Community characterisitics, social service allocation, and child maltreatment reporting. *Child Abuse and Neglect, 41,* 136–145.

Beresford, P. (2014). What service users want from social workers. *Community Care*, 1–8. Retrieved from www.communitycare.co.uk/2012/04/27/what-service-users-want-from-social-workers (accessed 30 March 2015).

Berland, C., Cardinal-Stone, W., Chewka, D. and Schroder-Prince, M. (2011). Trauma and Iyiniw people. In R. Boder (ed.) *Indigenous social work practice: Creating good relationships* (pp. 19–46). Edmonton, Alberta: McCallum Printing Group.

Bernard, C. and Gupta, A. (2008). Black African children and the child protection system. *British Journal of Social Work*, 38(3), 476–492.

Bessant, J. (2013). History and Australian child welfare policies. *Policy Studies*, 34(3), 310–325.

Bevan, G. and Hood, C. (2006). What's measured is what matters: Targets and gaming in the English public health care system. *Public Administration*, 84(3), 517–538.

Bilson, A. (2007). International issues of children's participation and protection. *Child Abuse Review*, 16, 349–352.

Bilson, A., Cant, R. Harries, M. and Thorpe, D. (2013). A longitudinal study of children reported to the Department of Child Protection in Western Australia. *British Journal of Social Work*, 45(3), 767–770.

Blackstock, C., Trocmé, N. and Bennett, M. (2004). Child maltreatment investigations among Aboriginal and non-Aboriginal families in Canada: A comparative analysis. *Violence Against Women*, 10(8), 901–916.

Bourdieu, P. (1999). *The weight of the world: Social suffering in contemporary society.* Cambridge: Polity.

Bozalek, V., Henderson, H., Lambert, W., Collins, K. and Green, S. (2007). Social services in Cape Town, South Africa: An analysis of the perspectives of service providers from the political ethics of care. *Social Work/Maatskaplike Werk*, 43(1), 31–44.

Bradshaw, J. (2011). *The well-being of children in the UK* (3rd edn). Bristol: Policy Press.

Brodie, K., Paddock, C., Gilliam, C. and Chavez, J. (2014). Father involvement and child welfare: The voices of men of color. *Journal of Social Work Values and Ethics*, 11(1), 1–33.

Bromfield, L. and Higgins, D. (2005). *National comparisons of child protection systems: Child abuse prevention issues.* Melbourne, VIC: National Child Protection Clearing House, Australian Institute of Family Studies.

Bronfenbrenner, U. (1979). *The ecology of human development.* Cambridge, MA: Harvard University Press.

Bronfenbrenner, U. (1986). Ecology of the family as a context for human development: Research perspectives. *Developmental Psychology*, 22(6), 723–742.

Brown, C. and Augusta-Scott, T. (2007). *Narrative therapy: Making meaning, making lives.* Thousand Oaks, CA: Sage Publications.

Brown, I., Chaze, F., Fuchs, D., Lafrance, J., McKay, S. and Thomas Prokop, S. (2007). *Putting a human face on child welfare: Voices from the prairies.* Regina, Saskatchewan: Centre for Excellence for Child Welfare.

Brown, L., Callahan, M., Strega, S., Walmsley, C. and Dominelli, L., (2009). Manufacturing ghost fathers: the paradox of father presence and absence in child welfare. *Child and Family Social Work*, 14(1), 25–34.

Bruce, M. (2014). The voice of the child in child protection: Whose voice? *Social Sciences*, 3(3), 514–526.

Bruer, J. (1999). *The myth of the first three years.* New York: The Free Press.

Buber, M. (1958). *I and Thou.* New York: Scribner.

Buckley, H., Carr, N. and Whelan, S. (2011b). 'Like walking on eggshells': Service user views and expectations of the child protection system. *Child and Family Social Work*, 16, 101–110.

Buckley, H., Whelan, S., Carr, N. and Murphy, C. (2008). *Service users' perceptions of the Irish child protection system.* Dublin: Office of the Minister for Children and Youth Affairs.

Buckley, H., Whelan, S. and Carr, N. (2011a). Like waking up in a Franz Kafka novel: Service users' experiences of the child protection system when domestic violence and acrimonious separations are involved. *Children and Youth Services Review*, 1, 126–133.

REFERENCES

Burgess, C., Rossvoll, F., Wallace, B. and Daniel, B. (2010). 'It's just like another home, just another family, so it's nae different': Children's voices in kinship care: a research study about the experience of children in kinship care in Scotland. *Child and Family Social Work, 15*, 297–306.

Burke, B. and Harrison, P. (2009). Anti-oppressive approaches. In R. Adams, L. Dominelli and M. Payne (eds), *Critical practice in social work*. (2nd edn). (pp. 209–219). Basingstoke: Palgrave Macmillan.

Busch, M., Wall, J.R., Koch, S.M. and Anderson, C. (2008). Addressing the disproportionate representation of children of colour: A collaborative community approach. *Child Welfare, 87*(2), 255–278.

Butler, I. and Drakeford, M. (2005). *Scandal, social policy and social welfare* (2nd edn). Bristol: BASW/Policy Press.

Bywaters, P. (2015). Inequalities in child welfare: Towards and new policy, research and action agenda. *British Journal of Social Work, 45*(1), 6–23.

Bywaters, P., Brady, G., Sparks, T. and Bos, E. (2014). Child welfare inequalities: New evidence, further questions. *Child and Family Social Work*. Retrieved from http://bjsw.oxfordjournals. org/content/early/2013/05/02/bjsw.bct079.short?rss=1 (accessed 8 July 2015).

Cameron, G. and Freymond, N. (2006). Understanding international comparisons of child protection, family service and community caring systems of child and family welfare. In N. Freymond and G. Cameron (eds), *Towards positive systems of child and family welfare: International comparisons of child protection, family service, and community caring systems* (pp. 3–27). Toronto, ON: University of Toronto Press.

Cameron, G. and Freymond, N. (2015). Accessible service delivery of child welfare services and differential response models. *Child Abuse and Neglect, 39*, 32–40.

Carpenter, M. (2009). The capabilities approach and critical social policy: Lessons from the majority world? *Critical Social Policy, 29*(3), 351–373.

Carroll-Lind, J., Chapman, J., Gregory, J. and Maxwell, G. (2006). The key to the gate-keepers: Passive consent and other ethical issues surrounding the rights of children to speak on issues that concern them. *Child Abuse and Neglect, 30*, 979–89.

Carter, V. and Myers, M. (2007). Exploring the risks of substantiated physical neglect related to poverty and parental characteristics: A national sample. *Child and Youth Services Review, 29*(1), 110–121.

Child Trends. (2012). Child maltreatment. Retrieved from www.childtrends. org/?indicators=child-maltreatment (accessed 30 March 2015).

Christensen, D., Todahl, J. and Barrett, W. (1999). *Solution-focused casework: An introduction to clinical and casework management skills in casework practice*. New York: Walter de Gruyter.

Claiborne, N., Auerbach, C., Lawrence, C., Liu, J., McGowan, B., Fernendes, G. and Magnano, J. (2011). Child welfare agency climate influence on worker commitment. *Children and Youth Services Review, 33*, 2096–2102.

Clapton, G., Cree, V. and Smith, M. (2013). Moral panics, claims-making and child protection in the UK. *British Journal of Social Work, 43*(4), 803–812.

Clark, C. (2006a). Moral character in social work. *British Journal of Social Work, 36*, 75–89.

Clark, C. (2006b). Against confidentiality? Privacy, safety and the public good in professional communications. *Journal of Social Work, 6*(2), 117–136.

Clark, T. with Heath, A. (2014). *Hard times*. New Haven, CT: Yale University Press.

Cleaver, H. and Freeman, P. (1995). *Parental perspectives in cases of suspected child abuse*. London: HMSO.

Clifford, D. and Burke, B. (2009). *Anti-oppressive ethics and values in social work*. Basingstoke: Palgrave Macmillan.

Collins, S. (2008). Statutory social workers: Stress, job satisfaction, coping, support and individual differences. *British Journal of Social Work, 38*, 1173–1193.

Commission to Inquire into Child Abuse. (2009). *Final report*. Dublin: Commission to Enquire into Child Abuse. Retrieved from www.childabusecommission.ie/publications/index.html (accessed 30 March 2015).

Congress, E. (1999). *Social work values and ethics: Identifying and resolving professional dilemmas*. Chicago, IL: Nelson-Hall.

Congress, E. (2010). Codes of ethics. In M. Gray and S.A. Webb (eds), *Ethics and value perspectives in social work* (pp. 19–30). London: Routledge.

Congress, E. and McAuliffe, D. (2006). Professional ethics: Social work codes in Australia and the United States. *International Social Work*, 49(2), 165–176.

Connolly, M. and Ward, T. (2008). *Morals, rights and practice in the human services*. London: Jessica Kingsley.

Cooper, K. and Stewart, K. (2013). *Does money affect children's outcomes? A systematic review*. York: Joseph Rowntree Foundation.

Corley M., Minick P., Elswick R. and Jacobs, M. (2005). Nurse moral distress and ethical work environment. *Nursing Ethics*, 12(4), 381–390.

Coulter, M. (2013). Strength to change. Paper presented at Safeguarding and Domestic Violence Conference, Durham, UK, 21 May.

Council of Australian Governments (COAG). (2009). *Protecting children is everyone's business: National Framework for Protecting Australia's Children 2009–2020*. Canberra, ACT: FaHCSIA. Retrieved from www.dss.gov.au/our-responsibilities/families-and-children/publications-articles/protecting-children-is-everyones-business/protecting-children-is-everyone-s-business-national-framework-for-protecting-australia-s-children-2009-2020-annual-report-2010-11 (accessed 30 March 2015).

Crittenden, P. (1999). Child neglect: Causes and contributors. In H. Dubowitz (ed.), *Neglected children: Research, practice and policy* (pp. 47–69). Thousand Oaks, CA: Sage.

Cross, J., Dickmann, E., Newman-Gonchar, R. and Fagan, J. (2009). Using mixed-method design and network analysis to measure development of interagency collaboration. *American Journal of Evaluation*, 30(3), 310–329.

Crowe, J. and Toohey, L. (2009). From good intentions to ethical outcomes: The paramountcy of children's interests in the Family Law Act. *Melbourne University Law Review*, 33, 391–414. Retrieved from www.law.unimelb.edu.au/files/dmfile/33_2_3.pdf (accessed 30 March 2015).

Culpitt, I. (1999). *Social policy and risk*. London: Sage.

Cummins, P., Scott, D. and Scales, B. (2012). *Report of the Protecting Victoria's Vulnerable Children Inquiry*. Melbourne, VIC: Department of Premier and Cabinet. Retrieved from www.childprotectioninquiry.vic.gov.au/report-pvvc-inquiry.html (accessed 30 March 2015).

Curtis, C. and Denby, R. (2011). African American children in the child welfare system: Requiem or reform. *Journal of Public Child Welfare*, 5(1), 111–137.

Dale, P. (2004). Like a fish in a bowl: Parents perceptions of child protection services. *Child Abuse Review*, 13, 137–157.

Dalrymple, J. (2005). Constructions of child and youth advocacy: Emerging issues in advocacy practice. *Children and Society*, 19, 3–15.

Daly, M. and Lewis, J. (2003). The concept of social care and the analysis of contemporary welfare states. *British Journal of Sociology*, 51(2), 281–298.

Daniel, B. and Taylor, J. (2001). *Engaging fathers in health and social care*. London: Jessica Kingsley Publishers.

Daniel, B., Taylor, J. and Scott, J. (2010). Recognition of neglect and early response. *Child and Family Social Work*, 15, 248–257.

Davies, H. (2009). Ethics and practice in child protection. *Ethics and Social Welfare*, 3(3), 322–328.

REFERENCES

Davion, V. (1993). Autonomy, integrity, and care. *Social Theory and Practice, 19*(2), 161–182.

D'Cruz, H. and Gilligan, P. (2014). Improving child protection services: Australian parents' and grandparents' perspectives on what needs to change. *Practice: Social Work in Action, 26*(4), 239–257.

de Boer, C. and Coady, N. (2007). Good helping relationships in child welfare: Learning from stories of success. *Child and Family Social Work, 12*, 32–42.

Devaney, J. (2004). Relating outcomes to objectives. *Child and Family Social Work, 9*, 27–38.

Dickey, B. (1986). *No charity there: A short history of social welfare in Australia*. Sydney, NSW: Allen and Unwin.

Dickson. D.T. (2009). When law and ethics collide: Social control in child protective services. *Ethics and Social Welfare, 3*(3), 264–283.

Dingwall, R., Eekelaar, J.M. and Murray, T. (1983). *Protecting children, controlling parents: State intervention and family life*. Oxford: Basil Blackwell.

Dolgoff, F., Loewenberg, F. and Harrington, D. (2009). *Ethical decisions for social work practice* (8th edn). Belmont, CA: Thomson, Brooks Cole.

Drake, B., Jolley, J., Lanier, P., Fluk, J., Barth, R. and Jonson-Reid, M. (2011). Racial bias in child protection: A comparison of competing explanations using national data. *Pediatrics, 127*(3), 471– 478.

Dubowitz, H. (2007). Understanding and addressing the 'neglect of neglect:' Digging into the molehill. *Child Abuse and Neglect, 31*(6), 603–606.

Dubowitz, H. (2013a). Neglect in children. *Pediatric Annals, 42*(4), 73–77.

Dubowitz, H. (2013b). (ed.). *World perspectives on child abuse*. Aurora, CO: International Society for the Prevention of Child Abuse and Neglect.

Dumbrill, G. (2003). Child welfare: AOP's nemesis. In W. Shera (ed.), *Emerging perspectives on anti-oppressive practice* (pp. 101–119). Toronto, ON: Canadian Scholars Press.

Dumbrill, G. (2006). Parental experience of child protection intervention: A qualitative study. *Child Abuse and Neglect, 30*(1), 27–37.

Dumbrill, G. (2010). Power and child protection: The need for a child protection service users' union or association. *Australian Social Work, 63*(2), 194–206.

Dumbrill, G. and Lo, W. (2007). Bridging service users and service providers' knowledge systems: Issues of power. Paper presented at Canadian Association of Schools of Social Work Conference, Saskatchewan, May.

Dunk-West, P. and Verity, F. (2013). *Sociological social work*. Farnham: Ashgate.

Durrant, J.E. (2006). From mopping up the damage to preventing the flood: The role of social policy in the prevention of violence against children. *Social Policy Journal of New Zealand, 27*, 1–17.

Ellis, C. (2007). Telling secrets, revealing lives: Relational ethics in research with intimate others. *Qualitative Inquiry, 13*(1), 3–29.

Endres, B. (1996). Habermas and critical thinking. *Philosophy of Education Archive*. Retrieved from http://ojs.ed.uiuc.edu/index.php/pes/article/view/2259/954 (accessed 9 July 2015).

Esping-Andersen, G. (1990). *The three worlds of welfare capitalism*. Princeton, NJ: Princeton University Press.

Eurochild. (2010). *Children in alternative care: National Surveys* (2nd edn). Retrieved from www.crin.org/docs/EuroChild%20Children%20in%20Alternative%20Care.pdf (accessed 30 March 2015).

Faludi, S. (1992). *Backlash: The undeclared war against women*. London: Chatto and Windus.

Fargion, S. (2014). Synergies and tensions in child protection and parent support: Policy lines and practitioners' cultures. *Child and Family Social Work, 19*(1), 24–33.

Featherstone, B. (2001). Where to for feminist social work? *Critical Social Work, 2*(1). Retrieved from http://www1.uwindsor.ca/criticalsocialwork/where-to-for-feminist-social-work (accessed 30 March 2015).

Featherstone, B. (2004). *Family life and family support: A feminist analysis*. Basingstoke: Palgrave Macmillan.

Featherstone, B. (2009). *Contemporary fathering: Theory, policy and practice*. Bristol: Policy Press.

Featherstone, B. (2010). Ethic of care. In M. Gray and S.A. Webb (eds), *Ethics and value perspectives in social work* (pp. 73–84). Basingstoke: Palgrave Macmillan.

Featherstone, B. and Fraser, C. (2012a). 'I'm just a mother: they're all professionals': Advocacy for parents as an aid to parental engagement. *Child and Family Social Work*, 17(2), 244–53.

Featherstone, B. and Fraser, C. (2012b). Working with fathers and domestic violence: Contemporary debates. *Child Abuse Review*, 21, 255–263.

Featherstone, B. and Gupta, A. (2014). Relationship-based practice in an unequal society: dilemmas and possibilities. Paper presented at the Conference on Relationship based practice, University of Central Lancashire, UK, 8 January.

Featherstone, B. and White, S. (2006). Fathers talk about their lives and services. In C. Ashley Ashley, B. Featherstone, C. Roskill, M. Ryan and S. White (eds), *Fathers matter* (pp. 69–81). London: Family Rights Group.

Featherstone, B., Fraser C., Ashley, C. and Ledward P. (2011). Advocacy for parents and carers involved with children's services: Making a difference to working in partnership? *Child and Family Social Work*, 16(3), 266–275.

Featherstone, B., Morris, K. and White, S. (2014a). A marriage made in hell: alliance of early intervention and child protection. *British Journal of Social Work*, 44, 1735–1749.

Featherstone, B., Rivett, M. and Scourfield, J. (2007). *Working with men in health and social care*. London: Sage.

Featherstone, B., White, S. and Morris, K. (2013). From the individual to the relational: Child protection re-imagined. *Relational Welfare*. Retrieved from www.relationalwelfare.com (accessed 30 March 2015).

Featherstone, B., White, S. and Morris, K. (2014b). *Reimagining child protection: Towards humane social work with families*. Bristol: Policy Press.

Ferguson, H. (2004). *Protecting children in time: Child abuse, child protection and the consequences of modernity*. Basingstoke: Palgrave Macmillan.

Ferguson, H. (2005). Trust, risk and child protection. In S. Watson and A. Moran (eds), *Trust, risk and uncertainty* (pp. 89–106). Basingstoke: Palgrave Macmillan.

Ferguson, H. (2014). What social workers do in performing child protection work: Evidence from research into face-to-face practice. *Child and Family Social Work*. Retrieved from http://onlinelibrary.wiley.com/doi/10.1111/cfs.12142/abstract (accessed 8 July 2015).

Ferguson, H. and Hogan, F. (2004). *Strengthening families through fathers*. Dublin: Family Support Agency.

Fernandez, E. (2014). Child protection and vulnerable families: Trends and issues in the Australian context. *Social Sciences*, 3, 785–808.

Fischer, J. (1978). *Effective casework practice: An eclectic approach*. New York: McGraw Hill.

Flyvbjerg, B. (2001). *Making social science matter*. Cambridge: Cambridge University Press.

Folgheraiter, F. (2004). *Relational social work: Toward networking societal practices*. London: Jessica Kingsley Publishers.

Folgheraiter, F. (2007). Relational social work: Principles and practices. *Social Policy and Society*, 6(2), 265–274.

Folgheraiter, F. and Raineri, N.L. (2012). A critical analysis of the social work definition according to the relational paradigm. *International Social Work*, 55(4), 473–487.

Fook, J. and Gardiner, F. (2012). *Critical reflection in context: applications in health and social care*. New York: Routledge.

Ford, J.L. (2008). *Doing the right thing: Relational ethics in institutional caregiving for veterans*. Dissertation, Virginia Polytechnic Institute and State University, Blacksburg, Virginia.

Fostering Network. (2011). Crisis looms for foster care in 2012. Retrieved from www.fostering.net/news/2011/crisis-looms-foster-care-in-2012 (accessed 30 March 2015).

Fox Harding, L. (1996). *Family, state and social policy*. Basingstoke: Macmillan Press.

Fox Harding, L. (1997). *Perspectives in child care policy*. (2nd edn). Harlow: Longman.

REFERENCES

Freymond, N. (2003) *Mothers and child welfare: Mothers' everyday realities and child placement experiences*. Research report presented at the 'Finding a Fit' Conference, Waterloo, 27 August.

Freymond, N. and Cameron, G. (eds). (2006). *Towards positive systems of child and family welfare: International comparisons of child protection, family service, and community caring systems*. Toronto, ON: University of Toronto Press.

Frost, P. and Hoggett, P. (2008). Human agency and social suffering. *Critical Social Policy*, 28(4), 438–60.

Fuller, T., Ellis, R. and Murphy, J. (2014). *Examining outcomes of differential response: Results from three randomized controlled trials in Colorado, Illinois, and Ohio*. Urbana, IL: Children and Family Research Center, School of Social Work, University of Illinois at Urbana-Champaign. Retrieved from http://cfrc. illinois.edu/pubs/pt_20140501_ExaminingOutcomesOfDifferentialResponseResults FromThreeRandomizedControlledTrialsInColoradoIllinoisAndOhio.pdf (accessed 30 March 2015).

Fuller, T., Nieto, M. and Zhang, S. (2013). *Differential response in Illinois: Final evaluation report*. Urbana, IL: Children and Family Research Center, School of Social Work, University of Illinois at Urbana-Champaign.

Fuller, T., Paceley, M. and Schreiber, J. (2015). Differential response family assessments: Listening to what parents say about service helpfulness. *Child Abuse and Neglect, 39*, 7–17.

Gabriel, L. (2001). A matter of ethical literacy. *Counselling and Psychotherapy Journal, 12*, 14–15.

Gabriel, L. (2005). *Speaking the unspeakable: The ethics of dual relationships in counselling and psychotherapy*. London: Brunner-Routledge.

Gabriel, L. and Casemore, R. (2009). *Relational ethics in practice: Narratives from counselling and psychotherapy*. Routledge: New York.

Gadd, D. (2004). Evidence led or policy led evidence: Cognitive behavioural programmes for men who are violent towards women, *Criminal Justice, 4*, 173–197.

Gallagher, M. and Smith, M. (2010). *Engaging with involuntary service users in social work: Literature Review 1 – context and overview*. Retrieved from www.socialwork.ed.ac.uk/__ data/assets/pdf_file/0016/44224/review_1_context_and_overview.pdf (accessed 30 March 2015).

Gardiner, H., Mutter, J. and Kosmitzki, C. (1998). *Lives across cultures: Cross-cultural human development*. Boston, MA: Allyn and Bacon.

Germain, C. and Gitterman, A. (1980). *The life model of social work practice*. New York: Columbia University Press.

Ghaffar, W., Manby, M. and Race, T. (2012). Exploring the experiences of parents and carers whose children have been subject to child protection plans. *British Journal of Social Work, 42*, 887–905.

Ghate, D. and Hazel, N. (2002). *Parenting in poor environments: Stress, support and coping*. London: Jessica Kingsley Publishers.

Giddens, A. (1998). *The third way: The renewal of social democracy*. Cambridge: Polity.

Gilbert, N. (1997). (ed.). *Combatting child abuse: International perspectives and trends*. New York: Oxford University Press.

Gilbert, N., Parton, N. and Skivenes, M. (eds). (2011). *Child protection systems: International trends and orientations*. Oxford: Oxford University Press.

Gilbert, R., Fluke, J., O'Connell, M., Gonzalez-Izquierdo, A., Brownell, M., Gulliver, P., Janson, S. and Sidebotham, P. (2012). Child maltreatment: Variations in trends and policies in six developed countries. *The Lancet, 379*, 758–772.

Gilbert, R., Kemp, A., Thoburn, J., Sidebotham, P., Radford, L., Glaser, D. and Macmillan, H.L. (2009a). Recognising and responding to child maltreatment. *The Lancet, 373*(9658), 167–180.

Gilbert, R., Widom, C., Browne, K., Fergusson, D., Webb, E. and Janson, S. (2009b). Burden and consequences of child maltreatment in high-income countries. *The Lancet, 373*, 68–81.

Gillespie, K., McCosker, L., Lonne, B. and Marston, G. (2014). Australian print media reporting of mandatory reporting. *Communities, Children and Families Australia, 8*(2), 13–28.

Gillespie, J., Whitford, D. and Abel, M. (2010). Community networking: A policy approach to enhance Aboriginal child welfare in off-reserve communities. *Indigenous Policy Journal, 21*(3), 1–19.

Gilligan, C. (1982). *In a different voice: Psychological theory and women's development.* Cambridge, MA: Harvard University Press.

Gilligan, P. (2010). Faith-based practice. In M. Gray and S.A. Webb (eds), *Ethics and value perspectives in social work* (pp. 60–70). London: Routledge.

Gillingham, P. (2011). Decision making tools and the development of expertise in child protection practitioners: Are we 'just breeding workers who are good at ticking boxes'? *Child and Family Social Work, 16*(4), 412–421.

Gillingham, P. and Humphreys, C. (2010). Child protection practitioners and decision making tools: observations and reflections from the frontline. *British Journal of Social Work, 40*(8), 2598–2616.

Gimmler, A. (n.d.). The discourse ethics of Jürgen Habermas. Retrieved from http://caae.phil.cmu.edu/Cavalier/Forum/meta/background/agimmler.html (accessed 30 March 2015).

Gladstone, J., Dumbrill, G., Leslie, B., Koster, A., Young, M. and Ismaila, A. (2012). Looking at engagement and outcome from the perspectives of child protection workers and parents. *Children and Youth Services Review, 34*(1), 112–118.

Gladstone, J., Dumbrill, G., Leslie, B., Koster, A., Young, M. and Ismaila, A. (2014). Understanding worker–parent engagement in child protection casework. *Child and Youth Services Review, 44*, 56–64.

Glisson, C. and Hemmelgarn, A. (1998). The effects of organizational climate and interorganizational coordination on the quality and outcomes of children's service systems. *Child Abuse and Neglect, 22*(5), 401–421.

Goldner, V., Penn, P., Sheinberg, M. and Walker, G. (1990). Love and violence: Gender paradoxes in volatile attachments, *Family Process, 29*(4), 343–64.

Goldstein, H. (1983). Starting where the client is. *Social Casework: The Journal of Contemporary Social Work, May*, 267–275.

Goldstein, H. (1987). The neglected moral link in social work practice. *Social Work, 32*(3), 181–187.

Goldstein, H. (1999). The limits and art of understanding in social work practice. *Families in Society: The Journal of Contemporary Human Services, 80*(4), 385–395.

Gondolf, E. (2002). *Batterer intervention systems.* Thousand Oaks, CA: Sage.

Gordon, L. (1989). *Heroes of their own lives.* London: Virago.

Gray, M. (2010a). Moral sources and emergent ethical theories in social work. *British Journal of Social Work, 40*(6), 1794–1811.

Gray, M. (2010b). Postmodern ethics. In M. Gray and S.A. Webb (eds), *Ethics and value perspectives in social work* (pp. 120–132). London: Routledge.

Gray, M. (2010c). Social development and the status quo: Professionalisation and Third Way cooptation. *International Journal of Social Welfare, 19*(4), 463–470.

Gray, M. (2011). Back to basics: A critique of the strengths perspective in social work. *Families in Society, 92*(1), 5–11.

Gray, M. (2014). The swing to early intervention and prevention and its implications for social work. *British Journal of Social Work, 44*(7), 1750–1769.

Gray, M. and Gibbons, J. (2007). There are no answers, only choices: Teaching ethical decision making in social work. *Australian Social Work, 60*(2), 222–238.

Gray, M. and Lovat, T. (2006). The shaky high moral ground of postmodernist ethics. *Social Work/Maatskaplike Werk, 42*(3/4), 201–212.

REFERENCES

Gray, M. and Lovat, T. (2007). Horse and carriage: Why Habermas's discourse ethics gives virtue a *praxis* in social work. *Ethics and Social Welfare*, 1(3), 310–328.

Gray, M. and McDonald, C. (2006). Pursuing good practice? The limits of evidence-based practice. *Journal of Social Work*, 6(1), 7–20.

Gray, M. and Stofberg, J. (2000). Social work and respect for persons. *Australian Social Work*, 53(3), 55–61.

Gray, M. and Webb, S.A. (eds). (2010). *Ethics and value perspectives in social work*. Basingstoke: Palgrave Macmillan.

Gray, M., Coates, J. and Yellow Bird, M. (eds). (2008). *Indigenous social work around the world: Towards culturally relevant education and practice*. Aldershot: Ashgate.

Gray, M., Kreitzer, L. and Mupedziswa, R. (2014). The enduring relevance of indigenisation in African social work: A critical reflection on ASWEA's legacy. *Ethics and Social Welfare*, 8(2), 101–116.

Greenfield, B. (2015) Parents under investigation for neglect after allowing kids to walk to playground. Retrieved from www.yahoo.com/parenting/parents-under-investigation-for-neglect-after-108180228512.html (accessed 30 March 2015).

Gupta, A., Featherstone, B. and White, S. (2014). Reclaiming humanity: From capacities to capabilities in understanding parenting in adversity. *British Journal of Social Work*. Retrieved from http://bjsw.oxfordjournals.org/content/early/2014/11/22/bjsw.bcu137. abstract (accessed 8 July 2015).

Habermas, J. (1996). *Between facts and norms: Contributions to a discourse theory of law and democracy*. Cambridge, MA: MIT Press.

Hall, S. (2011). The neoliberal revolution. *Soundings*, 48, 9–27.

Hamilton, S. and Braithwaite, V. (2014). *Complex lives, complex needs, complex service systems: Community worker perspectives on the needs of families involved with ACT care and protection services*. Regulatory Institutions Network, Occasional Paper 21, Australian National University, Canberra, ACT. Retrieved from www.finvic.org.au/resources/HAMILTON%20BRAITHWAITE%2015%20JULY%202014.pdf (accessed 30 March 2015).

Hansen, P. and Ainsworth, F. (2007). Parent blaming in child protection and health settings: A matter for concern. *Children Australia*, 32(2), 29–35.

Harber, A. and Oakley, M. (2012). *Fostering aspirations: Reforming the foster care system in England and Wales*, Research Note. London: Policy Exchange. Retrieved from www.policyexchange.org.uk/images/publications/fostering%20ambitions%20-%20jan%2012.pdf (accessed 30 March 2015).

Harries, M. (2008). *The experiences of parents and families of children and young people in care*. Perth, Western Australia: Centre for Vulnerable Children and Families.

Harries, M. and Clare, M. (2002). *Mandatory reporting of child abuse: Evidence and options*. Report for the Western Australian Child Protection Council. Perth, Western Australia: University of Western Australia, Discipline of Social Work and Social Policy. Retrieved from www.celt.uwa.edu.au/__data/assets/pdf_file/0009/1102131/MRFinalReport.pdf (accessed 30 March 2015).

Harries, M., Cant, R. Bilson, A. and Thorpe, D. (2015). Responding to information about children in adversity: Ten years of a differential response model in Western Australia. *Child Abuse and Neglect*, 39, 61–72.

Harries, M., Lonne, B. and Thomson, J. (2007). Protecting children and caring for families: Re-thinking ethics for practice. *Communities, Children and Families Australia*, 2(1), 39–48.

Harris, N. (2008). Governing beyond command and control: A responsive and nodal approach to child protection. In M. Deflem (ed.), *Surveillance and governance: Crime control and beyond* (pp. 329–346). Bingley, UK: Emerald Group Publishing.

Harris, N. (2011). Does responsive regulation offer an alternative? Questioning the role of formalistic assessment in child protection investigations. *British Journal of Social Work* 41, 1383–1403.

Harrison, C., Harries, M. and Liddiard, M, (2014). The perfect storm: Politics, media and child welfare policy making. *Communities, Children and Families Australia*, 8(2), 29–45.

Harvey, D. (2005). *A short history of neoliberalism*. Oxford: Oxford University Press.

Hayes, D. and Houston, S. (2007). Lifeworld, system and family group conferences: Habermas' contribution to discourse in child protection. *British Journal of Social Work*, 37, 987–1006.

Hegge, M. (2012). Navigating ethical whirlwinds in nursing practice. *Dakota Nurse Connection*, 10(2), 21–26.

Held, V. (ed.). (1995). *Justice and care: Essential readings in feminist ethics*. Boulder, CO: Westview Press.

Held, V. (2006). *The ethics of care: Personal, political, and global*. New York: Oxford University Press.

Herman, B. (1993). *The practice of moral judgment*. Cambridge, MA: Harvard University Press.

Higgins, D.J. (2011). Unfit mothers … unjust practices? Key issues from Australian research on the impact of past adoption practices. *Family Matters*, 87, 56–67. Retrieved from www.aifs. gov.au/institute/pubs/fm2011/fm87/fm87g.html (accessed 30 March 2015).

Hill, D. (2007). The forgotten children: Fairbridge Farm School and its betrayal of Australia's child migrants. Sydney, NSW: Random House Australia.

Hinton, T. (2013). *Parents in the child protection system*. Hobart, Tasmania: The Social Action and Research Centre, Anglicare.

HM Government. (2004). *Every child matters: Change for children*. London: Her Majesty's Stationery Office.

Hoggett, P. (2005). Radical uncertainty: Human emotion and ethical dilemmas. In S. Watson and A. Moran (eds), *Trust, risk and uncertainty* (pp. 13–26). Basingstoke: Palgrave Macmillan.

Holland, S. (2014). Trust in the community: Understanding the relationships between formal, semi-formal and informal child safeguarding in a local neighbourhood. *British Journal of Social Work*, 44, 384–400.

Holland, S. and Scourfield, J. (2004). Liberty and respect in child protection. *British Journal of Social Work*, 34(1), 21–36.

Holland, S., Burgess, S., Grogan-Kaylor, A. and Delva, J. (2011). Understanding neighbourhoods, communities and environments: New approaches for social work research. *British Journal of Social Work*, 41, 689–707.

Holland, S., Scourfield, J., O'Neill, S. and Pithouse, A. (2005). Democratising the family and the state? The case of family group conferences. *Journal of Social Policy*, 34(1), 59–77.

Hollis, M. and Howe, D. (1986). Child death: Why social workers are responsible. *Community Care*, 5 June, 20–21.

Hollis, M. and Howe, D. (1987). Moral risks in social work. *Journal of Applied Philosophy*, 4(2), 123–133.

Hooper, C-A., Gorin, S., Cabral, C. and Dyson, C. (2007). *Living with hardship 24/7: The diverse experiences of families in poverty in England*. London: The Frank Buttle Trust.

Horwath, J. (2007). The missing assessment domain: Personal, professional and organisational factors influencing professional judgements when identifying and referring child neglect. *British Journal of Social Work*, 37, 1285–1303.

Howarth, J. and Morrison, T. (2007). Collaboration, integration and change in children's services: Critical issues and key ingredients. *Child Abuse and Neglect*, 31, 55–69.

Houston, S. (2003). Establishing virtue in social work: A response to McBeath and Webb. *British Journal of Social Work*, 33, 819–824.

Houston, S. (2010). Discourse ethics. In M. Gray and S.A. Webb (eds), *Ethics and value perspectives in social work* (pp. 95–107). Basingstoke: Palgrave Macmillan.

Howe, D. (2009). Psychosocial work: An attachment perspective. In R. Adams, L. Dominelli and M. Payne (eds), *Critical practice in social work* (2nd edn) (pp. 137–146). Basingstoke: Palgrave Macmillan.

REFERENCES

Howe, D. (2011). Attachment theory and social relationships. In V. Cree (ed.), *Social work: A reader* (pp. 73–81). London: Routledge.

Howe, D., Dooley, T. and Hinings, D. (2000). Assessment and decision making in child abuse cases: An attachment perspective. *Child and Family Social Work*, 5, 143–155.

Hudson, K. (2008). *Involving young children in decision making: An exploration of practitioners' views.* Murdoch, WA: Centre for Social and Community Research, Murdoch University.

Hughes, R., Rycus, J., Saunders-Adams, S., Hughes, L. and Hughes, K. (2013). Issues in differential response. *Research on Social Work Practice*, 23(5), 493–520.

Hugman, R. (2005). *New approaches in ethics for the caring professions: Taking account of change for caring professions.* Basingstoke: Palgrave Macmillan.

Hugman, R. and Smith, D. (eds). (1995). *Ethical issues in social work.* London: Routledge.

Human Rights and Equal Opportunity Commission (HREOC). (1997). *Bringing them home: Report of the National Inquiry into the Separation of Aboriginal and Torres Strait Islander Children from Their Families.* Canberra, ACT: Commonwealth of Australia.

International Federation of Social Workers. (IFSW). (2014). Global definition of social work. Retrieved from http://ifsw.org/policies/definition-of-social-work (accessed 30 March 2015).

Ivec, M. (2013). *A necessary engagement: An international review of parent and family engagement in child protection.* Hobart, TA: Social Action and Research Centre, Anglicare.

Ivec, M., Braithwaite, V. and Harris, N. (2012). 'Resetting the relationship' in Indigenous child protection: Public hope and private reality. *Law and Policy*, 34(1), 80–103.

Jack, G. (2004). Child protection at the community level. *Child Abuse Review*, 13, 368–83.

Jack, G. (2012). Ecological perspective. In M. Gray, J. Midgley and S.A. Webb (eds), *Sage Handbook of Social Work* (pp. 129–142). London: Sage.

Jack, G. and Gill, O. (2010). The role of communities in safeguarding children and young people. *Child Abuse Review*, 19, 82–96.

Janczewski, C.E. (2015). The influence of differential response on decision-making in child protective service agencies. *Child Abuse and Neglect*, 39, 50–60.

Jarmon, B., Mathieson, S., Clark, L., McCulloch, E. and Lazear, K. (2000). *Florida foster care recruitment and retention: Perspectives of stakeholders on the critical factors affecting recruitment and retention of foster parents.* Tampa, FL: Lawton and Rhea Chiles Center for Healthy Mothers and Babies.

Jenson, J. and Saint-Martin, D. (2001). Changing citizenship regimes: Social policy strategies in the social investment state. *Workshop on Fostering social cohesion: A comparison of new policy strategies*, Université de Montréal, 21–22 June.

Johnson, M. (1995). Patriarchal terrorism and common couple violence: Two forms of violence against women. *Journal of Marriage and the Family*, 57, 43–59.

Jones, R. (2014). *The untold story of Baby P: Setting the record straight.* Bristol: Policy Press.

Jonsen, A. and Toulmin, S. (1988). *The abuse of casuistry: A history of moral reasoning.* Berkeley, CA: University of California Press.

Jonson-Reid, M., Drake, B. and Zhou, P. (2013). Neglect subtypes, race and poverty: Individual, family and service characteristics. *Child Maltreatment*, 18(1), 30–41.

Kaplan, K. (2013) Child welfare involvement among parents with mental illness. *CW 360° The Intersection of Child Welfare and Disability: Focus on Parents.* Retrieved from http://cascw. umn.edu/wp-content/uploads/2013/12/Fall2013_CW360_WEB.pdf (accessed 10 June 2015).

Kapland, C. and Merkel-Holguin, L. (2008). Another look at the national study on differential response in child welfare. *Protecting Children*, 23(1–2), 5–21.

Kapp, S. and Vela, R. (2004). The unheard client: Assessing the satisfaction of parents of children in foster care. *Child and Family Social Work*, 9, 197–206.

Keddell, E. (2014). Current debates on variability in child welfare decision-making: A selected literature review. *Social Sciences*, 3, 916–940.

Kelemen, M. and Peltonen, T. (2001). Ethics, morality and the subject: The contribution of Zygmunt Bauman and Michel Foucault to 'postmodern' business ethics. *Scandinavian Journal of Management, 17*, 151–166.

Keller, J. (1997). Autonomy, relationship, and feminist ethcs. *Hypatia, 12*(2), 152–164.

Kempe, H., Silverman, F., Steele, B., Droegemueller, W. and Silver, H. (1985). The battered-baby syndrome. *Child Abuse and Neglect, 9*, 143–154.

Kemshall, H. (2002). *Risk, social policy and welfare.* Buckingham: Open University Press.

Kennedy, R., Richards, J. and Leiman, T. (2013). *Integrating human services law, ethics and practice.* South Melbourne, VIC: Oxford University Press.

Kenny, P., Higgins, D., Soloff, C. and Sweid, R. (2012). *Past adoption experiences: National research study on the service response to past adoption practices* (Research report no. 21). Melbourne, VIC: Australian Institute of Family Studies.

Kenny, P., Higgins, D., Sweid, R. and Soloff, C. (2013). Past adoption experiences: Impacts, insights and implications for policy and practice. *Communities, Children and Families Australia, 7*(1), 35–46.

Kester, G.H. (2004). *Conversation pieces.* Berkeley, CA: University of California Press.

Kilpatrick, A. and Holland, T. (2009). *Working with families: An integrative model by level of need.* Boston, MA: Pearson.

Kimborough-Melton, R. and Campbell, D. (2008). Strong communities for children: A community-wide approach to prevention of child abuse and neglect. *Family and Community Health, 31*(2), 100–112.

King, M. (2014). 'It's about belonging'. *Person-centred care forum.* Perth, Western Australia: Alliance for Children at Risk. Retrieved from www.allianceforchildren.com.au/index.php/the-media/newsroom/54-it-s-about-belonging-says-michael-king (accessed 30 March 2015).

Kirkman, E. and Melrose, K. (2014). *Clinical judgement and decision making in children's social work: An analysis of the 'front door' system.* London: Department for Education. Retrieved from www.gov.uk/government/uploads/system/uploads/attachment_data/file/305516/RR337_-_Clinical_Judgement_and_Decision-Making_in_Childrens_Social_Work.pdf (accessed 30 March 2015).

Kirton, D. (2013). 'Kinship by design' in England: Reconfiguring adoption from Blair to the coalition. *Child and Family Social Work, 18*, 97–106.

Kleinman, A. and Kleinman, J. (1991) Suffering and its professional transformation: Towards an ethnography of interpersonal experience. *Culture, Medicine and Psychiatry, 15*(3), 275–301.

Koehn, D. (1998). *Rethinking feminist ethics: Care, trust and empathy.* London: Routledge.

Kojan, B. and Lonne, B. (2012). A comparison of systems and outcomes for safeguarding children in Australia and Norway. *Child and Family Social Work, 17*(1), 96–107.

Kyte, A., Trocmé, N. and Chamberland, C. (2013). Evaluating where we are at with differential response. *Child Abuse and Neglect, 37*(2–3), 125–132.

Laliberte, T. and Lightfoot, E. (2013) Parenting with disability: What do we know? *CW360° The Intersection of Child Welfare and Disability: Focus on Parents.* Retrieved from http://cascw.umn.edu/wp-content/uploads/2013/12/Fall2013_CW360_WEB.pdf (accessed 10 June 2015).

Landau, J. (2011). Communities that care for families: The LINC Model for enhancing individual, family and community resilience. *American Journal of Orthopsychiatry, 80*(4), 516–524.

Larcher, V. (2007). Ethical issues in child protection. *Clinical Ethics, 2*(4), 208–212.

Lavarch, M. (1995). *Bringing them home: National inquiry into the separation of Aboriginal and Torres Strait Islander children from their families*, Sydney, NSW: Human Rights and Equal Opportunities Commission, NSW.

Leeson, C. (2007). My life in care: Experiences of non-participation in decision-making processes. *Child and Family Social Work, 12*, 268–277.

Levi, B.H. (2008). Child abuse and neglect. In P. A. Singer and A.M. Viens (eds), *The Cambridge textbook of bioethics* (pp.132–140). Cambridge: Cambridge University Press.

REFERENCES

Lévinas, E. (1998). *Entre nous: On thinking of the Other* (Tr. M.B. Smith and B. Harshav). New York: Columbia University Press.

Lindley, B. and Richards, M. (2002). *Protocol on advice and advocacy for parents (child protection)*. Cambridge: Centre for Family Research.

Lindsay, J. and Dempsey, D. (2012). *Families, relationships and intimate life*. South Melbourne, VIC: Oxford.

Lister, R. (2006). Children (but not women) first: New Labour, child welfare and gender. *Critical Social Policy*, 26(2), 315–336.

Little, M. (2010). Looked after children: Can existing services ever succeed? *Adoption and Fostering*, 34(2), 3–7.

Littlechild, B. (2005). The nature and effects of violence against child-protection social workers: Providing effective support. *British Journal of Social Work*. 35(3), 387–401.

Loewenberg, F.M. and Dolgoff, R. (2000). *Ethical decisions for social work practice* (6th edn). Itasca, IL: F.E. Peacock Publishers.

Loman, L. A. and Siegel, G.L. (2015). Effects of approach and services under differential response on long term child safety and welfare. *Child Abuse and Neglect*, 39, 86–97.

Lonne, B. (2003). *Submission by Dr Robert (Bob) Lonne to the Crime and Misconduct Commission Inquiry into Abuse of Children in Foster Care in Queensland*. Retrieved from www.childprotectioninquiry.qld.gov.au/__data/assets/pdf_file/0003/161481/Lonne_Bob_with_attachments.pdf (accessed 30 March 2015).

Lonne, B. (2015). Mandatory reporting and the difficulties in identifying and responding to risk of severe neglect: A response requiring a rethink. In B. Mathews and D. Bross (eds), *Mandatory reporting laws and the identification of severe child abuse and neglect* (pp. 245–275). New York: Springer.

Lonne, B. and Gillespie, K. (2014). How do Australian print media representations of child abuse and neglect inform the public and system reform? *Child Abuse and Neglect*, 38(5), 837–850.

Lonne, B. and Parton, N. (2014). Portrayals of child abuse scandals in the media in Australia and England: Impacts on practice, policy and systems. *Child Abuse and Neglect*, 38(5), 822–836.

Lonne, B., Brown, G., Wagner, I. and Gillespie, K. (2015). Victoria's Child FIRST differential response system: Progress and issues. *Child Abuse and Neglect*, 39, 41–49.

Lonne, B., Harries, M. and Lantz, S. (2012). Workforce development: A pathway to reforming child protection systems in Australia. *British Journal of Social Work*, 43(8), 1630–1648.

Lonne, B., McDonald, C. and Fox, T. (2004). Ethical practice in the contemporary human services. *Journal of Social Work*, 4(3), 345–367.

Lonne, B., Parton, N., Thomson, J. and Harries, M. (2009). *Reforming child protection*. London: Routledge.

Lovat, T. and Gray, M. (2008). Towards a proportionist social work ethics: A Habermasian perspective. *British Journal of Social Work*, 38, 1100–1114.

MacLaurin, B., Trocmé, N., Fallon, B., McCormack, M., Pitman, L., Forest, N., Banks, J., Shangreaux, C. and Perrault, E. (2005). *Alberta incidence study of reported child abuse and neglect, AIS-2003: Major Findings*. Calgary, AB: University of Calgary.

Maitra, B. (2005). Culture and child protection. *Current paediatrics*, 15, 253–259.

Manahan, C. and Ball, J. (2007). Aboriginal fathers support groups: Bridging the gap between displacement and family balance. *First Peoples Child and Family Review*, 3(4), 42–49.

Mansell, J., Ota, R., Erasmus, R. and Marks, K. (2011). Reframing child protection: A response to a constant crisis of confidence in child protection. *Children and Youth Services Review*, 33(11), 2076–2086.

Marcellus, L. (2005). The ethics of relation: Public health nurses and child protection clients. *Journal of Advanced Nursing*, 51(4), 414–420.

Marmot, M. (2005). The social determinants of health inequalities. *The Lancet*, 365, 1099–104.

Mason, B. (2005). Relational risk-taking and the training of supervisors. *Journal of Family Therapy*, 27, 298–301.

Mathews, B. (2012). Exploring the contested role of mandatory reporting laws in the identification of severe child abuse and neglect. In M. Freeman (ed.), *Law and childhood studies: Current legal issues* (pp. 302–338). Oxford: Oxford University Press.

Mathews, B. and. Bross, D. (eds). (2015). *Mandatory reporting laws and the identification of severe child abuse and neglect*. New York: Springer.

Mathews, B. and Kenny, M.C. (2008). Mandatory reporting legislation in the United States, Canada, and Australia: A cross-jurisdictional review of key features, differences, and issues. *Child Maltreatment*, 13(1), 50–63.

McAuliffe, D. (1999). Clutching at codes: Resources that influence social work decisions in cases of ethical conflict. *Professional Ethics: A Multidisciplinary Journal*, 17(3–4), 9–24.

McAuliffe, D. (2010). Ethical decision making. In M. Gray and S.A. Webb (eds), *Ethics and value perspectives in social work*. Basingstoke: Palgrave Macmillan.

McBeath, G. and Webb, S.A. (2002). Virtue ethics and social work: Being lucky, realistic, and not doing one's duty. *British Journal of Social Work*, 32, 1015–1036.

McConnell, D. (2013) The out-of-home placement of children born to parents with intellectual disability. *CW360° The Intersection of Child Welfare and Disability: Focus on Parents*. Retrieved from http://cascw.umn.edu/wp-content/uploads/2013/12/Fall2013_CW360_WEB.pdf (accessed 10 June 2015).

McConnell, D. and Llewellyn, G. (2005). Social inequality, 'the deviant parent' and child protection practice. *Australian Journal of Social Issues*, 40(4), 553–566.

McCosker, L., Lonne, B., Gillespie, K. and Marston, G. (2014). Feature article coverage of Australian out-of-home care: Portrayals and policy reform. *American Journal of Orthopsychiatry*, 84(3), 257–265.

McDonald, C. (2006). *Challenging social work: The context of practice*. Basingstoke: Palgrave Macmillan.

McDonald, M. and Rosier, K. (2011a). *Interagency collaboration – Part A: What is it, what does it look like, when is it needed and what supports it?* Melbourne, VIC: Australian Institute of Family Studies.

McDonald, M. and Rosier, K. (2011b). *Interagency collaboration – Part B: Does collaboration benefit families? Exploring the evidence*. Melbourne, VIC: Australian Institute of Family Studies.

McDonald, C., Harris, J. and Wintersteen, R. (2003). Contingent on context? Social work and the state in Australia, Britain, and the USA. *British Journal of Social Work*, 33, 191–208.

McDonell, J. and Melton. G. (2008). Toward a science of community intervention. *Family and Community Health*, 31(2), 113–125.

McDougall, S. and Gibson, C. (2014). Advancing the visibility of the child in adult and child and family services. *Communities, Children and Families Australia*, 8(1), 21–35.

McHugh, M. and Pell, A. (2013). *Reforming the foster care system in Australia*. Sydney: UNSW Social Policy Research Centre.

McLaren, H. (2007). Exploring the ethics of forewarning: Social workers, confidentiality and potential child abuse disclosures. *Ethics and Social Welfare*, 1(1), 22–40.

McLeigh, J. (2013). How to form alliances with families and communities. *Child Abuse and Neglect*, 37(S), 29–40.

McRoy, R. (2004). The color of child welfare policy. In K. Davis and T. Bent-Goodley, (eds), *The color of social policy* (pp. 37–64). Washington, DC: Council on Social Work Education.

McRoy, R. (2008). Acknowledging disproportionate outcomes and changing service delivery. *Child Welfare*, 87(2), 205–210.

Meagher, G. and Parton, N. (2004). Modernising social work and the ethics of care. *Social Work and Society*, 2(1), 10–27.

Melton, G.B. (2005). Mandated reporting: A policy without reason. *Child Abuse and Neglect*, 29(1), 9–18.

REFERENCES

Melton, G.B. (2010a). It's all about relationships! The psychology of human rights. *American Journal of Orthopsychiatry, 80*(2), 161–169.

Melton, G.B. (2010b). Angels watching over us: Child safety and family support in an age of alienation. *American Journal of Orthopsychiatry, 80*(1), 89–95.

Melton, G.B. (2014). Strong communities for children: A community-wide approach to prevention of child maltreatment. In J. Korbin and R.D. Krugman (eds), *Handbook of child maltreatment* (pp. 329–339). New York: Springer.

Melton, G.B. and Anderson, D. (2008). From safe sanctuaries to strong communities: The role of communities of faith in child protection. *Family and Community Health, 31*(2), 173–185.

Melton, G.B., Holoday, B. and Kimbrough-Melton, R. (2008). Community life, public health and children's safety. *Family and Community Health, 31*(2), 84–99.

Melton, G.B, Thompson, R. and Small M. (eds). (2002). *Toward a child-centred, neighborhood-based child protection system: A report on the consortium on children, families and the law.* Westport, CT: Praeger.

Merkel-Holguin, L., Hollinshead, D., Hahn, A., Casillas, K. and Fluke, J.D. (2015). The influence of differential response and other factors on parent perceptions of child protection involvement. *Child Abuse and Neglect, 39,* 18–31.

Montserrat, C. (2014). The child protection system from the perspective of young people: Messages from 3 studies. *Social Sciences, 3,* 687–704.

Morris, K. (ed.). (2008). *Social work and multi-agency working: Making a difference.* Bristol: Policy Press.

Morris, K. and Burford, G. (2007). Working with children's existing networks: Building better opportunities? *Social Policy and Society, 6*(2), 209–217.

Morris, K. and Featherstone, B. (2010). Investing in children, regulating parents and supporting whole families. *Social Policy and Society, 9*(4), 557–86.

Mullaly, B. (2007). *The new structural social work.* Oxford: Oxford University Press.

Munford, R. and Sanders, J. (2005).Working with families: Strengths-based approaches. In M. Nash, R. Mumford and K. O'Donoghue (eds), *Social work theories in action* (pp. 158–173). London: Jessica Kingsley Publishers.

Munro, E. (2004). The impact of audit on social work practice. *British Journal of Social Work, 34,* 1075–1095.

Munro, E. (2007). Confidentiality in a preventive child welfare system. *Ethics and Social Welfare, 1,* 41–55.

Munro, E. (2011). *The Munro review of child protection: A child-centred system.* London: UK Department for Education.

Murdoch, I. (1970). *The sovereignty of good.* London: Routledge and Kegan Paul.

Murphy, S., Hunter, A. and Johnson, D. (2008). Transforming caregiving: African American custodial mothers and the child welfare system. *Journal of Sociology and Social Welfare, 35*(2), 67–89.

Nandy, S., Selwyn, J., Farmer, E. and Vaisey, P. (2011). *Spotlight on kinship care.* Bristol: Hadley Centre and University of Bristol. Retrieved from www.bristol.ac.uk/hadley (accessed 30 March 2015).

National Council on Crime and Delinquency. (n.d). Structured decision making model. Retrieved from http://nccdglobal.org/assessment/structured-decision-making-sdm-model (accessed 30 March 2015).

National Society for the Prevention of Cruelty to Children (NSPCC). (2012). Factsheet: An introduction to child protection legislation in the UK. Retrieved from www.safenetwork. org.uk/news_and_events/news_articles/Pages/child-protection-legislation-factsheet.aspx (accessed 30 March 2015).

Neckoway, R., Brownlee, K., Jourdain, L. and Miller, L. (2003). Rethinking the role of attachment theory in child welfare with Aboriginal people. *Canadian Social Work Review, 20*(1), 105–119.

Neuberger, J. (2005). *The moral state we're in: A manifesto for 21st century society*. London: HarperCollins Publishers.

Noddings, N. (2003). *Caring: A feminine approach to ethics and moral education* (2nd edn). Berkeley, CA: University of California Press.

Nussbaum, M.C. (2000). *Women and human development: The capabilities approach*. Cambridge: Cambridge University Press.

Nussbaum, M.C. and Dixon, R. (2012). *Children's rights and a capabilities approach: The question of special priority*. Public Law and Legal Theory Working Papers No. 384.

Nussbaum, M.C. and Sen, A. (eds). (1993). *The quality of life*. Oxford: Clarendon Press.

O'Donoghue, K. and Maidment, J. (2005). The ecological systems metaphor in Australasia. In M. Nash, R. Mumford and K. O'Donoghue (eds), *Social work theories in action* (pp. 32–49). London: Jessica Kingsley Publishers.

Office for National Statistics (ONS). (2014). *Intimate personal violence and partner abuse*. London: ONS. Retrieved from www.ons.gov.uk/ons/dcp171776_352362.pdf (accessed 30 March 2015).

Oliver, C. and Charles, G. (2015). Which strengths-based practice? Reconciling strengths-based practice and mandated authority in child protection work. *Social Work*. Retrieved from http://sw.oxfordjournals.org/content/early/2015/01/19/sw.swu058 (accessed 8 July 2015).

Orme, J. (2002). Social work: Gender, care and justice. *British Journal of Social Work*, 32, 799–814.

Orme, J. (2008). Feminist social work. In M. Gray and S.A. Webb (eds), *Social work theories and methods* (pp. 65–75). London: Sage.

Orme, J. (2009). Feminist social work. In R. Adams, L. Dominelli and M. Payne (eds), *Critical practice in social work* (2nd edn) (pp. 199–208). Basingstoke: Palgrave Macmillan.

Osborn, A. and Bromfield, L. (2007). *Outcomes for children and young people in care, Research Brief No. 3*. Melbourne: National Child Protection Clearinghouse, Australian Institute of Family Studies (AIFS).

Osborn, A., Delfabbro, P.H. and Barber, J.G. (2008). The psychosocial functioning and family background of children experiencing significant placement instability in Australian out-of-home care. *Children and Youth Services Review*, 30, 447–460.

Owen, C. and Statham, J. (2009). *Disproportionality in child welfare: The prevalence of black and minority ethnic children within the 'looked after' and 'children in need' populations and on child protection registers in England*. London: UK Department of Children, Schools and Families.

Parkinson, P. (2000). Child protection law in Australia. In M. Freeman (ed.) *Overcoming child abuse: A window on a world problem* (pp. 15–38). Dartmouth, UK: Ashgate.

Parliament of Australia Senate Community Affairs Committee. (2004). *Forgotten Australians: A report on Australians who experienced institutional or out-of-home care as children*. Canberra: Commonwealth of Australia.

Parliament of Australia Senate Community Affairs Committee. (2012). *Commonwealth Contribution to Former Forced Adoption Policies and Practices*, Canberra: Commonwealth of Australia. Retrieved from www.nla.gov.au/openpublish/index.php/aja/article/viewFile/2342/2806 (accessed 30 March 2015).

Parton, N. (1985). *The politics of child abuse*. Basingstoke: Palgrave Macmillan.

Parton, N (1991). *Governing the family, child care, child protection and the state*. Basingstoke: Palgrave Macmillan.

Parton, N. (2003). Rethinking professional practice: The contributions of social constructionism and the feminist 'ethics of care'. *British Journal of Social Work*, 33, 1–16.

Parton, N. (2006a). Social work, risk and 'the blaming system'. In N. Parton (ed.), *Social theory, social change and social work* (pp. 98–114). London: Routledge.

Parton, N. (2006b). *Safeguarding childhood: Early intervention and surveillance in a late modern society*. Basingstoke: Palgrave Macmillan.

REFERENCES

Parton, N. (2014). *The politics of child protection: Contemporary developments and future directions*. Basingstoke: Palgrave Macmillan.

Parton, N. and O'Byrne, P. (2000). *Constructive social work: Towards a new practice*. Basingstoke: Macmillan Press.

Parton, N., Thorpe, D. and Wattam, C. (1997). *Child protection: Risk and the moral order*. Basingstoke: Macmillan Press.

Pawlukewicz, J. and Ondrus, S. (2013). Ethical dilemmas: The use of applied scenarios in the helping professions. *Journal of Social Work Values and Ethics*, 10(1), 1–12.

Payne, M. (2005). *The origins of social work: Continuity and change*. Basingstoke: Palgrave Macmillan.

Payne, M. (2014). *Modern social work theory* (4th edn). Basingstoke: Palgrave Macmillan.

Pecora, P., Whittaker, J., Maluccio, A. and Barth, R. (eds) (2007). *The child welfare challenge: Policy, practice and research* (2nd edn). Piscataway, NJ: Transaction Publishers.

Pelton, L.H. (1989). *For reasons of poverty: A critical analysis of the public child welfare system in the United States*. Westport, CT: Praeger Publishers.

Pelton, L.H. (2011). Concluding commentary: Varied perspectives on child welfare. *Children and Youth Services Review*, 33, 481–485.

Pelton, L.H. (2014). The continuing role of material factors in child maltreatment and placement. *Child Abuse and Neglect*. Retrieved from www.sciencedirect.com/science/article/pii/S0145213414002786 (accessed 8 July 2015).

Pence, E. and Paymar, M. (1993). *Education groups for men who batter*. New York: Springer.

Penglase, J. (2005). *Orphans of the living: Growing up in care in twentieth century Australia*. Fremantle, WA: Curtin University Press.

Phoca, S. and Wright, R. (1999). *Introducing postfeminism*. Cambridge, MA: Icon.

Pithouse, A., Broadhurst, K., Hall, D., Peckover, S., Wastell, D. and White, S. (2011). Trust, risk and the (mis)management of contingency and discretion through new information technologies in children's services. *Journal of Social Work*, 12(2), 158–178.

Platt, D. and Turney, D. (2014). Making threshold decisions in child protection: A conceptual analysis. *British Journal of Social Work*, 44(6), 1472–1490.

Poole, E., Speight, S., O'Brien, M., Connolly, S. and Aldrich, M. (2013). *Fatherhood in the UK: What do we know about non-resident fathers?* Retrieved from www.modernfatherhood.org/wp-content/uploads/2014/05/BSA-presentation.pdf (accessed 3 June 2015).

Putnam, R. (2000). *Bowling alone: The collapse and revival of American community*. New York: Simon and Schuster.

Queensland Child Protection Commission of Inquiry. (2013a). *Discussion Paper*. Brisbane, QLD: Queensland Child Protection Commission of Inquiry. Retrieved from www.childprotectioninquiry.qld.gov.au/publications/discussion-paper-individual-chapters (accessed 30 March 2015).

Queensland Child Protection Commission of Inquiry. (2013b). *Taking responsibility: A roadmap for Queensland child protection*. Brisbane, QLD: Queensland Child Protection Commission of Inquiry. Retrieved from www.childprotectioninquiry.qld.gov.au/__data/assets/pdf_file/0017/202625/QCPCI-FINAL-REPORT-web-version.pdf (accessed 30 March 2015).

Queensland University of Technology (QUT) and Social Research Centre (SRC). (2013). *The child and family services outcomes survey 2012 final report*. Melbourne, VIC: Department of Human Services. Retrieved from www.dhs.vic.gov.au/about-the-department/documents-and-resources/reports-publications/the-child-and-family-services-outcomes-survey (accessed 30 March 2015).

Quinton, D. (2004). *Supporting parents: Messages from research*. London: Jessica Kingsley Publishers.

Radford, D. (2013). NSPCC project working with mothers and children in the context of domestic abuse. Paper presented at Conference on Domestic Violence and Safeguarding, Durham, UK, 21 May.

Radford, L., Corral, S., Bradley, C., Fisher, H., Bassett, C. Howat, N. and Collishaw, S. (2011). *Child abuse and neglect in the UK today*. London: NSPCC.

Rasmussen, D.B. and Den Uyl, D.J. (1991). *Liberty and nature: An Aristotelian defense of liberal order*. La Salle, IL: Open Court Publishing Company.

Reading, R., Bissell, S., Goldhagen, J., Masson, S., Parton, N., Pais, M.S., Thoburn, J. and Webb, E. (2009). Promotion of children's rights and prevention of maltreatment. *The Lancet, 373*, 332–343.

Reamer, F. (2001). *The social work ethics audit: A risk management tool*. Washington, DC: NASW Press.

Reder, C. and Lucey, P. (1995). *Assessment of parenting: Psychiatric and psychological contributions*. London: Routledge.

Reder, P. and Duncan, S. (2001). Abusive relationships, care and control conflicts and insecure attachments. *Child Abuse Review, 10*, 411–427.

Reder, P., Duncan, S. and Gray, M. (1993). *Child abuse tragedies revisited*. London: Routledge.

Redshaw, S. (2012). Understanding the needs of children and young people in care: Towards a taxonomy of needs. *Communities, Children and Families Australia, 6*(1), 13–19.

Reisch, M. and Jani, J.S. (2012). The new politics of social work practice: Understanding context to promote change. *British Journal of Social Work, 42*(6), 1132–1150.

Respect (2010). Statement on Caring Dads programme. Retrieved from http://caringdads.org/pros/res/ap/130-response-to-respect (accessed 10 June 2015).

Revans, L. (2009). Lurking in the shadows. *Community Care, 9*, 18–21.

Reynolds, T. (2009). Exploring the absent/present dilemma: Black fathers, family relationships, and social capital in Britain. *ANNALS of the American Academy of Political and Social Science, 624*, 12–28.

Ridge, T. (2013). 'We are all in this together': The hidden costs of poverty, recession and austerity policies on Britain's poorest children. *Children and Society, 27*, 406–17.

Rivett, M. (2010). Working with violent male carers (fathers and step-fathers). In B. Featherstone, C-A. Hooper, J. Scourfield and J. Taylor (eds), *Gender and child welfare in society* (pp. 195–223). Chichester: John Wiley and Sons.

Robb, M., Featherstone, B., Ruxton, S. and Ward, M. (forthcoming). *Boys talk about relationships with welfare workers*. London: ESRC.

Roberts, D. (2002). *Shattered bonds: The color of child welfare*. New York: Basic Civitas Books.

Roberts, D. (2008). The racial geography of child welfare: Toward a new research paradigm, *Child Welfare, 87*(2), 125–150.

Robinson, W. and Reeser, L.C. (2000). *Ethical decision-making in social work*. Boston, MA: Allyn and Bacon.

Rooney, R. (ed.). (2013). *Strategies for work with involuntary clients*. New York: University Press.

Rorty, R. (1999). *Philosophy and social hope*. London: Penguin.

Roskill, C., Featherstone, B., Ashley, C. and Haresnape, S. (2008). *Fathers Matter, 11*. London: Family Rights Group.

Ross, T. (2009). *Child welfare: The challenges of collaboration*. Washington, DC: The Urban Institute Press.

Rossiter, A. (2006). The 'beyond' of ethics in social work. *Canadian Social Work Review, 23*(1–2), 139–144.

Rossiter, A., Prilleltensky, I. and Walsh-Bowers, R. (2000). A postmodern perspective on professional ethics. In B. Fawcett, B. Featherstone, J. Fook, J. and A. Rossiter (eds), *Practice and research in social work* (pp. 83–103). London: Routledge.

Ruch, G. (2005). Relationship-based practice and reflective practice: Holistic approaches to contemporary child care social work. *Child and Family Social Work, 10*, 111–123.

Ruch, G., Turney, D. and Ward, A. (2010). *Relationship-based social work: Getting to the heart of practice*. London: Jessica Kingsley Publishers.

Saari, C. (2005). The contribution of relational theory to social work practice. *Smith College Studies in Social Work*, 75(3), 3–14.

Saleebey, D. (2009). *The strengths perspective in social work practice*. Boston, MA: Allyn and Bacon.

Salveron, M. and Arney, F. (2013). Understanding the journey of parents whose children are in out-of-home care. In F. Arney and D. Scott (eds), *Working with vulnerable families: A partnership approach* (2nd edn) (pp. 213–234). New York: Cambridge University Press.

Sanders, R. and Mace, S. (2006). Agency policy and the participation of children and young people in the child protection process. *Child Abuse Review*, 15(2), 89–109.

Saunders, E., Nelson, K. and Landsman, M. (1993). Racial inequality and child neglect: Findings in a metropolitan area. *Child Welfare*, 72(4), 341–354.

Schön, D. (1990). *Educating the reflective practitioner*. San Francisco, CA: Jossey-Bass Publishers.

Scott, D. (2006). Towards a public health model of child protection in Australia. *Communities, Families and Children Australia*, 1(1), 9–16.

Scott, D. (2013). Child protection at the crossroads: Where to from here? Paper presented at the Child Protection Practitioners Association of Queensland Limited, Brisbane, 13 September.

Scott, D. (2014). *Understanding child neglect*. Melbourne, VIC: Australian Institute of Family Studies. Retrieved from www.aifs.gov.au/cfca/pubs/papers/a146596/index.html (accessed 30 March 2015).

Scott, D. and O'Neil, D. (2003). *Beyond child rescue*. Sydney, NSW: Allen and Unwin.

Scott, E. (2006). From family crisis to state crisis: The impact of overload on child protection in New South Wales. Paper presented at 16th ISPCAN International Congress on Child Abuse and Neglect, Children in a Changing World: Getting it Right, York, UK.

Scott, K. and Crooks, C. (2004). Effecting change in maltreating fathers. *Clinical Psychology: Science and Practice*, 11, 95–111.

Scourfield, J. (2003). *Gender and child protection*. Basingstoke: Palgrave Macmillan.

Scourfield, J. (2006). The challenge of engaging fathers in the child protection process. *Critical Social Theory*, 26(2), 440–449.

Segal, E. (2013). Beyond the pale of psychoanalysis: Relational theory and generalist social work practice. *Clinical Social Work Journal*, 41(4), 376–386.

Sen, A. (1985). *Commodities and capabilities*. Oxford: Oxford University Press.

Sen, A. (1999). *Development as freedom*. Oxford: Oxford University Press.

Sen, A. (2005). Human rights and capabilities. *Journal of Human Development*, 6(2), 151–66.

Sennett, R. (2003). *Respect: The formation of character in an age of inequality*. London: Penguin Books.

Sevenhuijsen, S. (1998). *Citizenship and the ethics of care*. London: Routledge.

Sevenhuijsen, S. (2000). Caring in the Third Way: The relation between obligation, responsibility and care in Third Way discourse. *Critical Social Policy*, 20(1), 5–37.

Sevenhuijsen, S. (2003). Principle ethics and the ethic of care: Can they go together? *Social Work/ Maatskaplike Werk*, 39(4), 393–399.

Sewpaul, V. (2004). Emancipatory citizenship education in action: Discourse ethics and deconstruction (Part 1), *Social Work/ Maatskaplike Werk*, 40(3), 218–231.

Shireman, J. (2003). *Critical issues in child welfare*. New York: Columbia University Press.

Shoesmith, S. (2013). Social workers should not be blamed for child murders. *Guardian Professional*, 13 December. Retrieved from www.theguardian.com/social-care-network/2013/dec/13/sharon-shoesmith-social-workers (accessed 30 March 2015).

Simmons, R. and Birchall, J. (2005). A joined-up approach to user participation in public services: Strengthening the 'participation chain'. *Social Policy and Administration*, 39(3), 260–283.

Sinclair, I. (2010). Looked after children: Can existing services ever succeed? A different view. *Adoption and Fostering, 34*(2), 8–13.

Sinclair, I., Baker, C., Lee, J. and Gibbs, I. (2007). *The pursuit of permanence: A study of the English care system*. London: Jessica Kingsley Publishers.

Sinclair, T. (2005). Mad, bad or sad? Ideology, disturbed communication and child abuse prevention. *Journal of Sociology, 41*(3), 227–246.

Sinha, V., Trocme, N., Fallon, B., MacLaurin, B., Fast, E., Prokop, S. and Others. (2011). *Kiskisik Awasisak: Remember the children. Understanding the overrepresentation of First Nations children in the child welfare system*. Thunder Bay, ON: Assembly of First Nations. Retrieved from www.fncaringsociety.com/sites/default/files/docs/FNCIS-2008-report.pdf (accessed 30 March 2015).

Smith, C. (2001). Trust and confidence. *British Journal of Social Work, 31*, 287–305.

Smith, D. (2005). *Values and practices in children's services*. Basingstoke: Palgrave Macmillan.

Smith, L. (2014). Editorial. The toxic work environment: A question of ethics. *Journal of Social Work Values and Ethics, 11*(1), 1. Retrieved from http://jswve.org/download/2014-1/JSWVE-11-1-final-all%20text.pdf (accessed 30 March 2015).

Smolin, D. and Smolin, D. (2012). The aftermath of abusive adoption practices in the lives of adoption triad members: Responding to adoption triad members victimized by abusive adoption practices. Presented as Plenary Presentation, Annual Symposium, Joint Council on International Children's Services, April, New York. Retrieved from http://works.bepress.com/david_smolin/12 (accessed 30 March 2015).

Spratt, T. and Callan, J. (2004). Parents' views on social work interventions in child welfare cases. *British Journal of Social Work, 34*(2), 199–224.

Stalker, K. (2010). Surveillance or reflection: Professional supervision in the risk society. *British Journal of Social Work, 40*, 1279–1296.

Stanley, J. and Goddard, C. (2002). *In the firing line: Violence and power in child protection work*. Chichester: John Wiley and Sons.

Steen, J. and Duran, L. (2014). Entryway into the child protection system: The impacts of child maltreatment reporting policies and system structures. *Child Abuse and Neglect, 38*, 868–874.

Steering Committee for the Review of Government Service Provision. (2013). *Report on government services 2014*. Canberra: Productivity Commission.

Steinberg, K., Levine, M. and Doueck, H. (1997). Effects of legally mandated child-abuse reports on the therapeutic relationship: A survey of psychotherapists. *American Journal of Orthopsychiatry, 67*(1), 112–122.

Stevens, M. and Higgins, D. (2002). The influence of risk and protective factors on burnout experienced by those who work with maltreated children. *Child Abuse Review, 11*(5), 313–331.

Stoltenborgh, M., Bakermans-Kranenburg, M. and van Ijzendoorn, M. (2013). The neglect of child neglect: A meta-analytic review of the prevalence of neglect. *Social Psychiatry and Psychiatric Epidemiology, 48*, 345–355.

Strega, S. and Carriere, J. (eds). (2009). *Walking this path together: Anti-racist and anti-oppressive child welfare practice*. Toronto, ON: Fernwood Press.

Swift, K. (1995). *Manufacturing bad mothers: A critical perspective on child neglect*. Toronto, ON: University of Toronto Press.

Tanner, K. and Turney, D. (2003). What do we know about child neglect? A critical review of the literature and its application to social work practice. *Child and Family Social Work, 8*, 25–34.

Tascón, S. (2010). Ethics of responsibility. In M. Gray and S.A. Webb (eds), *Ethics and value perspectives in social work* (pp. 85–94). Basingstoke: Palgrave Macmillan.

Tew, J. (2006). Understanding power and powerlessness: Towards a framework for emancipatory practice in social work. *Journal of Social Work, 6*(1), 33–51.

REFERENCES

Thompson, I., Melia, K. and Boyd, K. (2006). *Nursing ethics* (5th edn). Edinburgh: Churchill Livingstone.

Thomson, J. and Thorpe, R. (2004). Powerful partnerships in social work: Group work with parents of children in care. *Australian Social Work, 57*(1), 46–56.

Tilbury, C. (2009). The over-representation of Indigenous children in the Australian child welfare system. *International Journal of Social Welfare, 18*(1), 57–64.

Tobin, B. (1994). Codes of ethics: Why we also need practical wisdom. *Australian Psychiatry, 2*(2), 55–57.

Tobis, D. (2013). *From pariahs to partners: How parents and their allies changed New York City's child welfare system.* Oxford: Oxford University Press.

Trevithick, P. (2014). Humanising managerialism: Reclaiming emotional reasoning, intuition, the relationship, and knowledge and skills in social work. *Journal of Social Work Practice, 28*(3), 287–311.

Tronto, J.C. (1993). *Moral boundaries: A political argument for an ethic of care.* New York: Routledge.

Truax, C.B. and Carkhuff, R.R. (1967). *Toward effective counseling and psychotherapy.* Chicago, IL: Aldine.

Turnell, A. and Edwards, S. (1999). *Signs of safety: A solution and safety oriented approach to child protection casework.* New York: W.W. Norton and Co.

UK Department of Health. (1995). *Child protection: Messages from research.* London: HMSO.

Ungar, M. (2004). Surviving as a postmodern social worker: Two Ps and three Rs of direct practice. *Social Work, 49*(3), 488–496.

United Nations High Commissioner for Refugees (UNHCR). (2013). *Global Report 2013.* Retrieved from www.unhcr.org/gr13/index.xml (accessed 30 March 2015).

Urek, M. (2005). Making a case in social work: The construction of an unsuitable mother. *Qualitative Social Work, 4*(44), 451–467.

US Department of Health and Human Services. (2013). *Child maltreatment 2012.* Retrieved from www.acf.hhs.gov/programs/cb/research-data-technology/statistics-research/child-maltreatment (accessed 30 March 2015).

US Department of Health and Human Services. (2014). *Child welfare information gateway.* Retrieved from www.childwelfare.gov/systemwide/laws_policies (accessed 30 March 2015).

Uttal, W. (2011). *Mind and brain: A critical appraisal of cognitive neuroscience.* Cambridge, MA: MIT Press.

van den Bersselaar, O.D. (2005). *Virtue-ethics as a device for narratives in social work: The possibility of empowerment by moralising.* Lectoraat Reflectie op het handelen. Retrieved from www.reflectietools.nl/documentatie/Virtue_Ethics_VvdB.pdf (accessed 30 March 2015).

Varela, F.J. (1999). *Ethical know-how: Action, wisdom and cognition.* Stanford, CA: Stanford University Press.

Vis, S.A., Holtan, A. and Thomas, N. (2012). Obstacles for child participation in care and protection cases – why Norwegian social workers find it difficult. *Child Abuse Review, 21*(1), 7–23.

Wallace, D. (2013). *Decision-making technologies: A benefit or threat to ethical professional practice?* Unpublished doctoral dissertation. Sydney, NSW: Macquarie University.

Wallcraft, J., Schrank, B. and Amering, M. (eds). (2009). *Handbook of service user involvement in mental health research.* Chichester: John Wiley and Sons.

Walsh, J. (2010). *Theories for direct social work practice.* Belmont, CA: Wadsworth Cengage Learning.

Wan, H.K. (2007). Conflict management behaviours of welfare practitioners in individualistic and collectivist culture. *Administration in Social Work, 31*(1), 49–65.

Warner, J. (2014). *The emotional politics of social work and child protection.* Bristol: Policy Press.

Warnke, G. (1995). Discourse ethics and feminist dilemmas of difference. In J. Meehan. (ed.), *Feminists read Habermas* (pp. 247–262). London: Routledge.

Wastell, D. (2011). *Managers as designers in the public services: Beyond technomagic*. Axminster: Triarchy Press.

Wastell, D. and White S. (2012). Blinded by neuroscience: Social policy, the family and the infant brain. *Families, Relationships and Society*, 1(3), 397–414.

Waterhouse, L. and McGhee, J. (2009). Anxiety and child protection–implications for practitioner–parent relations. *Child and Family Social Work*, 14(4), 481–490.

Watson, S. (2005). Attachment theory and social work. In M. Nash, R. Mumford and K. O'Donoghue (eds), *Social work theories in action* (pp. 208–222). London: Jessica Kingsley Publishers.

Webb, S.A. (2006). *Social work in a risk society: Social and political perspectives*. Basingstoke: Palgrave Macmillan.

Westcott, H.L. and Davies, G.M. (1996). Sexually abused children's and young people's perspectives on investigative interviews. *British Journal of Social Work*, 26(4), 451–474.

Wexler, R. (2003). *The road less travelled by: Towards real reform of child welfare in Missouri* (2nd edn). Alexandria, VA: The National Coalition for Child Protection Reform.

White, K. and Wu, Q. (2014). Application of the life course perspective in child welfare research. *Child and Youth Services Review*, 46, 146–154.

Whiting, P. (2010). Christianity and ethics. In M. Gray and S.A. Webb (eds), *Ethics and value perspectives in social work* (pp. 196–206). Basingstoke: Palgrave Macmillan.

Wilkinson, R. and Pickett, K. (2009). *The spirit level: Why greater equality makes societies stronger*. New York: Bloomsbury Press.

Winkworth, G. and White, M. (2010). May do, should do, can do: Collaboration between commonwealth and state service systems for vulnerable children. *Communities, Children and Families Australia*, 5(1), 5–20.

Winkworth, G., McArthur, M., Layton, M., Thomson, L. and Wilson, F. (2010). Opportunities lost: Why some parents of young children are not well connected to the service systems designed to assist them. *Australian Social Work*, 63(4), 431–445.

Winokur, M., Ellis, R., Drury, I. and Rogers, J. (2015). Answering the big questions about differential response in Colorado: Safety and cost outcomes from a randomized controlled trial. *Child Abuse and Neglect*, 39, 98–108.

Withington, T., Burton, J. and Lonne, B. (2013). Placement trajectory: Mapping the journeys of children and young people in out-of-home care. *Communities, Children and Families Australia*, 7(1), 21–34.

Wood Inquiry. (2008). *Report from the Special Commission of Inquiry into Child Protection Services in NSW*. Sydney, NSW: State of New South Wales. Retrieved from www.dpc.nsw.gov.au/publications/news/stories/?a=33796 (accessed 30 March 2015).

Woolfson, R.C., Heffernan, E., Paul, M. and Brown, M. (2009). Young people's views of the child protection system in Scotland. *British Journal of Social Work*, 40, 2069–2085.

Worrall, J. (2005). *Grandparents and other relatives raising kin children in Aotearoa, New Zealand Auckland*. Auckland: Grandparents Raising Children Charitable Trust.

Wrennall, L. (2010). Surveillance and child protection: De-mystifying the Trojan Horse. *Surveillance and Society*, 7(3/4), 304–324.

Wulczyn, F., Kogan, J. and Harden, B. (2003). Placement stability and movement trajectories. *Social Service Review*, 77(2), 212–236.

Index

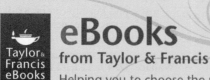

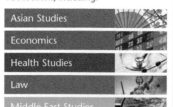